Professionalism, Boundaries and the Workplace

Edited by Nigel Malin

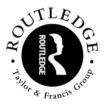

London and New York

First published 2000
by Routledge
11 New Fetter Lane, London EC4P 4EE

Simultaneously published in the USA and Canada
by Routledge
29 West 35th Street, New York, NY 10001

Routledge is an imprint of the Taylor & Francis Group

Typeset in Bembo by The Running Head Limited,
www.therunninghead.com
Printed and bound in Great Britain by
Biddles Ltd, Guildford and King's Lynn

British Library Cataloguing in Publication Data
A catalogue record for this book is available
from the British Library

Library of Congress Cataloging in Publication Data
Professionalism, boundaries, and the workplace / edited by Nigel
   Malin.
      A collection of 15 chapters by university contributors.
      Includes bibliographical references and index.
      1. Social workers–Great Britain.   2. Social workers–Professional
   ethics–Great Britain.   3. Social service–Great Britain.   4. Human
   services personnel–Professional ethics–Great Britain.   5. Medical
   personnel–Professional ethics–Great Britain.   6. Counselors–
   Professional ethics–Great Britain.   7. Counseling–Great Britain.
   I. Malin, Nigel.
   HV10.5.P74   2000
   361.3′2′0941–dc21   99–17035   CIP

ISBN 0–415–19262–5 (hbk)
ISBN 0–415–19263–3 (pbk)

Contents

Contributors

Reva Berman Brown is Professor of Management in the Faculty of Management and Business at University College Northampton. She has published in the areas of her research interests, which embrace management issues in the NHS, organisational culture, the problems of time, emotion, competence and professionalism in management practice, and management education.

Sharon C. Bolton is a Research Fellow in the Department of Sociology, University of Manchester, and was previously an ESRC-funded research student in the School of Management at the University of Lancaster. Her chapter is based upon her doctoral thesis concerning emotion management in the workplace.

Mary Buck is undertaking doctoral research in the Department of Education, Politics and Social Science, South Bank University. She has conducted research in a number of areas and also worked as a lecturer in sociology and social policy.

Helen Cameron is a Tutor at Westminster College, Oxford, on ministerial development programmes in Applied Theology and Work and Vocational Consultancy. Her chapter on the social action of the local church is based upon her doctoral research undertaken at the Centre for Voluntary Organisation, London School of Economics. Her research interests include the role of local churches as membership organisations in a changing civil society. She also practises as a consultant in educational policy.

Katie Deverell is a senior consumer scientist at Unilever Research. She is currently carrying out research in various countries in the area of household care. Prior to this she worked for eight years in the field of HIV prevention research in academic and public sector organisations. Her Ph.D. 'Sex, Work and Professionalism' was awarded in 1997, from Keele University. She has published widely on issues related to sexuality, identity and HIV prevention; she is currently a Visiting Research Fellow at Southbank University.

Tina Eadie is a Lecturer in Social Work in the Centre for Social Work at the University of Nottingham. She worked as a Probation Officer and Senior

Probation Officer for a number of years, including a Joint Appointment for five years shared between Derbyshire Probation Service and the University of Nottingham. Her publications have addressed the teaching of law to social work students (*Social Work Education* 14(2), 1995) and the changes in probation officer training (*Critical Social Policy* 17(1), 1997).

Valérie Fournier is a Lecturer in Human Resource Management and Organisation Studies at Keele University. Her research interests centre around critical perspectives on management and organisations and, in particular, on subjectivity at work. She has recently written about the making and disciplinary effects of the professions, 'new career' discourse in organisations, and identity work in family businesses.

Matthew Gorton is a Lecturer in the Department of Agricultural Economics and Food Marketing at the University of Newcastle. His main area of research concerns the contribution of small and medium-sized enterprises to rural development and the creation of appropriate public sector support networks. He has contributed to *Entrepreneurship and Regional Development*, *Panorama* and *Philosophy and Geography*.

Steve Killigrew is a Senior Lecturer in Radiotherapy and Oncology at the University of Derby. Additionally as a qualified hypnotherapist and shiatsu practitioner, his research and teaching interests also include complementary therapies. Currently he is undertaking a Ph.D. investigating holism in complementary therapies from the perspective of patients receiving traditional Chinese medicine.

Mark Lymbery has been a Lecturer in Social Work at the Centre for Social Work, University of Nottingham, since 1995. He is a qualified social worker, with 18 years' work experience within social services departments, including three years as Community Care Implementation Officer in Nottinghamshire SSD. He has researched and published in the areas of care management, the history and development of social work, and on social work in primary health care.

Sean McCartney is a Lecturer in Accounting in the Department of Accounting, Finance and Management at the University of Essex. He is a Fellow of the Institute of Chartered Accountants in England and Wales, and worked in practice and industry before becoming an academic. He has published a number of papers in the areas of auditing and accounting and management education. His current research interests also include aspects of accounting theory and nineteenth-century British business history.

Steve McNally is a Lecturer Practitioner with Oxford Brookes University and the Oxfordshire Learning Disability NHS Trust. He also acts as a professional facilitator for the Royal College of Nursing. After having trained originally as a psychiatric nurse, since 1980 he has been committed to supporting people with a learning disability. His research interests are primarily concerned with advocacy and empowerment strategies for service users and support for families. He is currently developing a B.A. (Hons) Community Learning Disability Nursing option with UKCC Specialist Practitioner award at Oxford Brookes.

Nigel Malin is Professor of Community Care and Divisional Research Co-ordinator (Health and Social Care) at the University of Derby. He is the author or editor of seven books, including (with Jill Manthorpe, David Race and Stephen Wilmot) *Community Care for Nurses and the Caring Professions* (Open University Press, 1999). His main teaching has been in the field of social policy on health and social work programmes. He is currently undertaking research on clinical supervision and practice ethics in learning disabilities' services. He is Director of the Community and Social Care Research Forum in Southern Derbyshire.

Tim May is a Professor of Sociology at the University of Salford. He obtained his Ph.D. in 1990 and then worked at the Universities of Plymouth and Durham, before moving to Salford in 1999. He has published books on organisational change, social theory, philosophy and social research; he has co-edited books on ethnography, work with offenders, philosophy, social theory and methodology. His current work includes editing an international collection on qualitative research (Sage), writing a book on reflexivity (Sage), editing an international book series (Open University Press) and continuing his research interests on management, power and organisational transformation.

Ruth Pinder is Associate Research Fellow at Brunel University, and Research Fellow at Queen Mary College Westfield, University of London, where her research interests also include the sociology of ageing, and disability. She teaches social science and disability studies to medical students at the Royal Free Hospital, University of London, and runs teaching, training and development workshops for doctors and health care professionals within the British Postgraduate Medical Federation.

Richenda Power has practised as a naturopath and osteopath since 1983, working in the private and the public sectors, and in urban and rural settings. She has been working as a clinical tutor at the British School of Osteopathy since 1997. She is also a sociologist, currently teaching the Open University foundation module for the Masters in Social Science, and has just completed her first book, *A Question of Knowledge* (Longman, forthcoming).

Ursula Sharma trained in both sociology and social anthropology. She has carried out extensive research on social aspects of complementary medicine. Her most recent book, written jointly with Sarah Cant, is *A New Medical Pluralism? Alternative Medicine, Doctors, Patients and the State* (UCL Press, 1999). She is employed as Professor of Comparative Sociology at the University of Derby.

Introduction

Nigel Malin

Professionalism, Boundaries and the Workplace looks at professionalism as a set of workplace practices where boundaries have been redefined in response to socio-economic and cultural pressures. It uses examples principally from fields of health and social welfare, with the majority of chapters presenting new research findings. Different scenarios are depicted as a response to factors embedded in contemporary culture such as commercialism, credentialism and enterprise. The changed nature of professionalism is viewed also as a response to pressures from the Left and from the user movement. Partnerships and participation are taken as appropriate goals for professionalism, including desirability of extending service-user involvement into broader occupational groupings of caring professionals. Research studies contained in separate chapters are based on probation, social work, community care, NHS, small business and church settings. They address a number of issues including: the relationship between personal and professional values, changing professional–client relationships, definitions of 'being professional', conflicts arising from different understandings of professionalism, and the construction of professional boundaries.

The sociological literature on professions has largely treated the values associated with professionalism – altruism, personal detachment, public service, etc. – as part of the rhetoric by which professionalising groups support their claims to status. But we can also look at professionalism as a set of workplace practices, in modes of interacting with clients which stress the containment of subjective feelings (positive or negative) which a doctor, social worker, teacher, etc. might entertain for a patient/client/pupil. Professional training often provides ways in which over-identification with the client is avoided or managed, and codes of ethics which purport to police the boundaries between the personal and the professional. In some professions, boundaries are particularly hard to maintain.

For example, social and community workers, healers and counsellors can be overwhelmed by the problems their clients bring to them – resulting in 'burn out'. Chapter 2 by Katie Deverell and Ursula Sharma shows how some kinds of professional work, characteristics or experiences which are shared with the client group may be a major qualification for the job (black workers taken on to work with black client groups, gay male workers employed to work with gay males, etc.). In such cases the professional worker may need to develop strategies to deal with the ambiguity of the boundary between 'work' and 'non-work'. The very private and relatively unsupervised nature of certain kinds of professional–client relationship may make it easier for detachment to be abandoned, as, for example, where sex takes place 'in the forbidden zone' between (say) therapist and patient, teacher and student.

The nature of professional practice, as it relates to scope, competence, level of discretion and power, has been linked to organisational culture within the wider UK and global economy. A notable example of the need for boundary redefinition arises from current links between professionalism and market/enterprise culture. The discourse of enterprise challenges occupational, functional and professional segmentation, monopoly and division; instead it celebrates integration and flexibility, the deregulation of professions and monopolies of competence. The collapse of barriers between occupations and functions within organisations means that members of different occupational groups are now required to work in multi-functional teams. This has given rise to the 'organisational professional', with a shift from productive behaviour, or inputs to productive behaviour, to a different emphasis on the total behaviour, attitudes and self-understanding of the individual employees. Managerialism's role in clipping the wings of professional groups has been backed by the previous Conservative Government's obsessive insistence that serious improvement can only be brought about by management. As such, managerialism has come to dom-inate professional culture by extending the 'technical' role of professions, including downgrading, de-skilling and task fragmentation.

The book explores the constitution of the professional field of expertise, how re-delineation of boundary contours has come about and how workplace practices have become substitutes for conventionally preconceived professional functions. The issue of professionalism as a set of workplace practices is considered within the following subcategories: professionalism and shared user identification (e.g. user self-advocacy), professionalism and enterprise culture, professionalism and new managerialism, professionalism and credentialism, and professionalism and emotion management.

In the caring services sector, professionalism and volunteerism can be seen as interacting in defining types of work, spheres of competence and modes of interaction between sectors. For instance, activities falling within the broad term 'caring' encompass the contribution of professional (i.e. paid) workers employed by non-governmental organisations, as well as the contribution of volunteers attached to any number of statutory and non-governmental agencies. This issue is explored in Part I, chapter 1, in relation to community and social care within the formal sector. Caring, when subjected to analysis, is often found to be about measuring the unmeasurable. When caring occupations are subjected to managerial-style review the different aspects of their identity often go unrecognised; this places unseen stresses on professional workers and may hamper their contributing to any struggle for power as a prerequisite to attaining a credible public identity. Moves towards multi-professionalism taking place within caring services may seem unpopular among single professional disciplines, despite rhetoric from politicians viewing such an objective as a fulfilment and culmination of a planned process. Chapter 3 by Steve McNally considers the ascendance of user self-advocacy and the challenge this poses to professional groups.

Part II, concerned with professionalism and enterprise culture, examines the way market values and organised competition have achieved an overriding prominence in creating professional efficiency. For instance, chapter 4 by Valérie Fournier considers the constitution of the independent and self-contained field of knowledge of the profession, illustrated with the example of the medical field and the emergence of the body as a valid object of knowledge. Focusing upon the labour of division that goes into erecting and maintaining boundaries between the professions and various groups, the argument is that much of the boundary work central to the establishment of the professions may be eroded or challenged by the spreading discourse of enterprise and its celebration of 'boundarylessness' and flexibility.

This is a theme taken forward in subsequent chapters. Chapter 5 by Matthew Gorton refers to the world of small businesses and considers links between delivering high quality services and customer satisfaction, where the latter may not always be commensurate with assisting organisational long-term survival. Here professionalism between agencies is restricted by structural and financial barriers. Chapter 6 by Helen Cameron explores the challenge posed by enterprise culture by looking at the work of a profession, i.e. the clergy – described as on the margins of society – to see what workplace practices its members use to sustain their professional mode of interacting with their clients. It demonstrates that clergy reluctance to allow overt conflict in their organisational leader role may be an attempt to safeguard their professional pastoral role with church members.

Part III, concerned with professionalism and managerialism, focuses upon social work and care management. Chapter 7 by Mark Lymbery examines how community care reforms have set in train a process which redefines the nature of the social worker/care manager's relationship with the service user. The increasingly short-term nature of social work involvement, focused largely on the process of assessment, detaches social workers from this key element of their professional identity, and gives more credence to technical and procedural requirements. Chapter 8 by Tim May and Mary Buck is based upon a research project on organisational change in a social service department, involving interviews with team managers and frontline social workers. Using Weber's concept of formal and substantive rationality, it evaluates strategies adopted by social workers to construct legitimated boundaries, given the plethora of organisational change.

Part IV, on professionalism and credentialism, considers the relative merits of competences and professional skills, including the notion of 'info-normative' control that places emphasis on the total behaviour, attitudes and self-understanding of individual employees. Chapter 9 by Tina Eadie addresses the changed professional focus of probation services embracing ideas of punishment and control, and how the interaction with clients is increasingly determined by rules and procedures. Chapter 10 by Reva Berman Brown and Sean McCartney is based upon research findings covering attitudes and values of general managers and clinicians in the NHS with respect to differing definitions of what it means to be a professional. Because of such differences in values the interaction between, for example, medical consultants and managers is clouded by different conceptions of what a 'true' professional is, and whether he or she acts in a properly professional manner. Credentialism and women GPs is considered in chapter 11 by Ruth Pinder. This chapter looks at boundary issues around part-time working and the ambiguity and anxiety around blurring boundaries between different kinds of part-time statuses.

Part V examines emotional organisation in an enterprise culture, the extent to which professional attachment is valued and whether it crosses cherished boundaries. Chapter 12 by Sharon Bolton considers skills of the nursing profession necessary in managing situations in order to create the correct emotional climate and the different characteristics of various types of organisational emotionality. Chapter 13 by Richenda Power considers the 'fat envelope patient' and the implications for professional boundaries and emotion management which arise from those patients who are frequently referred through NHS channels to osteopaths, homoeopaths, etc. The patient as active agent in the construction and maintenance of such situations is explored, as it is in the last chapter by Steve Killigrew, which evaluates the professionalism concept in relation to complementary medicine, including ways used by practitioners to redefine the role of emotions in the therapeutic process.

Part I

Professionalism, boundaries and the health/social care context

1 Professionalism and boundaries of the formal sector

The example of social and community care

Nigel Malin

Introduction

This chapter focuses on policy directions for social and community care within the UK and assesses change and development for the caring professions. In part, the shifting, peripheral and unspecified nature of care in the community is blamed for the failure of groups to professionalise, gain control and achieve closure status. In addition the mixed economy of care has tended to emphasise the need for staff to possess appropriate values, skills and attitudes, and for this to have greater importance than forms of academic training. A drive to 'modernise' health and social care services led by central government in the late 1990s has been accompanied by the search for an underpinning knowledge-base, and also for greater professional and hierarchical accountability. The argument is that this is creating a challenge for caring professions and is leading to the development of different types of expertise within social care.

Policy origins and developments

Social and community care arose in part as an outcome of de-institutionalisation. The 1957 Royal Commission on the Law Relating to Mental Illness and Mental Deficiency had concluded that 'it is not now generally considered in the best interests of patients who are fit to live in the general community that they should be in large or remote institutions such as the present mental or mental deficiency hospitals' (Ministry of Health 1957: 17, para. 46). Yet the Commission's vision of community care was founded on provision of a range of centres offering training, occupation or social activity and residential accommodation in private, voluntary and local authority homes and hostels. The idea of community care was not advanced as a principle during the 1960s chiefly because of lack of attention from central government and poor – almost invisible – co-ordination of services at local level. Barham's (1992) book covering mental health policy states that 'the declarations of government policy in this period represented not so much a new departure as an assertive formulation of trends that were already taking place' (ibid.: 11). Social and community care were unspecified 'simply because the character of the ex-mental patient in the community remained to a large degree unspecified' (ibid.: 12).

Community care facilities at this time were envisaged as transitional stepping-stones between a brief period of hospitalisation and full re-integration into the community. A transitional period in a rehabilitation hostel or day centre, it was believed, would accomplish the mutation of former mental health patients into ordinary citizens, distinguishable from their associates only by their occasional attendances at out-patient clinics to review their prescriptions. The new-found psychiatric optimism about the major tranquillisers, coupled with protest about the indignities of mental hospital regimes, converged to suggest that the concept of community care did not require elaborate specification or commitment (Bennett and Morris 1983). In truth the community as a locus of care came to possess little value (Barham 1992: 14); it was neither seen as a therapeutic site nor as the arena for an interrogation of the moral crisis in the relations between people with mental health problems and the larger society, but just as the place to which people were to be returned after medicine had cured them.

A by-product of the continuing non-specification of the nature and purpose of social and community care was a failure to carve out a proper role for staff as carers, including methods of working, training and service objectives. Care work linked to the public services was seen as having professional orientation but as a subordinate partner to established medical and clinical professions. Health and Welfare (Ministry of Health 1963) provided a list of services to promote social care for elderly people, including provision of suitably adapted ordinary housing, warden-supervised housing, home helps, laundry services, provision of cooked meals, chiropody at home, friendly visiting and the availability of additional transport to help people to attend social events. Many of these ideas were also taken up for younger people with disabilities in the Chronically Sick and Disabled Persons Act 1970.

Social and community care policies arose later from the 'planning for priority groups' agenda in the 1970s. Such policies demonstrated a significant gap between aspiration and intent and the means of implementation. Most of the central government master-plans published during this period for user groups such as mental health, learning disabilities and the elderly took the view that community care could be planned rationally and incrementally through 'local agency collaboration' following general objectives and principles laid down by government. In retrospect this seems naive; the model for achieving change was 'simply inappropriate' (Lewis and Glennerster 1996: 20). The government had tried to adopt centralized, rational, comprehensive planning. It had produced a national budget and planning guidelines, and local districts and social service departments were intended to plan jointly to implement these guidelines. In practice, power in the National Health Service (NHS) and local authorities was so diverse and the competing bureaucratic interests so entrenched that such a model had little hope of success; setting achievable goals to create high quality or adequate social care within the community for vulnerable, dependent service users proved unrealistic.

Local service providers muddled through; in general they extended residential and day centre services but with the emphasis on providing basic physical care and occupation. This showed a failure to connect with any desired outcome: 'policy throughout the 1970s was not incisive and continued to straddle community-oriented and institutional positions' (Felce and Grant 1998: 25). It meant also that a distinction was being drawn between treatment function and the long-term supportive function of care services. Whereas the former retained a foothold in hospital provision linked to clinical skills, the latter, as located in the community, lacked a clear purpose despite eventually being seen as an alternative 'social' non-clinical form of care. Social care as an occupational identity was disadvantaged through its failure to organise as a corporate group, and through its dependence on a third party defining and mediating contracts between client and professional worker.

In the 1980s it was widely publicised that the majority of community care was provided by family members, mainly women. Community care policies were examined against the background of an increasingly ubiquitous carers' lobby. The nature of care and who provided it became issues subject to frequent, rigorous analysis. In its original form, community care policy had envisaged a significant role for public services in maintaining highly dependent people outside large institutions. By the early 1980s this was less clearly the case (Baldwin and Twigg 1991). Under the twin pressures of fiscal crisis and an ideologically driven commitment to reducing the role of the state in service provision, the original vision was replaced by a much stronger emphasis on the provision of care by 'the community' itself (Parker 1990).

It raised the question that if care in the community was being provided by unpaid non-professionals then where was the argument for professionalising other spheres of similarly provided social care in residential homes and day centres. Within the formal sector, the notion of care was perceived as having less active connotations than certain other concepts used to describe what professionals do to their clients or patients. Terms such as treatment or therapy suggest an active intervention by a professional who has undergone training and has particular skills which qualify her to use technologies designed to achieve particular outcomes (Barnes 1997: 13). In contrast to this, care is seen to be something which can be provided without the need for professional training: the job of 'care worker' which exists in residential homes, domiciliary settings or day centres is usually an unqualified post. The provision of 'care' can imply an absence of clinical intervention directed towards cure, and when not undertaken against a background of medical technology, for instance within a hospital setting, it can be seen as activity subordinate to the work undertaken by the professionals.

Since the 1980s the problem of who provides social and community care has been taken up as a gender issue. How to 'empower' carers was central to the gender-based debate. In April 1997 service users were given power to select and employ their own carers through direct payments legislation. Ungerson (1997) has described the double disadvantage of mainly women being employed as low paid carers working in relative isolation from mainstream services, where informal and illegal contractual arrangements were unlikely to provide them with employment rights.

Emphasis upon values and philosophy rather than forms of professional training

The intention of the community care initiative was to help long-stay hospital patients unnecessarily kept in hospital to return to the community. The 1981 Care in the Community consultative document (DHSS 1981) began with the phrase: 'most people who need long-term care can and should be looked after in the community. This is what most of them want for themselves and what those responsible for their care believe to be best' (ibid.: para. 1.1). The 'legal, administrative and financial framework within which health and local authorities operate' (ibid.: para. 1.2) was presented as the obstacle to their transfer.

The policy of the Conservative government was not to fund de-institutionalisation nationwide but to set up demonstration projects where lessons could be learned, particularly with respect to managing joint health–local authority finance. The real motive of government was to cut the formidable expense of long-term hospital care and later to promote more cost-effective, cost-efficient varieties of care through separating the role of purchaser of care from that of provider. The emphasis would be upon altering the means rather than the outcomes (unless cutting the overall state financial contribution counted as an outcome). In a 1983 circular, the government established a number of pilot projects to investigate ways of moving long-stay patients out of hospital (DHSS 1983). Twenty-eight demonstration projects were centrally funded for three years (13 in the first round which began in April 1984, and 15 in the second which commenced a year later). Most of the projects represented models of care for people with mental illness or learning difficulties, and for elderly or elderly mentally infirm people. Together these pilot projects expected to provide services which would enable about 900 hospital patients to move into the community (Renshaw *et al.* 1988: 34). As the Personal Social Services Research Unit (University of Kent) evaluation indicates, by March 1987, 456 people (only) had moved out to the community, from a planned total of 896 (ibid.: 173). The main problems concerned finance (for example, 'double funding' – transitional costs required to put a new service in place before the old one can be removed), timescales (nearly all projects found that every step took far longer than had been anticipated), and professional resistance.

Professional resistance included efforts by health service staff to slow down the pace of hospital closure, coupled with the failure to demonstrate approval for care being provided by non-clinically qualified personnel. For the majority of demonstration projects this initiative created an opportunity to begin formulating objectives for care in the community and in so doing, to recognise the significance of the philosophy of care and values held by staff. The success of any project was seen to hinge on the quality of staff (Renshaw *et al.* 1988: 134). Back in 1980 the King's Fund Centre project entitled 'An Ordinary Life' decided that skills for residential care 'are mainly very ordinary ones: because staff themselves live in society and do most of these activities for themselves every day, they have the skills already' (King's Fund Centre 1980: 33). This seminally influential report on planning localised provision for people with learning disabilities concluded that most tasks which staff undertake fell into one of two categories: 'teaching' and 'doing'. It identified that staff needed training in the techniques of identifying need, deciding priorities, setting programmes and teaching skills to clients, and that 'in many cases the formal qualifications of staff and programmes of training currently provided for them are quite irrelevant' (ibid.: 33).

The 1980s Care in the Community projects emphasised in-house training for staff and evaluations focused upon its function in providing support, boosting morale and in clarifying service values and objectives. The tendency was to distance training from professional agendas, to reinforce local ownership, for staff to become partners in a local project; hence across the country much of the staff training evolved in a fragmented fashion. The PSSRU studies reported: 'our research showed that in-service training was positively related to expressed job satisfaction' (PSSRU 1990: 15).

Brown's (1992) analysis of joint training (between nursing and social work) as it applies to learning disabilities demonstrated that such modes of training arose as a result of the marginalisation of learning disabilities from mainstream services and competition for ownership between the two main caring professions. For staff training in the field of learning disabilities this divide-and-rule mentality lessened their claims to professional status and competence. When in the early 1990s government increasingly questioned occupational boundaries and addressed workforce issues, including training, in ways that challenged traditional demarcation, such collaboration between nursing and social work have provided lessons of relevance to their professions as a whole. By looking for links within and among the training for caring professions, the result had been to undermine rather than to enhance any special claim for identity. In learning disabilities, much of this had its roots in the Jay Report (Jay Committee 1979), whose remit was to recommend patterns of training, but which largely sidestepped the issue of professional alliance and concentrated upon the nature of the care task in an arguably apolitical manner: 'we did, however, feel strongly that it was a central part of our remit to look at the essential nature of the tasks of caring, without being constrained by how that task is currently allocated between particular professions or agencies' (Jay Committee 1979: 35).

Ten years later, following the Griffiths Report (1988) on community care, the policy emphasis became more blatant, recommending staff training in skills fit for the task rather than focusing upon any single caring profession. The Audit Commission, in a survey of collaboration between health and social services on implementing community care, reported that staff training was weak, and that fewer than 20 per cent of authorities provided adequate training in moving service delivery 'from "caring for" to "enabling" clients' (Audit Commission 1989: 14). When 'care in the community' was introduced, the Green Paper consultative document (DHSS 1981) stated in a section on staffing implications that both 'health and local authority workers should be fully committed to the success of projects' (ibid.: para. 3.9) and that this should be the overriding concern in appointing staff. From this period on, policy documents focused upon how to bring about progressive new services and referred to staff having to learn new skills (see, for example, Sheffield Area Health Authority/District Council 1981; Guy's Health District 1981): 'it will be vital that staff attend specially-designed re-orientation courses' (Sheffield ibid.: para. 3.2.1).

The underlying sentiment was that professional background was less relevant than capacity and orientation to undertake the task in hand. This applied both to certain non-clinical and clinical areas, and in particular to various forms of residential care. The government-led 'care in the community' project demonstrated on a national scale the need for individual care plans, service flexibility and the removal of structural, professional barriers. It also demonstrated the importance of salient local leadership and need for government to take more responsibility if practice was to change radically.

Professionalism as applied to social and community care

As a sociologist, Macdonald (1995: 133) discusses factors which affect the position and the practice of caring professions, including mediation, knowledge, indeterminacy and patriarchy. He quotes Johnson's (1972) reference to caring professions as 'mediative'; that is, they operate in conditions where 'a third party mediates in the relation between producer and consumer, defining both the needs and the manner in which the needs are met' (ibid.: 46). Their activities are defined by the state – both the needs they are to deal with and the way in which those needs are to be met; and furthermore, their funds are provided by the state (Macdonald 1995: 134). This limits their power, their dealings with other occupational groups, and weakens their position in negotiating economic rewards. Where the product of their activities is not clearly defined, their position is weakened still further.

This latter point applies in particular to the wider community-focused, enabling role prescribed to social work following the Griffiths Report in 1988. This report followed in the tradition of the previous Barclay Report (1982) and Section 12 of the Social Work (Scotland) Act 1968 in advocating a role for social work and social services beyond that of client counselling and service provision. It appeared to implement the Barclay Report's recommendation that social work and social care were marginal to the provision of care in the community. Instead the role of social work was of a broker, an enabler, an assessor of individual needs who organised the design and delivery of care packages. The provision of care *per se* would be performed by others and be relatively mechanistic and undemanding of high levels of professional skill.

The problem of defining outcomes of caring professions relates to the issue of the knowledge-base (Macdonald's analysis refers to professions possessing esoteric knowledge). In the caring professions, however, there is a considerable body of opinion that holds that practice is actually the more important aspect (see MacKay 1990: 34). The emphasis on knowledge derives from 'trait' theory, which relied heavily on the delineation of the characteristics which were held to constitute a profession. This formed the dominant perspective in early studies of professionalism (Greenwood 1957; Carr-Saunders and Wilson 1962; Etzioni 1969; Toren 1972) and one which reflected the views of established professions. Each occupation to be considered as a candidate for the label 'professional' could be compared to the list of traits, and the degree to which it matched was then taken as an indication of the extent to which that occupation was professionalised.

Hugman (1991: 104) states that one of the principal reasons why the trait theorists identified nursing, social work and the remedial professions as 'semi professions' is that they do not appear to have developed dominance in discrete areas of knowledge. Hugman quotes Howe (1986: 96) in claiming that 'professional attributes are the symptom and not the cause of an occupation's standing'. According to this view, professionalism is thus limited by the success in gaining power over such factors as an area of knowledge and associated autonomy, rather than limited by the intrinsic nature of those factors.

Indeterminacy concerns the notion that the greater the element of judgement required in the exercise of professional knowledge, the less likely it is that the professional tasks will be open to routinisation and inspection. Both nursing and social work require considerable exercise of judgement in their practice. Macdonald (1995: 135) takes the view, however, that the exercise of judgement in these cases is on the basis of knowledge that both the lay public and adjacent professions may not see as being sufficiently esoteric to take it into the true realm of 'indeterminacy'; being 'everyday' rather than professional knowledge. This view is possibly too generalised and fails to take account of the body of theoretical work which now underpins professional practice. Regarding the specific domains of social and community care, for instance, residential, domiciliary and day care provision, the objectives are directed towards long-term promotion of client independence and rehabilitation.

The idea of patriarchy has been claimed as significant in influencing the identity of caring professions (Larkin 1983; Witz 1992; Macdonald 1995): the values of patriarchal society are built into institutions, and its practices shape and reinforce the belief among its members that they have a vested interest in maintaining such values. Aspects of nursing and social work tasks are already socially defined as appropriate for women. Those taking up these roles accept that their position within the organisation will be strengthened and secured by adhering to their predefined role. Early developments of occupational associations, e.g. nursing, were based upon a 'probationership' model as the means of acquiring occupational knowledge; consequently the emphasis (in nursing) is on dedicated caring and concern as opposed to academic training. Patriarchy is implicit within the managerialist, employer-led approach to training in social care which created a distinctive trend, challenging the historical predominance of profession-determined education, in the early 1990s.

The mixed economy of care: managerialism versus professionalism

The Griffiths Report, *Community Care: An Agenda for Action* (Griffiths 1988), was concerned with modernising the management of community care and placing 'responsibility (for care) as near to the individual and his carers as possible' (ibid.: para. 30). The report occurred within the context of a government drive to 'reform' and overhaul public sector services (for example, health and education) so as to make professionals employed there more accountable for the work they had undertaken. The method chosen was the improvement, and by necessity the increase, of overall management, as this was perceived as the essential solution.

The report stressed the mixed economy of care, arguing that it was not nec-essary for social services authorities to provide all services themselves, but simply to ensure that they were provided. They should act 'as the designers, organisers and purchasers of non-health care services and not primarily as direct service providers, making the maximum possible use of voluntary and private sector bodies to widen consumer choice, stimulate innovation and encourage effi-ciency' (ibid.: para. 1.3.4). Radical changes in the workforce were needed, involving significant changes in role for a number of professional and occupa-tional groups. There was a further argument taken up from the earlier Audit Commission report (1986), namely the creation of a new occupation of 'com-munity carer' to undertake 'the front-line personal and social support of de-pendent people' (Griffiths 1988: para. 8.4). This provided a case for developing new skills among existing staff to enable them to tackle the new tasks proposed, developing completely new roles and replacing those that no longer appeared to be necessary.

The White Paper *Caring for People* (DoH 1989) constitutes the government's response to Griffiths and this was followed by enactment of the NHS and Com-munity Care Act 1990. Wistow (1990) described the purpose of the White Paper as operating at three levels: the macro (or service system) level; the micro (or individual user) level; and the inter-agency level. Encouraging local author-ities to focus upon a needs approach was to be achieved through linking *planning* for the whole community with *planning* at individual client level. Wistow's model implies:

- the organisation of service systems based on the separation of purchaser and provider functions, the promotion of a mixed economy and the creation of new providers operating in an external market;
- the organisation of service delivery through systematic arrangements for assessment, care management, devolved budgeting and, hence, some de-gree of decentralised purchasing; and
- a re-emphasis on joint working through the clearer allocation of respons-ibilities for health and social care, combined with strengthened financial incentives for collaboration and a focus on planning outcomes rather than structures or processes.

One effect of community care policy reforms has been the de-professionalisation of the workforce: a reduction of professionally trained staff in hands-on care and in areas outside management and need assessment (see, for example, Hatfield and Mohamad 1996 on community mental health support teams). Sheppard (1995: 75) refers to the 'marginalisation of a core of tasks centred around senti-mental work such as interprofessional skills and reflective responses brought about by a different style of culture dominating health and social care'. As the Griffiths Report envisaged,

> the change in role of social service authorities might also allow them to make more productive use of the management abilities and experience of all their staff, including those who are not qualified social workers . . . the professional skills of community nurses and health visitors need to be effec-tively harnessed and their contribution in working with other professional groups fully recognised.
>
> (Griffiths 1988: paras 8.1, 8.3)

The separation of management from professional work dealing with clients – with the former dominating professional culture – has been accompanied by a belief that such management expertise is the sole legitimate criterion for decision making in public organisations.

Griffiths (ibid.: para. 8.4) recommended: 'the creation of a new occupation of "community carers" to undertake the frontline personal and social support of dependent people . . . such job descriptions [should] enable individual workers to provide the assistance required without demarcation problems arising'. There has since been some work supporting the claim that unqualified workers dem-onstrate greater flair and innovation in undertaking hands-on work (Cole and Perides 1995) and that 'quality' is more associated with workplace ethos than with training and qualifications of staff (Wilding 1994). The division between managerial and professional/quasi-professional tasks has had a knock-on effect of deconstructing traditional professional competence (or professionals' right of ownership) and substituting routinisation, rule-following and form-filling. Many professionals, for example clinicians, have traditionally enjoyed high levels of autonomy, reflecting both primacy of expertise over political control and the complexity of delivering services. The impact of managerialism and the growth in power of accountancy over health professionals have demonstrated how this autonomy and hegemony is now challenged, and there is evidence of de-skilling, task fragmentation and centralisation of work planning in both health and social care.

A further jolt to the 'cognitive superiority' argument used to recognise the essence of the professional claim (see Hughes 1971: 375) has been the impact of consumerism, where professionals are 'now being asked to share their knowl-edge with unqualified users and to join with these users in reaching care de-cisions' (Wilson 1995: 8). This has been interpreted as a form of devaluing professional training. The fact that consumers should be given considerably

Figure 1.1 An example of a competence-based approach

Methods of client assessment: A1

Element A1.1   Gather and collate information from sources other than client

Performance criteria
1   His/her role is established with the appropriate persons.
2   The purpose and methods of the assessment are established with the appropriate persons.
3   Available factual information and views relevant to the assessment are obtained from appropriate sources.
4   Information is checked for accuracy where necessary.
5   Information is noted accurately, collated and stored in an appropriate form.

Element A1.2   Observe and discuss with the client

Performance criteria
1   The client's behaviour is continuously observed and recorded and valid conclusions drawn from the evidence.
2   The client's views relevant to the purpose are obtained.
3   Relevant factual information is obtained from the client.
4   All information is summarised and agreed with the client, collated and stored in an appropriate form.

Source: Care Sector Consortium (1990).

greater say in defining their own needs 'firmly places [professionals'] area of work, at least in part, in the arena of matters of everyday concern and competence. The need for any particular expertise is concomitantly reduced' (Sheppard 1995: 77).

Consequences for training

Training policy in residential, domiciliary and day care became directed during the 1990s towards a competence-based approach, a method of behaviour and performance assessment using core performance descriptors. An example is given in Figure 1.1.

It was intended that evidence be collected through observation and oral questioning to gather 'proof' of a carer's skill acquisition. Together with other factors this signalled a pendulum shift away from 'indetermination' towards 'technicality' (see Jamous and Peloille 1970 for an explanation of indetermination–technicality ratio, where for example if there is insufficient indeterminacy, the occupation is likely to be perceived as a practical vocation). Despite the original antipathy of the nursing profession towards contributing to the development of competence-based training (Brown 1994), 'competence' became the currency in which training programmes were expressed. Employer-led training which challenged the historical predominance of profession-determined education was promulgated by central government (for example,

Figure 1.2 Levels of competence in nurse and social work training

---

Level 1 Occupational competence in performing a range of tasks under supervision.

Level 2 Occupational competence in performing a wider range of more demanding tasks with limited supervision.

Level 3 Occupational competence required for satisfactory, responsible performance in a defined occupation or range of jobs.

Level 4 Competence to design and specify defined tasks, products or processes and to accept responsibility for the work of others.

Source: Brown (1992: 362).

by involving employers at a regional level in training and enterprise councils (TECs), and in training health care and social workers). A question might arise as to whether a coherent staff training policy for community care existed. Implementing the reforms gave purchasers and providers the opportunity to reflect on staff training policies and the workforce infrastructure, which involved redeploying care staff and considering how staff might acquire new knowledge and skills. Some local authorities undertook a training need analysis of their workforce (e.g. Bradford and North Yorkshire Social Services Departments).

One reason for the move towards de-professionalisation was that the contractual environment meant that traditional patterns of service provision and training programmes were no longer sacrosanct. The discernible trend was for local managers to develop their own specific training courses rather than patronise courses offering a regional, if not national, expertise, thus granting a feeling of local ownership. This raises the issue of comparability in standards between courses in different localities. Professional training bodies, for example English National Board for Nursing, Midwifery and Health Visiting (ENB), Central Council for Education and Training in Social Work (CCETSW), were expected to take a back seat, as new National Vocational Qualifications (NVQs) were devised following the government White Paper *Working Together: Education and Training* (DoH 1986). In community care, the emphasis was to be on 'pre-qualifying' (Levels 1 to 4) in the context of nurse and social work training (see Figure 1.2).

New NVQs were devised to meet demands of needs-led assessment and care planning, involving wide-ranging consultation with users and carers. There have been studies illustrating how 'unqualified' (non-professional) staff 'appear to be working in appropriate ways' (Hatfield and Mohamad 1996: 217) and contribute significantly to the support of people with chronic psychotic illness living in the community; personal qualities have been seen as more important than training. As stated earlier, this has contributed to a perception in some quarters that anyone can perform a care task: this has been disempowering to staff trying to promote the professional training argument (see Key 1995).

Modernising social and community care

> Government can act in partnership with agencies in civil society to foster community renewal and development. The economic basis of such partnership is what I shall call the new mixed economy . . . The state should expand the role of the public sphere, which means constitutional reform directed towards greater transparency and openness, as well as the introduction of new safeguards against corruption.
>
> (Giddens 1998: 69, 73)

The Government White Paper entitled *Modernising Social Services: Promoting Independence, Improving Protection, Raising Standards* (DoH 1998) addressed the issue of raising standards, improving quality and devising a national framework. The focus was upon regulation, and while recognising that around 80 per cent of those employed in social care have no recognised qualifications or training, it recommended setting standards of practice and conduct in the workplace. The establishment of eight Commissions for Care Standards, taking inspection from local authority control, was intended to have a broader scope for regulation than the current regimes. The overall approach of the White Paper is on 'the quality of services experienced by, and outcomes achieved for, individuals and their carers and families' (ibid.: 1.7).

The device chosen by the Labour government is to create a General Social Care Council to regulate training and to set conduct and practice standards for all social services staff. A desired effect would be a general improvement in ethical standards in the workplace. Provider agencies are likely to be advantaged by the employment of more trained personnel who are able to defend workplace practices during inspection. The approach follows that adopted within the NHS on clinical governance referring to forms of administrative or regulatory capacities. Clinical governance entails:

> arrangements [which] secure that the highest clinical standards are embedded in the organisation's wider quality assurance systems, and that research and development and support for continuing professional development are aligned with priorities for quality improvement, [involving] well-established systems to monitor and audit clinical standards and programmes to identify and reduce clinical risks.
>
> (DoH National Health Service Executive 1998: 3.18)

Care provided by a trained and skilled workforce is one of a number of key principles identified by the White Paper which are designed to underlie a high quality and effective service (Davis 1999). Other themes include: protection, co-ordination, inflexibility, clarity of role, consistency, eligibility criteria and inefficiency. The emphasis within the New Labour programme is on defining objectives at national level and setting outcomes leaving local agencies to set an enabling framework. The government's modernisation programme for health

Figure 1.3 National social services targets

Local authorities will take the lead on meeting a series of tough targets on promoting the welfare of socially excluded children, inter-agency working and regulation.

Children's welfare

1   The number of looked after children who have had three or more placements in one year to be cut to no more than 16 per cent by 2001.
2   By 2001 at least half of the children who leave care at 16 or later must do so with a GCSE or GNVQ qualification. By 2003, three-quarters of the children should have obtained a qualification.
3   Between 1997 and 2002, authorities must have cut by 10 per cent the proportion of children who were re-registered on the child protection register.
4   Authorities must prove that the level of employment, training or education among care leavers aged 19 in 2001–2 is at least 60 per cent of the level of all young people the same age in their area.
5   Every child or young person entering the care system to receive a health assessment.

Inter-agency working

1   During next year, health and local authorities must show at least one 'significant initiative' related to the establishment of the new youth offending teams, the crime reduction strategy and the Sure Start partnerships.

Regulation

The social care White Paper will set out the government's plans to overhaul regulation of care services. Until then health and local authorities must ensure that they:

1   Carry out the number of inspections required by law.
2   Work together and share information, develop joint standards and carry out joint inspections of dually registered homes.
3   Carry out effective investigations into complaints, particularly those involving allegations of abuse.
4   Ensure openness and public access to inspection reports.

Source: DoH (1998b).

and social care requires both sectors to work jointly to meet a raft of detailed targets (DoH 1998). Social services are to take the lead role in improving services for children, inter-agency working and regulation (see Figure 1.3). Health is to lead on cutting waiting lists, improving primary care and reducing heart disease and cancer rates. Both sectors are to share responsibility for tackling health inequalities, promoting independence and improving mental health services (see Figure 1.4).

The detailed targets are based on quantitative rather than qualitative aspects of service delivery. They represent continuation of a bureaucratic, managerialist approach emphasising cost-effectiveness in commissioning rather than tailoring services to meet individual needs. The network of regulatory procedures

Figure 1.4 National joint health/social services targets

Local authorities will share lead responsibility with their health colleagues for improving mental health, promoting independence for adults and tackling health inequalities.

Mental health

1   To reduce by 17 per cent the number of deaths from suicide and undetermined injury from 1996 levels by the year 2010.
2   To ensure joint plans for implementing the National Health Service Framework for mental health, due out by April 1999, are included in health improvement plans by the end of next year. The plans are likely to include targets for 24-hour staffed accommodation and access to help during a crisis, early assessment and intervention services, accommodation for rehabilitation and residential care.
3   Reduce the rate of emergency psychiatric re-admission by 2 per cent from the 1997–8 baseline, by 2002.
4   Improve mental health services for children and adolescents and provide assessments and treatment in locally based or specialist settings.
5   Improve access to mental health services and increase public safety by supporting regional high and medium secure services. Systems to be in place in shadow form by 1 April 1991, and fully operational by 1 April 2000.

Promoting independence

1   Slow the growth of emergency admissions of people aged over 75 to an annual average of 3 per cent over the five years up to 2002–3.
2   Develop and target preventive services for adults including respite care. DoH to issue guidance in the first half of next year.
3   Identify patients and service users who are or have carers and provide them with support, services and information.
4   Implement the proposals in *Better Services for Vulnerable People – Maintaining the Momentum*, Annex B, Action 1.

Cutting health inequalities

1   Develop local targets and action plans to reduce local inequalities, for example, to cut the number of unwanted teenage pregnancies or ensure black and ethnic minority groups and socially excluded groups have access to services.
2   Reduce the accident rate by one fifth for children and older people by 2010.
3   Set local targets for cutting the number of people smoking.
4   Improve drug treatment and care services to reach targets set out in the government's *Tackling Drugs to Build a Better Britain* strategy.
5   Maintain or raise to 95 per cent the immunisation rate for childhood vaccinations at age two.

Source: DoH (1998b)

intruding into day-to-day practice could mean a substantial loss of professional autonomy (Langan 1999). The converse may be true also: setting practice standards releases a more knowledge-driven approach. Central to the modernisation programme is the collection and use of scientific knowledge as the basis of decision making to ensure the most effective and efficient delivery of care. The

General Social Care Council should deliver two key objectives (DoH 1998a: 5.15):

> to strengthen public protection by relevant and appropriate regulation of personnel which has the interests of service users and the public at its heart; to ensure through a coherent, well-developed and regulated training system that more staff are equipped to provide social care which allows and assists individuals to live their own lives, and offers practical help, based on research and other evidence of what works, and free of unnecessary ideological influences.

The White Paper points to a training strategy (ibid.: 5.35) involving 'targets for quantitative and qualitative improvements'. Workforce analysis, advanced in the same White Paper, would demand multi-method research design to address the process of matching jobs/tasks with skills/training.

The planned policies of modernisation impose greater regulation, inspection and accountability on staff in practice, yet there would appear another scenario where opportunities for greater professionalisation emerge from an *evidence-based* approach underpinning the work of caring services. In summary, evidence-based practice is 'the process of systematically finding, appraising and using contemporaneous research findings as the basis for clinical decisions' (Long and Harrison 1996: 11).

The surge of interest in evidence-based medicine (EBM) began during the 1990s with the arrival of the NHS research and development strategy in 1991. Hunter (1997: 75) has criticised the over-optimistic claims of EBM to alter medical practice and decision taking, suggesting that this ignores sociological and political realities, such as the choice of clinicians to act interpretively or intuitively in contrast to the research evidence. The NHS research and development strategy aims to create a knowledge-based health service in which clinical, managerial and policy decisions are based on sound information about research findings and scientific developments. It has spawned a new industry in the evaluation of health care and the production of information about the effectiveness of various interventions. Hunter (ibid.: 76) quotes Sheldon and Long (1994) in identifying a list of practical barriers to deploying the evidence-based analysis of clinical effectiveness. These include: clinical practice is uncertain, clinical effectiveness is one issue on a crowded agenda for doctors and managers, and risk of information overload. So far the evidence-based approach to social care has not received a similar level of interest. However, advancing claims to professionalism may provoke such an interest in the near future.

Conclusion

The complex pattern through which policies have emerged to shape social care and community care developments in the last decades of the twentieth century has impacted upon attempts to create a professional project. Early on, the closures of long-stay hospitals and asylums were characteristic of efforts to build more humane, holistic, people-centred services in non-clinical settings, i.e. an 'ordinary life' experience. However, an absence of purpose, direction and means for measuring achievements in social care disadvantaged claims to professional status. Some of the attempts to build care in the community were opposed by, for instance, clinicians on the grounds of lack of verification or absence of clinical presence and safeguards. The Conservative government's policies (or lack of them) during the 1980s indicated that they believed the community possessed null value. Such policies led to a questioning both of the basis of providing care through the state sector and the relative merits of care personnel possessing correct values, philosophy and attitudes, as opposed to professional training.

The ideology of the mixed economy has altered expectations within the provision of social and community care and has shifted the role of the state from being a central provider to being an enabler, purchaser and planner. The state may still define the activities of the caring professions and the needs that they are to deal with, and their funds are still provided largely by the state, but the nature of the social care economy has meant that the delivery of care is more fragmented and that professional-type association and organisation is more difficult to achieve. Improving skills and training of those providing 'hands-on' care has remained low down the scale of policy objectives; the mixed economy of the 1990s has resulted probably in less government interference in independent sector care provision than previously. This is in spite of much earlier rhetoric concerning needs for workforce planning and skills analysis.

Policies for modernising health and welfare appear to vacillate between the need to achieve a number of desired outcomes and stress upon factors such as inclusiveness and reluctance to impose set structures. There is some evidence that values based upon communitarian ideas, such as those concerned with co-operative enquiry, mutual responsibility and reform of power relations will continue to have a bearing on shaping the state's public services, for instance in relation to creating partnership between care professionals and service users. The requirement to integrate expertise with the best available external evidence from systematic research underlines the current concern to improve professional standards within the workplace. The decision to set and enforce standards of practice and conduct in social care through registration has been identified as the administrative vehicle for achieving this. Whether a merging of the twin processes – inspection, regulation and registration, and an attempt to create more enlightened practice based upon scientific rationality – is eventually conceivable, is not likely to be apparent for several years.

References

Audit Commission (1986) *Making a Reality of Community Care*, London: HMSO.
—— (1989) *Developing Community Care for Adults with a Mental Handicap*, Occasional papers, no. 9, London: HMSO.

Baldwin, S. and Twigg, J. (1991) 'Women and community care: reflections on a debate', in M. McLean and D. Groves (eds) *Women's Issues in Social Policy*, London: Routledge, pp. 91–113.

Barclay Report (1982) 'Social workers: their role and tasks', report of a working party, London: Bedford Square Press.

Barnes, M. (1997) *Care, Communities and Citizens*, Harlow: Longman.

Barnam, P. (1992) *Closing the Asylum: The Mental Patient in Modern Society*, London: Penguin.

Bennett, D. and Morris, I. (1983) 'Deinstitutionalisation in the UK', *International Journal of Mental Health* 11(4): 5–23.

Brown, J. (1992) 'Professional boundaries in mental handicap: a policy analysis of joint training', in T. Thompson and P. Mathias (eds) *Standards in Mental Handicap: Keys to Competence*, London: Baillière-Tindall, pp. 352–70.

—— (1994) 'The caring professions', in N. Malin (ed.) *Implementing Community Care*, Buckingham: Open University Press, pp. 85–96.

Care Sector Consortium (1990) *Residential, Domiciliary and Day Care: Project National Standards*, London: HMSO.

Carr-Saunders, A. and Wilson, P. (1962) *The Professions*, Oxford: Clarendon Press.

Cole, R. and Perides, M. (1995) 'Managing values and organisational climate in a multiprofessional setting', in K. Soothill, L. MacKay and C. Webb (eds) *Interprofessional Relations in Health Care*, London: Edward Arnold, pp. 62–74.

Davis, A. (1999) 'A missed opportunity', White Paper Series: Part 3, *Community Care* 18–24 March: 23.

Department of Health [DoH] (1986) *Working Together: Education and Training*, Cmnd 9823, London: HMSO.

—— (1989) *Caring for People: Community Care in the Next Decade and Beyond*, Cm 849, London: HMSO.

—— (1998a) *Modernising Social Services: Promoting Independence, Improving Protection, Raising Standards*, London: HMSO.

—— (1998b) *Modernising Health and Social Services: National Priorities Guidance 1999/ 2000–2001/02*, London: HMSO.

Department of Health National Health Service Executive (1998) *A Consultation on a Strategy for Nursing, Midwifery and Health Visiting*, HSC, 1998/045, London: HMSO.

DHSS (1981) *Care in the Community: A Consultative Document for Moving Resources for Care in England*, HC (81) 9, LAC (81) 9, LAC (81) 5, London: HMSO.

—— (1983) *Care in the Community*, HC (83) 6, LAC (83) 5, London: HMSO.

Etzioni, A. (1969) *The Semi-Professions and their Organisation: Teachers, Nurses and Social Workers*, New York: Free Press.

Felce, D. and Grant, G. (1998) *Towards a Full Life: Researching Policy Innovation for People with Learning Disabilities*, Oxford: Butterworth-Heinemann.

Giddens, A. (1998) *The Third Way: The Renewal of Social Democracy*, Cambridge: Polity Press.

Greenwood, E. (1957) 'Attributes of a profession', *Social Work* 2(3): 44–55.

Griffiths, R. (1988) *Community Care: An Agenda for Action*, London: HMSO.

Guy's Health District (1981) *Development Group for Services for Mentally Handicapped People, Report to the District Management Team*, January.

Hatfield, B. and Mohamad, H. (1996) 'Case management in mental health services: the role of community mental health support teams', *Health and Social Care in the Community* 4(4): 215–25.

Howe, D. (1986) *Social Workers and their Practice in Welfare Bureaucracies*, Aldershot: Gower.

Hughes, E. (1971) *The Sociological Eye: Selected Papers*, Chicago: Aldine Atherton.

Hugman, R. (1991) *Power in Caring Professions*, Basingstoke: Macmillan.

Hunter, D. (1997) *Desperately Seeking Solutions: Rationing Health Care*, Harlow: Longman.

Jamous, H. and Peloille, B. (1970) 'Professions or self-perpetuating systems? Changes in the French University hospital system', in J. Jackson (ed.) *Professions and Socialisation*, Cambridge: Cambridge University Press, pp. 56–72.

Jay Committee (1979) *Report of the Committee of Enquiry into Mental Handicap Nursing and Care*, vol. 1, Cmnd 7468, London: HMSO.

Johnson, T. (1972) *Professions and Power*, London: Macmillan.

Key, B. (1995) 'Assessing your assets', *Community Care* 5–11, Oct, 28–9.

King's Fund Centre (1980) 'An ordinary life', Project paper no. 24, London: King's Fund Centre.

Langan, M. (1999) 'The management myth', *Community Care* 28 Jan–3 Feb: 24–5.

Larkin, G. (1983) *Occupational Monopoly and Modern Medicine*, London: Tavistock Press.

Lewis, J. and Glennerster, H. (1996) *Implementing the New Community Care*, Buckingham: Open University Press.

Long, A. and Harrison, S. (1996) 'Evidence-based decision making', *Health Service Journal* 106 (11 January): 8–11.

Macdonald, K. (1995) *The Sociology of the Professions*, London: Sage.

MacKay, L. (1990) 'Nursing: just another job?', in P. Abbott and C. Wallace (eds) *The Sociology of the Caring Professions*, London: Falmer Press, 116–29.

Ministry of Health (1957) *Report of the Royal Commission on Mental Illness and Mental Deficiency*, Cmnd 169, London: HMSO.

—— (1963) *Health and Welfare: The Development of Community Care*, Cmnd 1973, London: HMSO.

Parker, G. (1990) *With Due Care and Attention: A Review of Research on Informal Care*, London: Family Policy Studies Centre.

PSSRU (1990) *Care in the Community: Lessons from a Demonstration Programme*, Newsletter, no 9 May, University of Kent.

Renshaw, J., Hampson, R., Thomason, C., Darton, R., Judge, K. and Knapp, M. (1988) *Care in the Community: The First Steps*, Aldershot: Gower.

Sheffield Area Health Authority/District Council (1981) *Strategic Planning of Services for the Mentally Handicapped*, December. Joint Team of Officers, Sheffield.

Sheldon, T. and Long, A. (1994) *Report of Workshop on Clinical Effectiveness*, NHS Centre for Reviews and Dissemination, York.

Sheppard, M. (1995) *Care Management and the New Social Work: A Critical Analysis*, London: Whiting and Birch.

Social Work (Scotland) Act 1968, London: HMSO.

Toren, N. (1972) *Social Work: The Case of a Semi-Profession*, London: Sage.

Ungerson, C. (1997) 'Give them the money: is cash a route to empowerment?', *Social Policy and Administration* 31(1): 45–53.

Wilding, P. (1994) 'Maintaining quality in human services', *Social Policy and Administration* 28(1): 57–72.

Wilson, G. (1995) *Introduction*, in G. Wilson (ed.) *Community Care: Asking the Users*, London: Chapman and Hall.

Wistow, G. (1990) *Community Care Planning: A Review of Past Experience and Future Imperatives, Caring for People Implementation Document* CC13, London: DHSS.

Witz, A. (1992) *Professions and Patriarchy*, London: Routledge.

2 Professionalism in everyday practice

Issues of trust, experience and boundaries

Katie Deverell and Ursula Sharma

Introduction

Much of the existing sociological work on professions and professionalism takes a structural approach (Macdonald 1995); the focus is on how groups of people professionalise, or how professionalism can be defined, which occupations count as 'true' professions (Johnson 1981). For this reason 'professionalism' is often dismissed as rhetoric. In order to achieve status and monopolistic position in the market for services of some kind, aspiring professionals are seen to stress the distinctness of their knowledge, the undoubted authenticity of their altruism and the responsibility of their members. When professionalism is considered purely as a trope perhaps this is a legitimate line to take. However, it can overlook the fact that professionalism can also be regarded as a set of boundary-setting practices. These practices no doubt contribute to status since they distance the professional from the client, but they may also benefit the client. For example, the practitioner may adopt a persona in which his or her emotions or prejudices are backgrounded and subordinated to the client's task in hand (Cant and Sharma 1998).

In some kinds of work, knowledge – considered as formal academic knowledge derived from training – is not the only qualification for the work. There are many kinds of work where it is either essential or deemed an advantage to belong to or be identified with the client group: for example you have to be Asian and speak an Asian language to be an Asian advocacy worker in the health service, or a gay man to work for a gay and bisexual youth group. Or perhaps there is no requirement to belong to the 'client group', but workers are in fact recruited from the client body and women's refuges (and universities!). In some forms of therapy, membership or past membership of the client group may not be an advantage at the stage of recruitment, but nevertheless trainee professionals are expected to undertake therapy themselves in order to be prepared to treat others. In all these situations the professional shares identities or experience with the client group, which is seen to be as, or more important than, professional qualifications. This situation also means that professionals may share certain characteristics which decrease, rather than increase, their social distance from clients. This is particularly the case in occupations that have emerged from voluntary work or community-based organisations.

In this chapter we use examples drawn from two separate studies to explore professionalism at a more micro-level. Through a brief exploration of the experiences of homoeopaths and HIV-prevention outreach workers we identify several common themes pertinent to professionalism and boundary making, including: the importance of personal experience and empathy; maintaining a separate personal life; working in non-traditional workplaces; the nature of professional qualifications; and the management of relationships with clients. Through a discussion of these issues we show how ideas about professionalism are learned through reflexive practice and are expressed through the development and maintenance of various kinds of boundaries. This highlights how understandings of appropriate professional behaviour guide practice on an everyday level, even for those in occupations not traditionally classed as professions.

HIV-prevention outreach workers

Professionalism and boundaries

In this part of the chapter we use examples from research conducted with HIV-prevention outreach workers (Deverell 1997) to raise some issues about professionalism and boundaries. The focus of the research was on the relationship between sex, work and professionalism; a key theme was the development of boundaries within work, and between work and other parts of people's lives. We will discuss why being professional was seen to be important but also problematic for these workers, and we will highlight key themes that will be developed later in the section on homoeopaths.

Most of the outreach work undertaken within HIV prevention follows what Rhodes *et al.* have defined as 'detached outreach':

> work undertaken outside any agency setting, for example, on the streets, station concourses, in pubs and cafes. This may aim either to effect risk reduction change 'directly' (in situ) in the community, or to facilitate change 'indirectly' by attracting individuals into existing treatment and helping services.
>
> (Rhodes *et al.* 1991: 3)

The main point of outreach is for workers to go to where the targeted communities are and deliver health promotion messages in culturally appropriate ways. Those interviewed were all involved in HIV-prevention work with gay, bisexual and other men who have sex with men, and their outreach work occurred in gay pubs, clubs and public sex environments. Workers would give safer-sex advice, hand out condoms and lubricants and undertake crisis counselling. Significantly most of those interviewed had been specifically employed because they were either gay or bisexual men. Although two women who undertook this work were interviewed, many projects would only employ gay or bisexual men to undertake outreach work of this kind. This was partly because it was felt that sexual skills were needed to make contact with service users, but also because gay and bisexual men's life experience was felt to give them the necessary expertise and empathy for the work (see Deverell 1997 for a discussion).

Although outreach workers did not see themselves as a profession an idea of professionalism was drawn upon for several reasons. These included: to provide a respectable image; to communicate the importance of the work; to guide relationships with service users; to minimise the effect of personal issues on the work; and to enable personal detachment. The emphasis placed on being seen to 'be professional' was linked to the fact that the workers were being paid to provide a service. This was particularly the case because, as part of the NHS, workers were involved in competition to provide services, which exerted a further pressure to be seen as skilled and competent. Significantly, the nature of the work itself was also felt to demand a professional image. Sexual health work with gay and bisexual men takes place in a political and cultural climate that is not favourable to this target group. For the workers there was always the possibility of a local scandal which could stop the work, so they felt the need to present a professional and respectable front:

> Because the work is very new and because of its highly sexual nature, and because of its titillating sort of bits to it, unless we are seen I think as acting in the upmost professionalism then the work will be undervalued completely and people will see us as, you know, as a couple of gay boys having a good time on the poll tax or whatever.

By 'being professional' workers felt that they could gain acceptance for their work and would be taken seriously by other professionals. This involved demonstrating that outreach was much more demanding than 'just hanging around with gay men in clubs', or 'being paid to go cruising'. The reliance by HIV workers on an image of professionalism is a phenomenon which has also been pointed out by Cain, in a Canadian context:

> A professional image can help . . . workers maintain a sense of competence and expertise in the face of the uncertainty surrounding the epidemic. It is hard to measure the success of their educational efforts, and in the absence of a cure for HIV, their support programs are often experienced as inadequate. By asserting that they are providers of a specialized and professional service, workers claim a status, which is more highly valued than that afforded lay practitioners and peer counsellors. This image allows them to interact with doctors and social workers on a more equal footing and helps them successfully compete in an increasingly crowded field of AIDS service providers.
>
> (Cain 1994: 52)

Notions of professional behaviour were employed in various ways among outreach workers and were often expressed through the construction of different types of boundaries. Boundaries were seen to be essential because they enabled workers to manage their interactions with users and maintain a separate personal life. The kinds of boundaries developed included using different places to work and socialise in, the use of time as a marker between work and personal life, the use of different clothing, an emphasis on forms of self-presentation, and rules about confidentiality and the control of information. Although the nature of outreach work may make personal and professional boundaries particularly important, many of the methods employed, such as using different places in which to socialise, changing clothes and maintaining time for leisure, can be seen to be common to most occupations.

Personal or professional qualifications?

One of the questions raised by studying outreach is the difference between taught knowledge and life experience. The former is classically seen to be a defining feature of professionals (Larson 1977, 1990; Torstendahl 1990); the latter was frequently mentioned as the primary qualification for those doing HIV-prevention work with gay men. Most of the male workers saw their sexual identity as crucially important, and talked about being employed because they were gay men, rather than in relation to other skills they might have. For this reason several cited their sexual identity as the most important job qualification: as one worker said, 'being gay is our expertise'. This is quite different from the usual idea of expertise gained through professional training and formal qualifications (Crompton and Sanderson 1990). In this occupation most interviewees felt that what qualified you to do the job was life experience and insights gained from a gay sexual identity.[1] This situation was seen to be positive because it recognised the importance of community-based work and the need for culturally appropriate and rooted HIV-prevention initiatives.

Having a similar sexuality to service users was felt to engender the understanding and empathy crucial to the success of outreach. For many of the gay workers, being part of the local community and being seen to have had similar experiences and difficulties was the way in which they built trust. This led some to suggest that there was a need for a new definition of professionalism, one which recognised the usefulness of shared experience.[2] Given the nature of the places they worked in, several workers also suggested that different definitions of what it meant to be professional needed to be adopted. For example, it was possible to be professional while being naked, wearing jeans, or drinking a pint of beer.

Although a close and empathic relationship with service users was beneficial in building trust, it was not without its drawbacks. Many of the workers felt that their professional and personal lives became inextricably linked and talked about 'living the job'. For example:

I think the nature of the work concerned, it's like, because you're working with men who have sex with men and you are yourself a man who has sex with men and so on, a lot of the issues . . . are issues that concern you as well not just because you're working . . . because a lot of the people who [you] come into contact with are like yourself, and there's a kind of obligation . . . it's almost like if you weren't being paid you'd feel this duty to do it, because it's about helping your own people.

One of the big issues for the workers was that they were often dealing with issues in work that also touched them personally. This led to a clear link between work and their personal lives. Indeed, a few interviewees suggested that as gay men they sometimes over-empathised with the community, which made drawing boundaries hard and caused their personal life to suffer. Although the closeness of their relationship to service users was at times very valuable, workers had to find ways to manage it and prevent themselves from feeling overwhelmed by work and associated issues.

Interestingly, there is a move in many of the semi-professions (health promotion, social work, nursing) towards a new understanding of professionalism. This has involved the challenging of expert knowledge and a recognition of the importance of the 'self' or personal qualities of the professional, most particularly their interpersonal skills and intuition (Williams 1993). The development of a new understanding, in which the personal is seen to be a potential resource for professionals, may make the adoption of a professional identity more comfortable for many semi-professionals. However, it still raises issues about how much the personal experiences, values and feelings of the worker should influence what is done.

Trust and empathy – emotional boundaries

For many of those interviewed, the primary reason for becoming involved in the field was to work with gay men, and their feelings of empathy with clients and service users meant that sometimes they did not feel a great distinction between themselves and those with whom they worked: as part of a community many wanted to emphasise their links to it. This meant not trying to create social distance between themselves and clients in the manner of some professionals, but developing a professional relationship which maintained their connections to other men who have sex with men:

The reason why I got into this job was because I had a keen interest in seeing HIV prevention done amongst gay men . . . and because politically I wanted to be involved in a job that had something to say to me personally, something that gave me some kind of personal fulfilment, and about which I knew a lot, because I've been involved in like, gay politics and gay organisations for a long time.

Many interviewees emphasised the importance of having community links and were concerned that a professional image might distance them from the men with whom they worked. There was a feeling that to do community-based work there was a need to draw on personal experience and motivation:

> I'm not just standing there spouting off about what the textbook says, um, I'm a real person, with real feelings and a real sex life. Um, and I think there can be too much detachment, which is why I'm always testing things out . . . things like lubricants, I'll always be able to recommend to people which ones I think are the best.

This sense of empathy meant that at times the workers' identity as a professional was less strong than other identities related, for example, to their sexuality or ethnicity. For this reason, their relationships with service users were very different from those considered to be the norm for other professionals. They were not interested in increasing distance between themselves and service users/ clients but in working on the basis of a shared sexual identity – or at least the shared experience of having sex with men. Indeed, the male workers were themselves part of the client group (see also MacLachlan 1992: 443). For outreach workers distinct tensions arose from working with members of a community with which they also identified. At times they felt more like a peer than a professional and had to work hard to establish a new basis for relating.

Communicating a professional role

Developing new services in a new occupational field meant workers had to find ways to communicate their role. This was particularly important given that they were often working in spaces defined as non-work by others (pubs, clubs and public parks). Outreach workers would often refer to being professional in these contexts in terms of behaviour, or role enactments. Thus when the context did not signal professionalism they felt they could still do this through their behaviour. Because the maintenance of boundaries was seen as a way to create a work atmosphere they felt it made boundaries particularly important when working outside the office:

> in outreach it's really difficult because the boundaries are really invisible. You don't have a building around you to kind of say: 'Once through this door you're entering another organisation, you're entering another set of rules.' You're on territory that is at best, from my point of view neutral, um, in my weakest of moments I was thinking: 'well actually this is their territory' . . . they're here selling sex, or socialising, or doing something that's part of their private world, and here I am proposing to support them but coming into their world to do it. Do you know?

This was a particular issue when working in cruising areas, where until they identified themselves as workers other men would assume they were looking for sex. This meant that workers had to find ways to communicate sexual boundaries to the men they contacted through their work. The lack of physical barriers and the fact that potentially it could be relatively simple to engage in sex meant that they had to work hard at maintaining boundaries, particularly where strong sexual feelings were involved. Boundaries were felt to be less of an issue in more structured interactions in offices because here the limits of the relationship with workers were more clearly understood by service users:

> I think when you are doing outreach on the scene and things like that people . . . see you as one of them. If you are doing it in an office, if somebody comes to you in an office, you are a professional worker; do you know what I mean? It's that difference. And the power structure seems different, the power relationship feels different, it seems you're on a more of an equal level if you are out in a club.

Boundaries between work and personal life

As members of the community they worked in, interviewees often found it hard to maintain boundaries between their work and private lives. One of the common ways this was manifested was being approached for advice or information when socialising:

> quite often problems are presented as urgencies, or, um, people are desperate, or they're just really depressed . . . Obviously it's difficult to turn that sort of person away . . . like I say it's not a job, it's a way of life really in the end.

Being part of the same community, workers would often meet service users when not working and so it was important to show discretion and confidentiality. Interviewees suggested that on the streets or in a venue they would not acknowledge a service user unless they acknowledged them first. Where they were approached in their own time workers often found it hard to turn people away or refuse to provide information. In this way their experiences were not unlike others doing community-based work (Cruikshank 1989: 41). Part of the problem was that they felt responsible to pass on information that could save people's lives:

> it's the emotive part, isn't it? That's what makes it difficult. The fact that if you don't answer that question that person may do something that's unsafe that night and that could be the, the one instance and he's HIV positive or whatever else . . . that's the biggest one for everyone.

The idea that it was important to be available and to provide support to service users could make it very hard to maintain a separate personal life, particularly where their professional identity marked them out within a community. For example:

> On one occasion [my co-worker] and I were working and we were in a club and there was a very distressed client. And like the bar staff were sort of begging and pleading for us to help this guy . . . and we had to get this guy admitted to psychiatric hospital for his own safety. Because he was sort of threatening to kill himself and he was very, very distressed. And we were like sort of ostensibly on duty from half seven to eleven, but at like two o'clock in the morning we're still sitting in this psychiatric hospital trying to persuade them to admit him . . . So there's sort of no predictability about it, so it's very difficult to make arrangements socially to do anything.

The pressure to be available was keenly felt by workers anxious to build trust and to develop an image of approachability. They feared that if they rejected people in their leisure time it would be hard to discuss safer-sex issues with them when they were working. Furthermore, the workers were aware that for many men who have sex with men existing services were felt to be difficult to use because of homophobia, or a lack of understanding and empathy shown by staff. Where men had had bad experiences with health workers in the past outreach workers were particularly concerned to present their service in a positive light. This meant that they had to find ways to juggle being available and approachable with a need for their own leisure time and a desire not to get burnt out. This situation was much more of an issue in smaller towns where workers had no choice but to work and socialise in the same places.

Where there was a small and closely networked gay scene a further issue was that workers felt their own sexual experiences had the potential to damage their professional identity. For this reason many felt a great pressure always to have safer sex. This was an area where they felt it was impossible to draw a personal and professional boundary; if it became known that they had unsafe sex, their professionalism would be seriously challenged.

Developing an understanding of professionalism

Despite the influence ideas about being professional had on their work and the making of boundaries, several workers felt ambivalent about being seen as professional. It is important to note that historically it has been 'the professions' that have criminalised and pathologised gay men. For example, it is not so long since homosexuality was categorised by the American Psychiatric Association as a mental disorder and as a sickness by the British Medical Association. It is perhaps therefore not surprising that many gay workers were also critical of professionalism and wary of describing themselves as professionals:

> I think professionalism is something that's not been available . . . to disenfranchised groups on the basis of who they are . . . and so I think a lot of people have an aversion to feeling that they are professional, and the service is professional, because it has all these connotations of elitism, of exclusion, of being an expert, and of being patronising.

This work relies on being more than professional . . . it's got to do with what I was saying about vocation, and I think you've got to do it with vigour and with enthusiasm and uh with passion . . . I see being professional as being a basic set of core, like ethical, being ethical if you like, um, but I don't think this work will succeed if you're just that.

In recent years this mistrust has at times been compounded by what has come to be described as the de-gaying of AIDS and the professionalisation of the HIV field (Patton 1990; King 1993a). The involvement of professionals in the field, and links with the statutory sector, have been seen by some to have had disastrous consequences for HIV-prevention work with gay men. Because for many gay men there is a clear link both between professionalism and discrimination, and professionalism and the neglect of gay men's needs, there can be profound tensions for those workers who, although having strong identities as gay men, also view themselves as professional. This situation is further complicated by the fact that many challenges to professionalism and expertise have occurred within the HIV/AIDS field, for example over the medicalisation of HIV, or the ways in which drug trials are undertaken (Kinsman 1992; Altman 1994). Throughout the epidemic, claims to expertise and professional knowledge have not been routinely accepted but frequently challenged. Hence despite an interest in appearing professional, the construct of professionalism was something that was questioned by many workers.

Because the workers were developing roles in a new occupational field they were to some extent caught up in a process of defining appropriate professional conduct. They did not usually receive training or socialisation into an agreed set of working practices when beginning the work, but through experience developed an understanding of what being professional meant:

> Being too professional is. There's two workers I know quite well [laughs], who will not allow any physical contact with them, from the rentboys for example. Um, you know whether that's a peck on the cheek, um, a hand on the knee while they're sat talking in Burger King, um, sometimes a cuddle . . . what I often see is that clients start rejecting 'em . . . they start treating 'em on this superficial: 'Oh you're the worker, I will only tell you what you need to know, and what you ask me.' Um, on the other side of that is the worker who wears inappropriate clothing that invites unwarranted advances of hands going up . . . his kilt . . . so it goes the other way. But for me it's [professional] about being in the middle, being flexible.

Guidelines were usually developed through reflective practice and discussion. Trying to do this in a field that has consistently challenged professional groups and notions of professionalism often proved hard. For some people boundaries were experienced as barriers that got in the way of relating to peers or made one's social life difficult, for example by limiting where and with whom they could have sex. Within the HIV-prevention field issues of professionalism and boundaries have been a hot topic in the past (King 1993b; Deverell 1997), with debates highlighting how notions of appropriate behaviour are tied into beliefs about the purpose of the work itself. For example, those who see their primary role as providing life-saving information to their peers often have very different ideas to those who see their role as being paid to provide health promotion and counselling to service users.

Boundaries as personal limits

One of the interesting things about seeing professionalism as a micro-relationship is that it encourages analysis of the professional–client relationship. Several writers have suggested that trust is at the core of professional relationships (Macdonald 1995), and Rueschmeyer (1993) has argued that where the professional relationship is itself the tool for work, trust takes on increased importance. For outreach workers this idea of trust was used to guide their relationships with service users. For example, guidelines about not having sex with clients drew on a notion of professional reputation and a concern not to abuse work relationships which was borrowed from a counselling/social work perspective. Many interviewees spoke about their guidelines in terms of ethics, and clearly saw professional boundaries as part of maintaining a relationship of trust. For example:

> it's an ethical question for me. About the potential influence you might have as somebody in this job with access to all kinds of privileged knowledge about people's, not just about people's sexual behaviour but about any emotional vulnerabilities as well, and how you could misuse that.

If workers had sex or made friends with some service users it was suggested that this could be seen as favouritism and they would no longer be seen as impartial. Minimising the influence of personal issues and feelings on the work was seen to be important to maintain a focus on the needs of service users, and not cloud the workers' judgement. For this reason a key aspect of professionalism which was felt to be important was not bringing personal issues into the work. This form of behaviour is frequently associated with the idea of being professional (Garfield 1994; McElhinny 1994) and was clearly internalised by some outreach workers, who felt that keeping their personal views and feelings out of work was key to maintaining integrity and effectiveness. For them, being seen to be professional involved maintaining a stance of consistency, neutrality and fairness. For example, interviewees were often keen to ensure that men did not become too attached to them:

> A good example is a guy who's a volunteer at the moment, who apparently is very like together, very sorted, is quite happy about talking to us and suddenly behind all this there came out all this shit, about he felt he didn't have any friends, he was very isolated, he found it difficult to meet friends

on the scene, he, he's got arthritis and so finds you know moving very difficult. Sometimes he's stuck in his flat and he hasn't got any money 'cos he's on the dole, so he hasn't got a phone, he hasn't got access to communications, transport. And then he started talking about how he feels suicidal sometimes, and how he doesn't practise safer sex . . . to me the first thing that signals for me is boundaries, in terms of how I relate to that person. Am I creating a false sense of friendship which isn't there on my part? . . . where their expectations of me are beyond what I am prepared to meet and therefore that is going to damage that individual?

In this way understandings of professionalism and boundaries served to communicate workers' roles and the limits of their relationships with service users.

In the next section we build on the issues identified through this brief discussion of outreach workers' experiences by discussing professionalism and boundaries in the context of British homoeopaths.

Holism and the 'wounded healer'

Holism as a therapeutic practice

Many complementary therapists aspire to holism of one form or another. That is, they see their model of the patient–practitioner relationship as radically different from that which is explicit or implicit in biomedical practice. We shall argue that this holistic model admits of much more permeable boundaries than is the case in the biomedical clinic, and to this extent can be problematic for the practitioner. We shall refer to a general study conducted by Sharma between 1988 and 1990 consisting of interviews with complementary practitioners of various kinds in a Midlands locality. More specifically we will consider the case of non-medically qualified (NMQ) homoeopaths, studied by Sharma over a number of years, using interviews, participation at professional conferences, and analysis of journals, newsletters and other professional literature emanating from their professional body, the Society of Homoeopaths.

Holism has many modes (Sharma 1995: 111ff), but usually involves the idea that bodily sickness is not simply a pathology of the body; healing involves the engagement of the healer with the patient's mind and emotions as well as physical symptoms, an understanding of their relationship with their inner self and social environment. The healer is therefore required to undertake an empathic exploration of many different facets of experience; the practitioner–patient relationship cannot be reduced to a subject–object relationship. The more pronounced forms of holism involve something nearer to a radical egalitarianism of healer and patient, in which the former assists and empowers the latter to effect their own healing. An idea that is commonly found in this kind of holistic discourse is that of the 'wounded healer'. This is both a *prescriptive* and a *descriptive* model of healing:

> A driven desire to heal the self is often the unconscious energy behind the initial impulse to want to help the 'other' . . . empathy for the other's suffering comes, more often than not, from an inner experience of similar suffering.
>
> (Danciger 1993: 130–1)

The practice of healing enables the healer to transcend his or her own wounds through treating others, as in the myth of the wounded centaur Chiron. Suffering therefore is essential to the healer, generating both the motivation and the actual capacity to heal. Writing of power in the practitioner–patient relationship, a well-known homoeopath argues that hierarchical authority should be avoided to prevent the therapist becoming

> at best a benign parent, at worst a punitive tyrant . . . It is surely more honest to talk not of patient and practitioner, rather of fellow sufferers. This non-hierarchisation of the therapeutic relationship is preferable if compassion is to arise and healing eventuate.
>
> (Norland 1998: 10)

The notion of holism is prescriptive to the extent that the healer ought to desire healing, ought to remember to 'take care of' him/herself. (The motto of the British Holistic Medical Association is 'Physician, heal thyself'.)

Some healers do attribute their desire to heal to early and profound illness experiences (see, for example, Moore and Stephenson 1962) but the notion of the wounded healer should probably not be taken too literally. The 'wound' need not refer to a physical illness, rather to a sense of incompleteness, a desire for healing. In this way healer and patient are identified (but not conflated): 'Thus, instead of thinking that any one person is *either* only-a-healer *or* only-a-patient, we can think of the inner healer in the patient and of the inner patient in the healer' (Mitchell and Cormack 1998: 131).

While conventional biomedical practice stresses that it is the scientific detachment and knowledge of physicians that qualify them to treat patients effectively, holism of this type stresses the commonalty of experience between patient and practitioner and the vulnerability of the latter.

The very communication and identification with the patient that makes holistic healing distinctive also seem to require an intimacy incompatible with detached professionalism. This could be particularly problematic in an area where in the quest for legitimacy practitioners are very conscious of the need to present their therapies as thoroughly professional. Increasingly, complementary therapy groups are making claims to greater professionalism, pointing to the greater length and academic formality of their training courses, the guarantees provided by their codes of ethics, the professional competence of their accredited members. Yet professionalism implies the capacity to control fairly well defined boundaries between work role and personal identity (see Cant and Sharma 1998), between professional and client. How do healers who claim to be holistic deal with the potential tension between claims to increasing 'professional-ism' and highly empathic practice?

Permeable boundaries: the stresses and strains of empathic practice

When so much of the work involves attending to and uncovering deep-seated emotional problems underlying layers of somatisation, hearing out and dealing with the patient's deep distress, it is no wonder that healers described this process as stressful. A metaphor which many of them used in describing this close and supportive attention was 'tuning in':

> You get really involved with people, you really tune into them, you listen, you take it in, you try to make a connection as much as you can. (NMQ homoeopath)

Tuning in to the patient involved 'feeling with' them, being sympathetic in the literal sense, being directly conscious of their emotions and pain:

> You have to become very sensitive to the patient, you have to tune in to people on a different level. Sometimes you get it wrong but most of the time I feel that if healing's anything then it is about the whole person, and I feel a responsibility to let them open at least some of those doors. (Masseur)

This largely intuitive process of opening doors and breaking down barriers between healer and patient was seen as necessary, but draining for the healer in the long run. How did healers deal with this?

A strategy which some healers took was to limit the number of patients to put strict boundaries around their work time. This would avoid 'burn out' arising from the relatively unbounded nature of their relation with patients, the need constantly to listen, receive and support:

> To do the job properly you can't have a full weight of people every day; the problems are so intense. (Acupuncturist)

> I cannot see more than 22 or 23 people a week, no, I don't want to see any more than that. I can only see so many . . . If I see five people in a day that, basically, for me is plenty. That is the amount of patients I can emotionally handle. Then I have time to do other things. Otherwise you get into the habit of just giving and it is important to be able to give to yourself or you have nothing left to give. (NMQ homoeopath)

This obviously creates a tension between the need to earn money (all the healers interviewed in the study were in private practice) and the need to retain some part of the self that was not immersed in the process of 'tuning in'. Some estab-lished healers manage this by dividing their time between treating patients and

teaching their therapy in training colleges, writing, researching or other activities connected with their healing work. Some established homoeopaths take
'sabbaticals', i.e. time spent out of clinical practice to write, travel and reflect,
but only practitioners with a very secure reputation can afford this; it is not an
option for the novice.

Among the NMQ homoeopaths there has been much discussion of the need
for emotional support for the healer so that the openness to the patient's demands does not become overwhelming, and so that the healer can retain that
detached capacity to unravel the patient's needs and sickness which should go
along with the emotional permeability. The Society of Homoeopaths set up a
helpline for recently qualified homoeopaths to deal with this and other problems experienced by new practitioners:

> The first three years after graduating is a very difficult time, emotionally
> and financially for many homoeopaths . . . It takes a long time to learn the
> subtleties of practice, how long to leave a patient between visits, whether or
> not to phone a patient, whether to answer the phone when it rings on
> Sunday morning.
>
> (*Newsletter* June 1994: 13)

Many of the healers interviewed in the general study claimed to draw on the
emotional support of other local healers, perhaps those with whom they shared
premises, or those who had studied at the same training college. One group of
healers had actually formed a local support group for each other. About a dozen
healers practising different kinds of therapy but with a common commitment to
holism met regularly for meditation and discussion. This was seen as contributing to the healers' responsibility to 'heal themselves':

> If there is someone that's in a high degree of pain and stress then we can
> dedicate the energy to that person. (Spiritual healer)

This dedication of energy could also be directed to patients whom the healers
found difficult to heal or whom they saw as being in crisis. The group had
devised a way of permitting a flow of emotional energy from other healers
without violating the principle of patient confidentiality.

Monitoring the boundaries of competence: ambiguities and limitations

Although therapies like homoeopathy are by no means new, many have only
recently standardised their training curricula and have been undergoing a process of collectively defining the limits of their professional competences (Cant
and Sharma 1999). The Society of Homoeopaths has certainly been very active
in this respect. From one point of view this is a political process, a matter for the
various training colleges and professional bodies to get together and agree on
what competences are to be expected of persons entitled to call themselves

homoeopaths, and what issues or conditions are beyond the scope of their competence. But until this is more clearly defined, and perhaps even once it is, defining competence remains a personal issue for practitioners when they deal with complex cases. Any therapy that is practised holistically can drift into very broad and deep waters. Many interviewees recognised that what they were doing was not unlike counselling, or had a component of counselling in it. But once the opening-up process has begun, how do therapists know when they are hearing material which either should not have been voiced in the first place, or which they are powerless or just not competent to do anything about? One experienced homoeopath explains that she enlists the support of a psychiatrist when she is faced with someone whose emotional problems appear to be beyond the scope of her healing competence:

> I always endeavour to find a possible route for any suffering individual who approaches me for help; I simply recognise that I am not always the person best fitted to give that help.
>
> (Thorley 1995: 10)

Another homoeopath recognises the same problem and warns:

> Empathetic case taking is therapeutic in its own right – placebo effect if you like! – but we are not counsellors or psychotherapists. There is a potentially dangerous boundary between what we need to know to find a simillimum [ideally matched homoeopathic remedy], and entering into the realms of counselling or psychotherapy.
>
> (Napper and Lacey-Smith 1996: 7)

This homoeopath also dealt with this problem by cultivating a good working relationship with other practitioners, such as counsellors, to whom such patients could be referred.

The individual practitioner is in the position of needing to identify and monitor the limits or boundaries of his/her own competence to protect both themselves and their patients – who may be just as unclear about what are the boundaries of a therapy they may never have used before, or who may just want something much more modest than what the healer wants for them:

> The danger is that we may not sense our own inadequacies and – desperate to fulfil the needs of our patients – we may try to play a role for which we have not been trained. This can contribute largely to the famous practitioner burn-out. We cannot, and must not, attempt to counsel patients without having trained in this area, acknowledging this gap in our training also needs self-awareness. There is a danger of creating an unhealthy dynamic when we play rescuer and want more for our patients than they want for themselves. We, as homoeopaths, owe it to our patients to recognise our limitations.
>
> (Pinto 1991: 83)

Boundaries between practitioner and client: empathic enquiry and the violation of the patient

There are other issues besides that of competence. The progress of the 'opening up' and 'tuning in' process may lead the patient to make revelations which they later regret. In the case of homoeopaths, the practitioner may probe into areas which the patient does not feel comfortable talking about. For example, the practitioner may see questions about the patient's sex life as normal and consistent with the need to explore every dimension of the problem and make an appropriate prescription, but some patients may experience this as abusive:

> Our sexuality is a private and vulnerable part of who we are. It deserves a special attitude . . . people are very sensitive in this area. People who have been shocked by the intrusiveness of a homoeopathic case taking say 'why did he need this information?'
>
> (Castro 1991: 41)

But the process may also be far from neutral for the practitioner. Castro describes how in listening to what a male patient had to say about his emotional life she recognised that in the past he had been betrayed or let down in some way by a person whom Castro was able to identify as an individual known to herself, by whom she herself had also been betrayed in the course of an intimate relationship far back in the past. This odd coincidence of lives unleashed unresolved emotions of her own and 'let loose a rising tide of attraction' to the patient. Associating this patient with her ex-lover, Castro projected these rekindled emotions on to him. She explained to the patient what had happened, saying that her professional principles as a homoeopath made it difficult for her to continue to treat him, and offered to refer him to another homoeopath. Castro was surprised to hear from the patient that he preferred her to continue to treat him if she could only 'take her feelings elsewhere'. She did so and 'healed a hurt that was long overdue'. Eventually this healing process in herself enabled her to treat the patient successfully (Castro 1991). The process of feeling *with* the patient holistically and the letting down of barriers which this involves can lead to the revisiting of painful old emotions on the part of the patient, and sometimes the healer also. This has to be resolved by some appropriate drawing up of new boundaries on the part of the healer, but is acknowledged by Castro as a very difficult business, requiring much self-examination and maturity.

The issue of sexual abuse, the violation of professional boundary keeping *par excellence*, has not been discussed very much among complementary practitioners, at least not in their public and official journals. This is in strong contrast to psychotherapy and counselling, where the issues are well rehearsed. Some psychotherapy groups have prohibited any kind of touching of the client by the therapist, to preclude the client accusing the therapist of abuse, or indeed to preclude the vulnerable client experiencing touch as abuse. In some complementary therapies (reflexology, massage) touch is an essential part of the treatment, and some of the healers whom I interviewed remarked that touch often facilitated the 'opening up' and 'tuning in' processes, assisting the flow of information from patients who might otherwise have found it difficult to talk about themselves.

Some healers are familiar with the concept of transference as used in psychoanalytic discourse. This idea provides a cognitive framework for understanding some of the emotions which the treatment (especially the 'opening up' and 'tuning in' parts) may unleash in the patient, but not all healers will have encountered this idea in the course of their training. They may therefore find themselves puzzled by some patient responses. One relatively inexperienced homoeopath revealed in a discussion group how he had been horrified when the simple gesture of putting his arm around the shoulder of a distressed patient had been interpreted as a sexual advance rather than empathy. The patient had felt attracted to the healer and the healer had then to disentangle himself from the situation.

Obviously treatment which can open up such emotional responses in the patient (and, as we have seen, sometimes in the practitioner also) raises problems about confidentiality. On the whole, holistic healing takes place within a framework which in many respects is not totally unlike the context in which doctors and patients interact in the biomedical clinic (and it must not be forgotten that some holistic practitioners are also biomedical doctors). That is, the relationship is conceived as individual and confidential; the practitioner does not have the right to reveal what the patient has said in the course of consultation except under very specific circumstances.

Yet there is an important sense in which a holistic understanding of sickness does not treat the patient as an 'individual' but as part of an interwoven set of relationships, embedded in a physical and social environment. Several practitioners whom I interviewed found that this contradiction sometimes generated a degree of frustration. One might become aware that much of the patient's suffering was a direct or indirect consequence of problematic relations with others; but one would not have access to those others or to their point of view. One ostoeopath pointed out that in some cases members of the same family might come to him as patients presenting different problems. Often he was aware that their problems were interconnected, but to treat the patients as other than individuals would be to violate important professional boundaries. Practising confidentiality with any seriousness meant not carrying information given by one patient into the treatment of another, related patient, putting boundaries around information. One reflexologist was aware that patients often 'opened up' to the extent that they made intimate revelations, and then they finished speaking and said: 'I don't know why I told you that.'

Though professionalism increasingly demands that practitioners keep systematic records of consultations, one practitioner said that when he heard such strange revelations

> They are locked within me. Sometimes I don't even write them down. [Patients] trust me and I don't abuse their trust. (Reflexologist)

Time and place: the boundaries of work

As we have seen, the lack of a well-defined 'workplace' was a problem for outreach workers. Some complementary therapists also had problems in avoiding over-accessibility. Interactions cannot always be limited to strictly scheduled appointments, and the support required by the patient in the journey towards wellness is not always predictable. In many forms of healing one hears reference to the idea of a 'healing crisis', a phase of treatment in which the patient's symptoms may worsen temporarily. In such a situation the patient may urgently require encouragement – which of course the healer will wish to provide, if only so that the patient does not simply give up the treatment. Homoeopaths in particular consider the healing process as highly likely to involve a reappearance of earlier symptoms; as the patient improves the symptoms are liable to reappear in the reverse order of their original appearance. This is regarded as normal, but the patient may not understand this and may require contact for immediate reassurance or support.

This is particularly problematic if, as is the case with many practitioners starting out, the practitioner is operating from his or her own home rather than a public consulting room. Several recently qualified homoeopaths described that they had had to work out for themselves strategies for maintaining a reasonable degree of accessibility for anxious patients while meeting their own needs for rest and privacy. Telephone technology provided a good answer for many. Putting a message on an answering machine – that requests for new appointments would be dealt with between, say, nine and ten in the morning, while queries from existing patients would be dealt with between five and six in the evening – cued the patients as to appropriate times to ring with their particular problem without making them wait a long time. Many holistic therapists do permit patients a degree of freedom of access which GPs may once have permitted but have now almost entirely abrogated. They juggle the wish to avoid the impersonality they associate with the biomedical clinic with the need to protect themselves from the emotional overloading and intolerable incursions into their own personal time that can lead to 'burn out'.

In this respect the homoeopaths resemble the outreach workers, having the same need to negotiate a way between over-identification with the client (on the one hand) and empathy and the practice of reflexive knowledge (on the other) so that they can be effective in their work. Claims to demonstrate 'professionalism' describe and legitimate the products of this juggling process.

Discussion

From some points of view the comparison of outreach workers with NMQ homoeopaths might seem strained. Outreach workers work in the community, while holistic healers work from the more ordered setting of a consulting room. Unlike NMQ homoeopaths, outreach workers do not have a representative professional body which is attempting to define a collectively acceptable professional practice; for them the responsibility of defining boundaries for themselves is more consciously and individually felt in everyday work.

On the other hand, there are some features of their work which both these groups share with some other new occupational groups who provide 'professional' services in non-bureaucratic or unconventional settings, especially those which have in one way or another challenged existing professional groups or dominant notions of professionalism. Both espouse a philosophy of client empowerment with a concomitant abnegation of hierarchical practitioner–client relations. Both holistic healers and outreach workers experience a tension between traditional ideas about professional detachment and working relationships that demand some degree of intimacy or closeness. In many other professions, using shared identification as a resource would be seen as over-involvement and therefore unprofessional. For example, Purtillo (1993) suggests that over-identification with clients can be very damaging, and Hanmer and Statham (1993) point out that while female social workers often experience links with their clients, they are not encouraged to recognise these for fear of over-involvement with the client.

Whatever the collective professional view, accounts of everyday practice show that many professionals find that in their everyday work with clients personal life experience is as important as formalised knowledge. For the outreach workers and the healers these areas of commonality were seen quite explicitly as a positive resource. While quite extensive formal professional training had been received by most homoeopath interviewees, both the outreach workers and the healers drew on life experience that could not, by its very nature, be conveyed through professional training. Yet in most accounts of professionalisation, the creation of a body of knowledge that can be conveyed through academic instruction is a key component of the claim to professionalism. Both the groups we have described experience this contradiction in the course of their everyday work in terms of an ongoing need to define boundaries between self and client, work self and non-professional persona. In the case of outreach workers there is also the strain of working in a setting where there are no physical boundaries to 'work space'. In the case of the healers there is the need to ring-fence their own personal time so that accessibility for clients does not lead to an invasion of private life. In both cases (though more especially in the case of the outreach workers), this requires an ongoing personal effort which can contribute to stress and even 'burn out'.

When outreach workers and healers refer to the notion of professionalism either as a problem or as an ideal to aspire to, they are not therefore simply using empty rhetoric, but referring to ideas they use to orient themselves when working in non-bureaucratic settings. While many accounts of professional work have contrasted the professional ethos with the bureaucratic ethos, we should not underestimate the extent to which many of the occupational groups who are regarded as undoubtedly 'professional' work within a bureaucratic setting even if they do not regard themselves as bureaucrats. As Freidson points out, the bureaucratic organisation to which they are subject is usually loose enough for their work to be recognisable as professional (Freidson 1986: 158ff). The accounts elsewhere in this book of tension between managerialism and professionalism can be understood as reflecting a tightening up of bureaucratic control in such formerly loosely organised groups. Yet healers outside the NHS have never had managers or bureaucratic superiors in the first place, and outreach workers conduct their everyday work in a space physically and culturally removed from those who manage them.

As they professionalise (and some do so with a profound sense of ambivalence, pointing to the medical profession as the self-interested collectivity *par excellence*), homoeopaths will struggle to retain the sense that personal experience and empathy are among their most valuable resources. And could the outreach workers ever retain the necessary identification with clients were their employment to depend mainly upon professional credentials? In the case of outreach workers it is possible that there is no way to reconcile professionalism (as they understand it) with professionalisation.

Notes

1 Because of the historical (and in some cases continued) discrimination by professions, formal qualifications are not necessarily going to be seen as signs of trust by gay and bisexual men (see King 1995). Indeed, it is more likely that trust will be signalled through shared identity or sexual practice, as well as through symbols that signify a link to sex with men and/or gay communities.

2 One of the reasons why interviewees might not have made reference to knowledge is that health promotion work may differ from other professionally associated occupations. Indeed, Macdonald (1995: 134) argues that the emphasis on the importance of practice, rather than knowledge, in the caring professions has devalued these occupations and made it harder for them to achieve professional status. This has been compounded by the expectation of objectivity as an aspect of professional practice. This causes problems for the caring professions because their work involves a degree of involvement which others would see as undermining their professionalism (p. 137). This is especially important in relation to the health services, and particularly work which is community based. In the last twenty years various social and political movements have led to the emergence of a 'new public health' which emphasises the need for a style of work that is needs led and owned by communities (Ashton and Seymour 1988). This has led to a style of health promotion which encourages professionals working in partnership with communities. This method of work profoundly challenges the traditional expert and pedagogical role of the health professional (see Williams 1993), who in this different role becomes an involved guide and advocate rather than a distant educator and expert. In this way outreach workers' challenges to ideas of professionalism can be seen as part of a wider move within health promotion to change the nature of working relationships.

References

Altman, D. (1994) *Power and Community. Organizational and Cultural Responses to AIDS*, London: Taylor and Francis.
Ashton, J. and Seymour, H. (1988) *The New Public Health*, Milton Keynes: Open University Press.

Cain, R. (1994) 'Managing impressions of an AIDS service organization: into the mainstream or out of the closet?', *Qualitative Sociology* 17(1): 43–61.

Cant, S. and Sharma, U. (1998) 'Reflexivity, ethnography and the professions (complementary medicine)', *Sociological Review* 46(2): 244–63.

—— (1999) *A New Medical Pluralism? Alternative Medicine, Doctors, Patients and the State*, London: UCL Press.

Castro, M. (1991) 'Sex in the consulting room', *The Homoeopath* 11(2): 39–44.

Crompton, R. and Sanderson, K. (1990) *Gendered Jobs and Social Change*, London: Unwin Hyman.

Cruikshank, J. (1989) 'Burnout: an issue among Canadian community development workers', *Community Development Journal* 24(1): 40–54.

Danciger, E. (1993) 'The wounded healer', *The Homoeopath* 51: 130–2.

Deverell, K.E. (1997) 'Sex, work and professionalism: a qualitative study of boundary construction by HIV prevention outreach workers', unpublished Ph.D. thesis, University of Keele.

Freidson, E. (1986) *Professional Powers: A Study of the Institutionalization of Formal Knowledge*, Chicago: University of Chicago Press.

Garfield, S. (1994) *The End of Innocence – Britain in the Time of AIDS*, London: Faber and Faber.

Hanmer, J. and Statham, D. (1993) 'Commonalities and diversities between women clients and women social workers', in J. Walmsley, J. Reynolds, P. Shakespeare and R. Woolfe (eds) *Health, Welfare and Practice: Reflecting on Roles and Relationships*, London: Open University/Sage.

Johnson, T. (1981) *Professions and Power*, London: Macmillan.

King, E. (1993a) *Safety in Numbers*, London: Cassell.

—— (1993b) 'Beating boundaries', *The Pink Paper* 17 September, 295: 14.

—— (1995) 'Stab in the dark', *The Pink Paper* 1 September: 8.

Kinsman, G. (1992) 'Managing AIDS organizing: "consultation", "partnership", and the national AIDS strategy', in W.K. Carroll (ed.) *Organizing Dissent: Contemporary Social Movements in Theory and Practice*, Canada: Garamond Press.

Larson, M.S. (1977) *The Rise of Professionalism: A Sociological Analysis*, London: University of California Press.

—— (1990) 'In the matter of experts and professionals, or how impossible it is to leave nothing unsaid', in R. Torstendahl and M. Burrage (eds) *The Formation of Professions: Knowledge, State and Society*, London: Sage.

Macdonald, K. (1995) *The Sociology of the Professions*, London: Sage.

MacLachlan, J. (1992) 'Managing AIDS: a phenomenology of experiment, empowerment and expediency', *Critique of Anthropology* 12(4): 433–56.

McElhinny, B. (1994) 'An economy of affect: objectivity, masculinity and the gendering of police work', in A. Cornwall and N. Lindisfarne (eds) *Dislocating Masculinity*, London: Routledge.

Mitchell, A. and Cormack, M. (1998) *The Therapeutic Relationship in Complementary Health Care*, London: Churchill Livingstone.

Moore, M. and Stephenson, J. (1962) 'A Motivational and Sociological analysis of homoeopathic physicians in the USA and UK', *British Homoeopathic Journal* 51: 297–303.

Napper, R. and Lacey-Smith, J. (1996) 'Psyche and remedy – a joint perspective', *Society of Homoeopaths Newsletter*, 7 March.

Norland, M. (1998) 'A few thoughts on taking the case', *The Homoeopath* 69: 10.

Patton, C. (1990) *Inventing Aids*, London: Routledge.

Pinto, G. (1991) 'Supervision and support in practice', *The Homoeopath* 11(3): 83–5.

Purtillo, R. (1993) 'Meaningful distances', in J. Walmsley, J. Reynolds, P. Shakespeare and R. Woolfe (eds) *Health, Welfare and Practice: Reflecting on Roles and Relationships*, London: Open University/Sage.

Rhodes, T., Holland, J. and Hartnoll, R. (1991) *Hard to Reach or Out of Reach? An Evaluation of an Innovative Model of HIV Outreach Health Education*, London: Tuffnell Press.

Rueschmeyer, D. (1993) 'Professional autonomy and the social control of expertise', in R. Dingwall and P. Lewis (eds) *The Sociology of the Professions*, London: Macmillan.

Sharma, U. (1995) *Complementary Medicine Today: Practitioners and Patients* (revised edition), London: Routledge.

Thorley, A. (1995) 'Psyche speaks in homoeopathy', *Society of Homoeopaths Newsletter* December: 10.

Torstendahl, R. (1990) 'Introduction: promotion and strategies of knowledge-based groups', in R. Torstendahl and M. Burrage (eds) *The Formation of Professions: Knowledge, State and Society*, London: Sage.

Williams, J. (1993) 'What is a profession? Experience versus expertise', in J. Walmsley, J. Reynolds, P. Shakespeare and R. Woolfe (eds) *Health, Welfare and Practice, Reflecting on Roles and Relationships*, London: Sage/Open University.

3 Professionalism and user self-advocacy

Steve McNally

Introduction

This chapter considers the nature and impact of self-advocacy by service users. Initially some key literature in this subject area will be reviewed; subsequently the chapter describes original research in the area of self-advocacy for people with a learning disability. The ways in which self-advocacy relates to professional boundaries will be explored, along with clients' views of service workers and the influence of these perceptions on professional roles. Implications for training, development and supervision of service professionals will be analysed in the light of research findings. While the chapter is relevant to a range of disciplines, the professional group referred to most often is nursing. Although the focus of the research is on people with a learning disability, implications for other groups of service users are also explored.

The chapter comprises three sections. First there is an overview of the concept of self-advocacy, followed by an initial discussion of professionals and the advocacy role. The second part draws on interviews with service users with a learning disability who participate in self-advocacy groups. The focus here will be on service users' perception of staff and staff roles. Finally, the connections between user self-advocacy and the client–professional relationship are considered, with particular reference to the impact on professional roles.

Self-advocacy

The concept of self-advocacy has gained prominence in recent years. It is a device which is particularly apposite for use by people who are disadvantaged in society, or who are at risk of such disadvantage. Self-advocacy provides a strategy by means of which members of a potentially vulnerable group – for example disabled people or users of mental health services – can redress this imbalance in society by securing their rights.

Advocacy is partly a device to influence the needs and rights of the group in favour of the needs and rights of individuals (Brandon 1995). Advocacy is a powerful mechanism for achieving empowerment. Several types of advocacy are concerned with representing another person's wishes. Self-advocacy is about people speaking for themselves and asserting their own rights, individually and in groups which share a common interest or face particular difficulties, for example stigma. It has been an important and influential idea for two decades, especially in services for people with learning disabilities.

Self-advocacy is associated with groups, there being different types with different objectives, for example service-linked groups and independent groups. What groups have in common is the capacity to provide a supportive, empathic environment in which a person belongs and is valued. Groups offer the individual the opportunity to learn skills and to develop confidence.

People with a learning disability have described self-advocacy as 'sticking up for yourself' (Simons 1992). Definitions of self-advocacy often refer to 'speaking up for yourself', 'standing up for your rights', 'taking action' and 'changing things' (Williams and Shoultz 1982). The core components of self-advocacy have been identified by Clare (1990) as being able to express thoughts and feelings with assertiveness, if necessary; being able to make choices and decisions; having clear knowledge about rights; being able to make changes. Any act of self-determination or choice can be seen as self-advocacy. *Everyone can take part in self-advocacy at some level, regardless of the severity of their disabilities* (Crawley 1987: 1). People with a severe learning disability can be and are involved in self-advocacy.

The importance of promoting self-advocacy for adults who have learning disabilities cannot be overstated; despite the emphasis on improving quality of life and access to the mainstream of the community, people with learning disabilities may still not enjoy full civil rights. From its origins in Sweden in the 1960s, People First – the international self-advocacy movement – began in the USA in 1973 when service users in Oregon wished to meet as peers. Self-advocates from the UK attended the inaugural People First international conference at Tacoma, Washington, USA in 1984. People First of London was established during the same year. Culturally, self-advocacy is well established in Western countries (Bramley and Elkins 1988). In other parts of the world, for example Pakistan, Western ideas of self-advocacy are considerably less relevant (Miles 1992).

The self-advocacy movement has developed rapidly in the UK in recent years. There is some empirical data which indicates an increase in the number of self-advocacy groups since the 1980s (Crawley 1987; Whittaker 1991). Groups have become established to encourage and support members to develop their skills and to assert their interests.

Self-advocacy could be seen as a potent medium through which the individual could have greater control in his or her life; as a means to achieving self-empowerment. The relationship between self-advocacy, empowerment and citizenship is strong.

Recent community care legislation (NHS and Community Care Act 1990) has emphasised the importance of representation of service users. A central policy aim of *Caring for People* (Department of Health 1989) was to give people more say in the services they use: 'promoting choice and independence underlies all the government's proposals' (ibid.: 4). Means and Smith (1994) cite subsequent Departmental guidance for practitioners which stresses the empowerment of users and carers as the rationale for community care reforms (ibid.: 71). Local authorities which provide social services are required to consult with service users and user organisations (Monach and Spriggs 1994). While it has been observed that the 'consumer' role of users of health and welfare services is a myth (Shemmings and Shemmings 1995), the voice of service users is considered crucial. This recognition is particularly significant for members of vulnerable groups.

Any serious discussion of self-advocacy must take account of empowerment (Beresford and Croft 1993: 85), given the close relationship between these concepts and the centrality of user and carer empowerment in recent community care legislation. Empowerment is a process which can be seen as a journey from personal needs to influencing and changing the attitudes and values, policy and practice that affect them (Croft and Beresford 1995). It is also an outcome (Gibson 1991). Self-advocacy can be regarded as a means of achieving empowerment.

The role which professionals play in the empowerment of service users has been the subject of much debate. While some argue that they have a crucial role in the empowerment of service users (Parsloe and Stevenson 1992), others take the view that this perspective is too cosy – for real empowerment to occur, users have to seize power for themselves rather than depend on benign professionals to give away some of their power (Jack 1995). There exist examples of studies which conclude that, although workers felt that they empowered users and carers through advocacy and assertiveness training, users reported frustration (Servian 1996).

Mental health service users have insisted on changes to services which have been characterised by reliance on institutional care, drug treatment and professional power (Braye and Preston-Shoot 1995). The growth of *Survivors Speak Out*, a network of psychiatric system survivors and allies, has been charted (Plumb 1993; Brandon 1995). By 1992, over 100 groups which could be described as self-advocacy or user groups were active in Britain (Wallcraft 1994). Plumb's (1993) paper considers the significance of *Survivors Speak Out* and the implications of the movement for practitioners and writers in the mental health field. In the United States, mental health associations have worked to prevent mental health problems through advocacy initiatives as well as by providing preventive intervention services. Banyay (1989) describes Project Share, a consumer-run, self-help advocacy programme in Pennsylvania. As is the case with learning disability, groups for people with mental health problems fall into a number of categories, including service linked, patients' councils or advocacy schemes, action groups concentrating on local service provision, and issues-based regional or campaigning groups. Provision of resources to implement self-advocacy for all users has been identified as a key issue. The greatest level of activity in the UK survivor movement has been reported to be self-advocacy *within* the mental health service system (Lindow 1995).

Recent research in the mental health field has investigated the views of people experiencing mental ill-health concerning self-advocacy. This was accomplished by means of focus group discussions to generate an interview schedule for use with individuals (Mawhinney and McDaid 1997). Service users were asked what encouraged them to speak up for themselves. Four categories emerged: strong emotion, relationships, knowledge, and encouragement and support.

Staff attitudes to self-advocacy were also explored. Overall, staff attitudes were positive about user self-advocacy. Concern was expressed about the possibility that the views of confident, assertive individuals would override the views of the less vocal. Some staff members felt that some service users would begin to complain constantly. This would best be handled by having a consistent, cohesive staff team.

Advocacy and nursing

It has been noted that recent years have seen an increase in publicity for the career of the nurse as patient advocate, with a preponderance of advocacy-related literature emanating from the United States and exerting influence on nursing in Britain (Mallik 1995). The most influential proponents of the nurse advocate role are probably Murphy and Gadow (Millette 1989). The advocacy role has been conceptualised as enabling and supporting the client (Murphy 1979). Murphy developed three models of advocacy in order to examine the barriers to the practice of such a role, namely the bureaucratic advocate, the physician advocate, and the client advocate model. Each model is distinguished by the influence of the salient factor, for example bureaucracy. In the client advocate model the person becomes the primary focus, with all health professionals working together to attain the client's self-determined goal. According to Murphy, it is the client advocate model which is most conducive to a positive nurse–patient relationship. While all three models may be employed at different times, it is the client advocate role which is the preferred model for the professional nurse.

Gadow characterised advocacy as the philosophical foundation of nursing. She sees freedom of self-determination as the most fundamental and valuable human right (Gadow 1979). Moreover, the nurse has a responsibility to assist the patient to achieve self-determination (Gadow 1980). A key principle is the egalitarian nature of the relationship, in which the nurse does not assume a superior or inferior position in relation to the client.

The nursing elite controlling the output of professional journals have supported this career of the nurse as patient advocate, as have professional organisations involved in national regulation and nurse education. Advocacy is a principle which underpins practice for nurses nationally and internationally (ICN 1973; UKCC 1992). Indeed, it is a requirement for practice in some parts of the USA (Mallik 1997).

Teasdale (1994: 94) summarises the advocacy debate thus:

> The main argument in favour of advocacy by nurses is the amount of contact they have with their patients, which potentially helps them to become

aware of the worries and wants of the vulnerable people in their care. Ranged against this is the argument that nurses may lack the independence and objectivity required of a true advocate.

The culture of the organisation and staff beliefs concerning their own role and their attitude towards clients are crucial. Nurses interviewed in an exploratory study of advocating for patients, working in general medical and surgical clinical areas, identified some key themes. The importance of the therapeutic relationship as the key to advocacy, the idea of nurse and patient sharing common humanity, and the cultural environment of care were prominent. Participants spoke of promoting humane care, characterised by equal nurse–patient relationships in an environment which they identified as 'having the potential to either enhance or limit their ability to advocate for patients' rights' (Snowball 1996: 72).

The role and purpose of learning disability nursing is concerned with promoting the empowerment of service users. Services for people with a learning disability have long been acknowledged as being at the forefront of developments designed to empower clients (Malin and Teasdale 1991). A recent Department of Health project on learning disability nursing concluded that nurses should place stronger emphasis on the support of initiatives that enable people with a learning disability to advocate for themselves, and that the DoH should support initiatives which develop better information for managers and professional staff on advocacy and self-advocacy (Kay *et al.* 1995). According to Gadow (1980) the nurse is in an ideal position to relate to the patient as a unique and complex individual, and she believes this to be a precondition for advocacy. Some writers are more circumspect about nurses as advocates but acknowledge that in certain circumstances it is desirable that they should take on this role (Gates 1994).

Group members' perspectives

Self-advocacy groups involved in the study identified a number of important issues in response to a postal survey. 'Relationships with staff' was cited as an important issue. Conducting staff interviews and training staff had also emerged as themes in the survey. The extracts used in this section are taken from a range of group interviews. Fifteen self-advocacy groups participated in this phase of the research, which used audiotaped semi-structured interviews. While the groups varied in type – from service-based, typically at a day centre, to completely independent – and character, some strong themes emerged. Relationships with staff was a crucial area for the self-advocates.

In some cases, groups were facilitated by accountable, independent advisers who were directly answerable to the group or employed by an independent body which had contracted to support groups and is subject to monitoring. Advisers were present during some group interviews, with the consent of group members.

An interview schedule was used as a framework but group members were able to say anything that they thought was relevant to self-advocacy. The researcher asked supplementary questions in order to explore themes emerging during the interviews. The questions used were mostly open. To help to generate ideas, it was necessary at times to use prompts, to pose the same question in a different way, making adjustments in the wording used according to the group giving the interview. Most of the groups, however, provided rich accounts of their experience of and views concerning self-advocacy, sometimes anticipating questions.

The purpose of the group

What is the group for?

For service users. It's all about rights, this group . . . it has helped us to make choices for ourself and speaking for ourselves.

We go and discuss it in a staff meeting and some staff don't like change.

The group is for helping to solve things that are difficult. Our rights and what we would like to do and things like that.

[A chair of group] I want to make things a bit more organised and stuff. We don't just talk about things, we like to do things as well.

We enjoy coming to the group and we enjoy getting involved in decision making.

How a service should be run – not the bosses telling us how it should be run.

We try to talk about things and we can't get anywhere.

What is self-advocacy?

It's about speaking up for yourself and sticking up for yourself, and about how everyone's got rights.

Speaking up for yourself. Making choices.

Do you speak up for yourself outside of the group?

You have to or otherwise you won't get anything done.

Effecting change

Effecting change is an issue for self-advocacy groups.

> We have changed the name of the centre.

> [About the council proposing cuts in services] Things have been taken away. They weren't really bothered with us. We went to meetings but they had already made up their minds.

The last two extracts illustrate the achievement and the frustration of attemping to bring about change. The process of trying, even if the desired change is not achieved, can be a valuable learning experience.

Peer advocacy

Peer advocacy is an area in which self-advocates express an interest. The person quoted below represents somebody who attends a different day service within the same urban area.

> I support . . . X . . . there is not much confidence there at all.

Role of the adviser

A particular role which carries the potential for boundary issues is that of facilitator to a self-advocacy group. It is said that individuals who facilitate groups should be entirely independent of the service settings which the group members use (Dowson and Whittaker 1993). There is indeed a strong rationale for this stance, given the tensions and conflicts which can arise if a service-employed group facilitator is compromised by their line manager or organisation.

In practice, many self-advocacy and user groups for people with a learning disability are facilitated by staff members. Independent advocacy workers are not always available; when they are – although they do not experience conflicting service users' and organisational agendas – questions about power and control still loom large. Ideally groups' members would take on the key roles without depending on the input of a non-disabled facilitator.

The groups had clear ideas about the adviser's role:

> *What should a good helper do in the group?*

> Advisers should not interrupt . . . We brought this up in a meeting, when we go to a conference meeting, any member of staff from any centre are not allowed to say anything while we are speaking.

> They should listen to both sides of the story.

Help you with any problems. She is very understanding.

You should make arrangements . . . You should acknowledge people. To prove that they are equal.

We thought it better to have someone from outside [of the day service].

We used to have it in the hall at one time. A great big mass meeting. It got too much so we had to go back to the old one.

Organising things like agendas. Take it in turns.

If there have been any major problems in the past we have had to see the manager to deal with them properly.

[To the adviser] You're there to help us make sure everything is all sorted out, such as the accounts, because we have our own bank for the funding.

There isn't an adviser for this group — we are all advisers and there isn't a supporter, we are all supporters.

[Adviser] This is a very open and honest group. If they are not happy with things, they say. Like the minute-writing wasn't good enough so we type it now.

They like minutes by almost return of post, so they have got the time to do it themselves on the computer.

They help us with very tricky things.

If we want to say something we put it how we said it.

Without X [an adviser who has a disability] we wouldn't get very far.

X is very good, pretty accurate [at recording minutes].

They should be smart at doing their job.

What should a good adviser be like?

Intelligent, helpful and cheerful.

Does the group help you?

Yes. I like being in the group. In a big group it's noisy but in a smaller group it's all right.

We have set jobs to do [representing others who use the service]. We have got an agenda.

I went on a 12-week course for committee skills – it was really great.

Some people are not confident to say something. You have to have some-body else speak up for them.

Some people in wheelchairs, they can't talk. Some can't speak properly so we speak for them.

[Adviser] That's like saying that all people in wheelchairs can't speak and that's not so, is it?

On groups having their own, accountable adviser

Do you think that having a worker is an idea that other groups might take up?

I think they should do.

What difference has it made to you, having a worker?

Well the difference is that if one of us did it we wouldn't catch up because we wouldn't be able to write down like you [SM].

If one of you lot [group] says something, and one of us wants to write something down we could keep up so that's what we asked — to do. She can write anything down and keep up with things.

On selecting staff

How long has the group had a worker? Is this a new thing?

We did interview people. We interviewed her [supporter] for the job and we asked her questions. Could you cope doing this whatever, you know, and then we finished the interview and we asked her to go out, didn't we, and we let her back in and asked her if she would take the job and that was it.

Another member of the same group

I did do some interviews . . . like this one here now, with the staff [at the day centre].

You actually interviewed them for their jobs?

To see if they were good enough.

What did the worker think about the selection process?

I was more nervous when I was interviewed by you lot because there were nine of you. It was the biggest interview panel I'd ever had.

We interviewed – and – for the job of self-advocacy woman. They brought back some really good stuff [in the interview]. That's what we like and it had some good points . . . If we didn't do that [the interview] we wouldn't have had them.

A member of this group, reflecting on being interrupted during the interview process:

I said 'Excuse me, we are here and we are interviewing somebody.' We had to get somebody higher up to make them sit out there.

In the near future we are going to do some interviews, when there's a job advertised [in a day service], pick somebody.

Relationships with staff

Some of them are OK but some of them are well . . . Some of them you can have a laugh and a chat with and some of them you like say something and then it gets back to management and gets you into trouble.

So when that happens what do you do about it?

We usually go to the manager himself.

Some staff are alright because they will listen to you and some of them won't listen to you, just don't want to know about things.

Do you go to the ones who will listen to you?

Yes. It upsets you an' all.

I went to a day centre . . . I was told what to do and when to do it. You had to do what they told you to do, and I got fed up with it. I went to see my social worker and asked them to find me something else . . .

> The thing about this group is that we are standing up for our rights. The staff listen to us more than they used to.

The above statements are quite forthright and illustrate the impact which staff responses may have upon service users. It is sometimes the case that people with a learning disability will perceive staff members as 'friends'. Friendship, literature suggests, is often based on similarity of social class, status, income group.

This need not be problematic if both parties are clear about the nature of the relationship and know where the boundaries lie. The context may be that the service user refers to the staff member as friend to denote a valued, trusted supporter whose company the person enjoys.

Self-concept

> I've got a learning disability.

> *People with a learning disability can still achieve a lot, can't they?*

> Yes. But we are a bit slower at it.

The above exchange is interesting because the group member said spontaneously that he has a learning disability. Evidence suggests that people tend to reject the label of 'mental handicap', a term still widely used, distancing themselves from the term and its implications (Booth and Simons 1989). The young man involved may have found 'learning disability' an acceptable term, possibly even taking a positive ownership of it (Szivos and Griffiths 1990). Self-esteem is an important aspect of self-concept; group membership can be a valuable source of information which the individual can use to build self-concept (Harris 1995). Those interested in examining the connection between individual identity – including for example, power and self-esteem – and membership of social groups may wish to refer to the work of Tajfel (1981).

Independence

> College is alright because the tutor don't tell you what to do, not like when you're at school. At school the teachers tell you off every five minutes.

> I like the course because it teaches you how to be independent . . . it teaches you that one day you could be independent for yourself and you won't be living at home.

> That's what we come here for, isn't it, to be independent?

> I'm looking forward to it [moving to a home of his own]. I've always had in my mind a big house and everything in it . . . very posh and a garage.

Reference to independence and living in their own home by the self-advocates quoted above is interesting. Self-advocates vary in how much of their self-advocacy group activities they share at home. Individuals may choose to separate aspects of their lives. The application of self-advocacy by a person and the encouragement and acceptance of this within the family could be said to represent the attainment of adulthood or the route towards it (Mitchell 1997).

Management

> If they are breaking the rules they have to be disciplined by the Management Committee meeting. [Committee is comprised of service users, staff members, a parent representative and a volunteer. Service users form the majority].

> Committee decides on new members.

> Taken in turns to chair.

> *What happens when someone breaks the rules?*

> It depends on how serious it is. Then we have an emergency meeting and decide. Usually people are sent away [excluded] for a few weeks. I've had that before.

Confronting racism

The benefits of a group for black and ethnic minority members:

> It makes me meet different people like Asian, like different religions. That's the best thing really.

On being abused verbally by another service user:

> I felt very angry and hurt. He shouldn't say things like that. Then . . . I went to see somebody to sort them out. [Went to see a staff member to explain what had happened.]

On council policy:

> Any form of racism is [reason for] exclusion for staff or trainees. A first offence is enough. If we can be sure that trainees understand that what they are saying is offensive, that's good enough reason.

The person speaking here – a supporter of self-advocacy – was on the staff of a unit that prepares trainees for open employment.

It has been recognised for some time that the diversity of people's needs, including those related to ethnicity and culture, tend to have been obscured by the label of 'learning disability' (Baxter *et al.* 1990).

The sociology of disability has developed in recent years, contributing to our understanding through the theorising of personal experience. The social model of disability has gained prominence. Dependency is created among disabled people, not because of the effects of functional limitations on their capacities for self-care, but because their lives are shaped by a variety of economic, political and social forces which produce it (Oliver 1990: 94). While the social model has enriched the sociology of disability (Chappell 1998), concern has been expressed at the lack of personal accounts by people with a learning disability. Key contributors to the social model of disability have a physical or sensory impairment but none with an intellectual impairment has yet emerged. This may not be surprising at one level, but it points perhaps towards a disability hierarchy which may conflict with the interests of disabled people.

Conclusion: implications for professional practice

It is a great irony that the era (since the 1980s) during which the self-advocacy movement has grown has also been marked by serious threats to services for vulnerable people. In many parts of the country, these threats have become an unpalatable reality, as service users have been caught in the political crossfire between the government and local authorities. Under pressure exerted by the community charge capping policy introduced by the Conservative government, many local councils have made dramatic cuts in the area of social service provision. This has meant that marginalised minorities have been hit hard by losses of services. Typically, resources such as day centres for older people, local authority mental health services and respite care centres for children with disabilities have been affected.

How is this paradox to be interpreted? A possible explanation is that cuts in services would have taken place on an even greater scale were it not for the lobbying and political action taken by self-advocates and user groups. There is no doubt that successive governments have welcomed self-advocacy and encouraged, at least in policy documents, the development of user self-advocacy and empowerment. The motivation here may have been that self-help is a laudable thing and, moreover, its influence would lead to citizens taking their own actions and initiatives, lessening the need for public funding. Self-advocacy fitted the agenda of consumerism promoted by the 'New Right' in the 1980s. Consumerism is, as Walker (1993) observes, a different phenomenon to advocacy. A consumer of a service has power through choice of how to spend his or her funds, but disadvantaged individuals, for example with a severe learning disability, tend not to have such power and options. Therefore 'market' is a misnomer in the context of human services and community care because the service users are not purchasing services directly.

Although there are examples of service changes brought about by individuals and user groups, it seems that the greatest impact of self-advocacy has been at the personal level. Group members report gains in confidence, assertiveness and communication skills.

User self-advocacy has also been a force driving change in local service provision, as some of the above interview extracts suggest. However, these changes, although important, would tend to be at a modest level in terms of resource commitment. Fundamentally, while self-advocacy influences systems and professionals, it is a minor lever for change in comparison to political factors. Decreasing allocation of resources has set an agenda in which there exists limited room for manoeuvre.

Professionals themselves may feel disempowered within service systems, and where this is the case it is likely to impact on relationships with clients. Service workers have been affected by the 'restructuring' or 'rationalisation' of social service departments and health Trusts, often with the concomitant prospect of redundancy. Professionals are increasingly finding that career paths and options are becoming limited as organisations move towards workforces consisting largely of unqualified support workers. Increased administrative demands have served to impact on professional roles, often to the detriment of time actually spent in face-to-face contact with clients. It is self-evident that, if professionals feel disempowered, they will not be in a strong position to promote user empowerment. They may perceive assertiveness on the part of service users as a further threat to their changing role. A major concern is that professionals may see empowerment in the context of their own assertiveness and ability to protect or restrict the independence of users.

It is important for professionals to recognise when it is appropriate for them to take on an advocacy role for a specific purpose. However, the potential for conflict must be borne in mind. They need to be aware of independent advocacy schemes locally and to make referrals to such schemes. Advocacy must be addressed in professional courses; there is evidence of a growing trend in this area. Professionals must identify user-advocacy needs and support those needs being met. Clearly there are strong conceptual and practical links between self-advocacy and empowerment. Self-advocacy can be characterised as a means towards achieving empowerment, having a greater degree of control in one's life. Empowerment is a multi-dimensional concept embracing a continuing process, not merely a goal.

Some would see the involvement of professionals as disempowering and at odds with user independence. The position of Oliver (1996), that professionals can help to create conditions for self-empowerment by disabled people, is a convincing and cogent one. There is evidence from professional groups, in this case occupational therapists, that they need to examine their own attitudes and communication about disability and to promote environmental change in order to increase opportunities for disabled people (Schlaff 1993).

Wallcraft (1994), writing about self-advocacy and empowerment from the perspective of a mental health services user, offers some constructive counsel to professionals. She states that self-determination is the key to empowerment;

power must come from within. A number of ways in which professionals can facilitate empowerment are described. Among the negatives to be avoided are the categorisation of clients, for example as 'manic', and the use of jargon and a condescending approach. The positive action Wallcraft (1994: 9) recommends includes:

- finding out about the national self-advocacy movement and passing on that information to service users locally;
- providing funding, for example for transport to meetings, and making a venue available;
- offering practical assistance, such as arranging training in the skills which the group members identify that they need – these might be committee skills, how to make meetings work, fund-raising, understanding health and social service structures, public speaking, running training workshops.

There are strong implications here for professional curricula. It has been acknowledged for some time that nurse and social work education must include competences in interpersonal skills, advocacy and empowerment, and working in partnership with service users (Malin 1992). Supporting self-advocacy should occupy a central position in professional education and be considered an essential, core skill.

Gates (1994) stresses the importance of a supportive environment as a condition of successful professional support for user self-advocacy. If service workers believe in the empowerment of people, they will be secure in encouraging users to voice their views. Peers will reinforce and value such support. Closed or hostile environments are contra-indications to professional support for self-advocacy; alternative forms of advocacy, such as legal advocacy or citizen advocacy, may be more appropriate.

Professionals need to be aware not only of the interface between their own role and the autonomy of service users but also of the contribution of other disciplines. Joint and shared approaches to training are becoming a feature of contemporary services. By the end of the 1980s joint training had developed to a greater extent in the learning disability field than in relation to any other client group. Moreover, it had become a vital part of government strategy to promote integrated community care services (Brown 1992). A major trend in learning disability nursing has been the movement towards community-based practice, as opposed to working with clients in segregated settings. Many registered nurses in this field will be part of a community team in which a number of disciplines are represented, including social work or care management, occupational therapy, physiotherapy, speech and language therapy, medicine, clinical psychology. Others will be leading teams of support staff who work with people in their own home and in the local community. The change of location for professional–client interaction will have implications for the nature of that contact.

The supportive skills and ability to develop independence practised by community psychiatric nurses and learning disability nurses have an invaluable role to play in meeting client and carer needs (Griffiths 1988). Professions are having to respond to a variety of pressures which have had a substantial impact on training. The modern era has been marked by a trend away from profession–determined towards employer-led education. Regional health authorities began to contract through regional education consortia in 1991 (Brown 1994).

An increase in joint and shared training initiatives will be a key theme in preparation for professional practice and will help to reduce territorial patterns of thinking. Multi-disciplinary team working in health and social care will become an even more crucial, central aspect of service delivery. While individual roles will continue to exist within the team setting, it will be vital to break down role boundaries or professional demarcation which can impede client care. Service users need to have access to appropriate support; skills in certain areas, for example counselling, are not the province of one particular discipline. The impact of self-advocacy on families is an area which is beginning to receive research attention (Mitchell 1997). Policy makers and professionals will need to respond appropriately to research findings.

Ways of including service users and carers in professional training in a meaningful way must be developed. Accounts exist of such initiatives at postqualifying level (Shears *et al.* 1998). The interface between user self-advocacy and professional roles will continue to change, and the challenge for professionals will be in striking the right balance between caring and encouraging autonomy. Effective supervision will be an essential element in the resolution of tensions and conflicts which may arise; peer supervision models have considerable potential here. Managers should encourage the sharing of good practice among peers, allowing practitioners the time for this activity. Forward-looking organisations will support professionals to encourage the self-empowerment of service users through advocacy approaches, whether self-, citizen or peer advocacy. Provider organisations in the statutory and independent sectors will increasingly develop partnership arrangements with bodies which seek to represent the collective interests of user groups. Indeed, commissioners of services will expect clear evidence of such good practice by providers. At individual level the client–professional relationship continues to be crucial; developing such relationships effectively is the foundation of professional practice. It is to be hoped that the balance of power will move towards the service user, leading to effective co-working, equality and genuine partnership.

References

Banyay, B. (1989) 'Prevention among mental health associations', *Prevention in Human Services* 6(2): 45–52.

Baxter, C., Poonia, K. and Nadirshaw, Z. (1990) *Double Discrimination*, London: King's Fund.

Beresford, P. and Croft, S. (1993) *Citizen Involvement – A Practical Guide for Change*, London: Macmillan.

Booth, T. and Simons, K. (1989) 'Whose terms?', *Community Care* 5 October 19–22.

Bramley, J. and Elkins, J. (1988) 'Some issues in the development of self-advocacy among persons with intellectual disabilities', *Australia and New Zealand Journal of Developmental Disabilities* 14(2): 147–57.

Brandon, D. (1995) *Advocacy – Power to People with Disabilities*, Birmingham: Venture Press.

Braye, S. and Preston-Shoot, M. (1995) *Empowering Practice in Social Care*, Buckingham: Open University Press.

Brown, J. (1992) 'Professional boundaries in mental handicap: a policy analysis of joint training', in T. Thompson and P. Mathias (eds) *Standards and Mental Handicap*, London: Baillière Tindall, pp. 352–70.

—— (1994) 'Demarcation and the public sector – the impact of the contract agenda upon mental health practice', in T. Thompson and P. Mathias, *Mental Health and Disorder*, London: Baillière Tindall, pp. 573–86.

Chappell, A. (1998) 'Still out in the cold: people with learning difficulties and the social model of disability', in T. Shakespeare (ed.) *The Disability Reader: Social Science Perspectives*, London: Cassell, pp. 211–20.

Clare, M. (1990) *Developing Self Advocacy Skills*, London: Further Education Unit.

Crawley, B. (1987) *The Growing Voice: A Survey of Self-advocacy Groups in Adult Training Centres and Hospitals*, London: CMH.

Croft, S. and Beresford, P. (1995) 'Whose empowerment? Equalizing the competing discourses in community care', in R. Jack (ed.) *Empowerment in Community Care*, London: Chapman and Hall, pp. 59–73.

Department of Health White Paper (1989) *Caring for People: Community Care in the Next Decade and Beyond*, London: HMSO.

Dowson, S. and Whittaker, A. (1993) *On One Side – The Role of the Adviser in Supporting People with Learning Difficulties in Self-advocacy Groups*, London: Values into Action/King's Fund Centre.

Gadow, S. (1979) 'Advocacy, nursing and new meanings of aging', *Nursing Clinics of North America* 14(1): 81–91.

—— (1980) 'Existential advocacy: philosophical foundation of nursing', in S. Spicker and S. Gadow (eds) *Nursing: Images and Ideals*, New York: Springer.

Gates, R. (1994) *Advocacy: A Nurse's Guide*, London: RCN/Scutari.

Gibson, C. (1991) 'A concept analysis of empowerment', *Journal of Advanced Nursing*, 16: 354–61.

Griffiths, R. (1988) *Community Care: An Agenda for Action*, London: HMSO.

Harris, P. (1995) 'Who am I? Concepts of disability and their implications for people with learning difficulties', *Disability & Society* 10(3): 341–51.

International Council of Nursing [ICN] (1973) *A Code for Nurses. Ethical Concepts Applied to Nursing*, ICN, Geneva.

Jack, R. (ed.) (1995) *Empowerment in Community Care*, London: Chapman and Hall.

Kay, B., Rose, S. and Turnbull, J. (1995) *Continuing the Commitment*, Report of the Learning Disability Nursing Project, London: Department of Health.

Lindow, V. (1995) 'Power and rights: the psychiatric system survivor movement', in R. Jack (ed.) *Empowerment in Community Care*, London: Chapman and Hall, pp. 203–21.

Malin, N. (1992) 'Community care and professional directions', in T. Thompson and P. Mathias (eds) *Standards and Mental Handicap*, London: Baillière Tindall, pp. 444–60.

Malin, N. and Teasdale, K. (1991) 'Caring versus empowerment: considerations for nursing practice', *Journal of Advanced Nursing* 16: 657–62.

Mallik, M. (1995) 'Advocacy in nursing: a study of the diffusion and interpretation of a concept', unpublished M.Phil. thesis, University of Nottingham, Nottingham.

—— (1997) 'Advocacy in nursing – a review of the literature', *Journal of Advanced Nursing* 25: 130–8.

Mawhinney, S. and McDaid, C. (1997) '"Having your say": self-advocacy and individuals experiencing meatal ill-health', *NT Research* 2(5): 380–9.

Means, R. and Smith, R. (1994) *Community Care Policy and Practice*, London: Macmillan.

Miles, M. (1992) 'Concepts of mental retardation in Pakistan: toward cross-cultural and historical perspectives', *Disability, Handicap and Society* 7(3): 235–55.

Millette, B. (1989) 'An exploration of advocacy models and the moral orientation of nurses', unpublished Ph.D. thesis, Massachusetts: University of Massachusetts.

Mitchell, P. (1997) 'The impact of self-advocacy on families', *Disability & Society* 12(1): 43–56.

Monach, J. and Spriggs, L. 'The consumer role', in N. Malin (ed.) *Implementing Community Care*, Buckingham: Open University Press, pp. 138–53.

Murphy, C. (1979) 'Models of the nurse–patient relationship', in C. Murphy and H. Hunter (eds) *Ethical Problems in the Nurse–Patient Relationship*, Boston, MA: Allyn and Bacon, pp. 8–26.

NHS and Community Care Act (1990) London: HMSO.

Oliver, M. (1990) *The Politics of Disablement*, Basingstoke, Macmillan and St Martin's Press.

—— (1996) *Understanding Disability: From Theory to Practice*, London: Macmillan.

Parsloe, P. and Stevenson, O. (1992) *Community Care and Empowerment*, York: Joseph Rowntree Foundation.

Plumb, A. (1993) 'The challenge of self-advocacy', *Feminism and Psychology* June 3(2): 169–87.

Schlaff, C. (1993) 'From dependency to self-advocacy: redefining disability', *American Journal of Occupational Therapy* October 47(10): 943–8.

Servian, R. (1996) *Theorising Empowerment – Individual Power and Community Care*, Bristol: Policy Press.

Shears, J., Ramon, S. and Conlon, E. (1998) 'Assessing learning outcomes in post-qualifying community care training', in S. Baldwin (ed.) *Needs Assessment and Community Care*, Oxford: Butterworth-Heinemann, pp. 209–18.

Shemmings, D. and Shemmings, Y. (1995) 'Defining participative practice in health and welfare', in R. Jack (ed.) *Empowerment in Community Care*, London: Chapman and Hall, pp. 43–58.

Simons, K. (1992) *Sticking up for Yourself – Self Advocacy and People with Learning Difficulties*, York: Joseph Rowntree Foundation.

Snowball, J. (1996) 'Asking nurses about advocating for patients: "reactive" and "proactive" accounts', *Journal of Advanced Nursing* 24: 67–75.

Szivos, S. and Griffiths, E. (1990) 'Consciousness raising and social identity theory: a challenge to normalization', *Psychology Forum* August: 11–15.

Tajfel, H. (1981) *Human Groups and Social Categories: Studies in Social Psychology*, Cambridge: Cambridge University Press.

Teasdale, K. (1994) 'Advocacy and the nurse manager', *Journal of Nursing Management* 2: 93–7.

United Kingdom Central Council [UKCC] (1992) *Code of Professional Conduct for the Nurse, Midwife and Health Visitor*, 3rd edn, London: UKCC.

Wallcraft, J. (1994) 'Empowering empowerment: professionals and self-advocacy projects', *Mental Health Nursing* 14(2): 6–9.

Walker, A. (1993) 'A community care policy: from consensus to conflict', in J. Bornat, C. Pereira, D. Pilgrim and F. Williams (eds) *Community Care: A Reader*, Basingstoke: Macmillan/Open University, pp. 204–26.

Whittaker, A. (1991) *How Are Self-advocacy Groups Developing?* London: King's Fund.

Williams, P. and Shoultz, B. (1982) *We Can Speak for Ourselves*, London: Souvenir Press.

Part II

Professionalism and enterprise culture

4 Boundary work and the (un)making of the professions

Valérie Fournier

Introduction

In the last few years it has become commonplace to question the future of the professions in the context of current trends of economic, technological and organisational change (for example Crompton 1990; Casey 1995; Sommerlad 1995; Randle 1996; Special issue of *Organisation Studies* 1996). These trends of change have been indexed under various labels, from flexibility to commercialism, enterprise, market liberalism, flexible accumulation, etc. However labelled, these new practices are said to challenge the legitimacy and foundations of the professions, and in particular, to erode the divisions central to the establishment of the professions. For example, it is argued (Kanter 1990; Casey 1995) that the boundaries between different professional groups are being blurred as professionals in organisations are asked to work in multi-functional teams in order to provide the 'flexibility' supposedly required to operate effectively in a 'turbulent environment'. The long-established division between managers and professionals (Gouldner 1957) also seems to be blurred as professionals are under increasing pressures from managerialism, partly by being required to take on some managerial responsibilities themselves, or to constitute themselves as entrepreneurs (Stanley 1991; Hanlon 1996). Finally, as the logic of the market is spreading its message across the professions, professionals' patients or clients are transformed into 'empowered customers' who, in their quest for choice and 'value for money', are questioning the authority and mystery surrounding the professions.

Concern over the future of the professions has also attracted much attention from the press; we are sometimes presented with images of declining respect, prospects and status conferred to professions such as medical doctors and teachers (Hattersley 1996; Mihill 1996), and a sense of nostalgia for the 'way it used to be':

> Young doctors don't want to face the prospect of a professional life in a branch of medicine where skills will wither, where credibility as a professional doctor is set to decline and their ability to add columns of figures and understand the jargon of contracting and purchasing is more important than clinical ability.
>
> (Mihill 1996: 8)

While some (for example Sommerlad 1995) deplore this state of affairs as signal-ling the colonisation of the public interest by the creeping logic of commercial-ism and the market, others (for example Kanter 1990) have celebrated the anticipated demise of the profession as the victory of flexibility and individual freedom over monolithic monsters. Yet others have been suspicious of this message of doom and do not anticipate current trends of change to lead to the death of the professions; the professions will survive (Ackroyd 1996), be it in a re-articulated or commercialised form (Hanlon 1996).

It is ironic that bureaucracy – often, if problematically, positioned as the antithesis of the new flexible, lean, market-driven organisation – was also said to be inimical to the survival of the professions. Although this opposition between the professions and bureaucracy has been refuted by some (for example Johnson 1972; Witz 1992; Armstrong 1993; Davies 1996), others have argued that bureaucratisation involved a process of rationalisation and codification of pro-fessional knowledge that would erode professional power (see the labour pro-cess debate on de-professionalisation, the proletarianisation of white-collar work and the commodification of professional labour, in for example Smith *et al.* 1991). Although the logics of bureaucracy and of the market are supposed to operate through different mechanisms – i.e. through the codification of professional knowledge for the former, and through direct attacks on pro-fessional monopolies for the latter – both have been declared to be fateful for the professions.

This brief and admittedly simplified overview of current debates on the fate of the professions suggests that these debates are rife with contradictions and paradoxes. Furthermore, the verdict of death or survival of the professions is often pronounced with little consideration as to what went into the making of the professions in the first place. Ultimately, it is not always clear how new organisational practices are eroding the (so far) robust institutions of the profes-sions. The 'fateful' effects of new practices on the professions seem to be predi-cated upon different, and sometimes conflicting, arguments. For some (for example Hanlon 1996), the logic of the market will lead to a 'corruption' of professional practice as the professions are required to reconstitute themselves along commercial rather than 'public interest' criteria. For others (for example Ackroyd 1996; Randle 1996), the spreading logic of the market serves to inten-sify the bureaucratic trend towards the commodification of professional knowl-edge. For yet another group – essentially managerialist writers (for example Kanter 1990) – the erosion of professional monopoly by the logic of the market involves the diffusion of 'expert knowledge' to customers, employees and the public at large; as such it opens up possibilities for a more 'empowering' distri-bution of knowledge.

While the chapter does not aim to resolve the contradictions outlined above, or to offer definitive conclusions regarding the future of the professions, it pro-poses to explore how current trends of change in organisational discourses and practices (in particular the spreading of market logic) may impact upon profes-sional projects, and to do so by first discussing what goes into the making of the professions. Here it is argued that the construction of boundaries ('boundary work') is central to the establishment and reproduction of the professions. The chapter discusses two processes of 'boundary work': the constitution of an 'independent and self-contained field of knowledge' as the basis upon which professions can build their authority and exclusivity; and the labour of division which goes into erecting and maintaining boundaries between the professions and various other groups. The second part of the chapter then discusses the effects of current practices and discourses of work and organisations – summarised under the 'logic of the market' – on the professions; it analyses the extent to which the processes central to the establishment and maintenance of the modern professions are challenged by new techniques and discourses of organisation.

The making of the professional project

The constitution of the professional field

Much of the literature on the professions has discussed the processes of exclusion and social closure central to the professional project; it has explored the various strategies professionals engage in to claim exclusive ownership and control over a particular field of knowledge and practice, and to establish their prestige and status (Larson 1977; Abbott 1988; Witz 1992; Macdonald 1995). These various strategies of social closure, ranging from credentialism to discursive strategies and to legalistic tactics, have already been well documented (see, for example, Larson 1977 and Witz 1992) and will not be reviewed in much detail here.

However, this emphasis on social closure in the analysis of the professional project, while valuable, overlooks an essential step in the formation of the profession: the constitution of the professional field of expertise. Much of the literature concentrates on how occupational groups appropriate a field, but not on how the field itself came to be constituted in the first place; the existence of identifiable fields or disciplines is treated as a 'given' and rarely seems to call for explanation.[1] The position taken in this chapter is that the professional project involves not only an occupational group appropriating a field as its exclusive area of jurisdiction and expertise, but also the making of this field into a legitimate area of knowledge of and intervention on the world.

The constitution of the professional field, or discipline, into an independent, autonomous and self-contained area of knowledge that is assumed to reflect some natural divisions and to be an autonomous object of analysis, is central to the making of the professions (Weber 1987). The professional system of knowledge needs to be established as isolated and self-contained, reposing on founding principles which naturally constitute the limits of the profession's jurisdiction and discipline and are based on an equally self-contained 'natural' state of things. ('Nature' here refers to the 'object' of the field, to the reference point on the basis of which the legitimacy and efficacy of the particularised knowledge can be established, for example the 'biological' body for the field of medicine.) Thus for the authority of the professionals to be recognised, their field of competence has to be established as essentially self-contained, in accordance with the self-identity of its objects; 'the professional sought to *isolate* in order to control' (Weber 1987: 27; emphasis in the original).

This autonomous and self-contained nature of the professional field and of the 'natural object' it is deemed to reflect, is not evident, given by nature or a product of technical rationalisation, but is achieved in the making of the professional project. Thus to understand the making of the professional project, it is not enough to concentrate on processes of social closure or 'turf wars' (Abbott 1995); we need to examine how the territories to be annexed and to be closed off came into existence, or became constituted as independent and recognisable entities. We need to explore how complex phenomena such as, for example, disease become isolated and contained into a 'medical problem' governed and remedied by laws which can best be understood in terms of a similarly isolated and self-contained area of knowledge such as medicine. The chapter does not argue that questions of social closure or 'turf wars' are irrelevant, but it concentrates on the question of the constitution of the independent field of professional knowledge as one which has been neglected.

The constitution of the 'independent field' as a process contingent upon social, historical, and economic conditions is illustrated through Foucault's analysis of the birth of medicine. The discussion below can in no way do justice to the breadth of Foucault's contribution but uses his work selectively (Foucault 1975, 1977, 1980) to illustrate the construction of the medical field. Foucault's work suggests that the growing concern with the health of populations and its problematisation in medical terms arose out of a combination of economic and demographic factors. Medicine, as an independent field of knowledge, only emerged in eighteenth-century Western Europe, at a time when under both economic and political pressures, the individual body was discovered as an object of knowledge, a valid target of control and intervention. Against this background of economic and demographic transformations, the establishment of medicine as an independent 'science' took place through two parallel and related mechanisms: first, the isolation of health from the general area of assistance, a process dictated by the economic concern to turn 'idle bodies' into productive ones; and second, the development of techniques of inscription of the individual body into a medical code, thus turning the individual body into a valid object of scientific knowledge.

With regard to the first point, Foucault (1980) shows that until the late seventeenth century, what would now be understood as health and medicine, was practised as part of the assistance given to the collective category of the 'sick poor' by various charitable organisations. However, from the eighteenth century, health became an isolated area of knowledge and intervention as the 'sick poor' became conceptualised in terms of their economic relevance rather than their need for assistance. The emerging importance of medicine as an independent field of knowledge and intervention can be attributed to the concern for the preservation and reproduction of the labour force. The general category of the 'pauper' gave way to a whole series of new distinctions between the 'good' and the 'bad' poor, the happily idle and the involuntarily unemployed, the 'able bodies' and the 'non-able bodies'. The problem of poverty and sickness became translated into a problem of health monitoring and improvement for economic management.

At the same time, various methods of observation, analysis and control of the body – which altogether would contribute to make the discipline of medicine – developed. The body became subjected to systematic observation, normalisation (i.e. measurement, comparison, analysis in terms of homogeneous norms to establish the body's normality), and examination (i.e. the reading and translation of the 'individual case' in terms of a homogeneous medical code of symptoms): the three components of disciplinary power (Foucault 1977). These three processes marked the entry of the individual (and no longer the species) into the field of knowledge of what might be generally called the 'clinical sciences' (Foucault 1975). These techniques of observation, normalisation, documentation, registration, constitution of files on individual cases, of noting individual differences, were decisive in the birth of a science of the individual. The individual body, translated into the 'medical case', became a valid object of scientific enquiry and knowledge which could be understood and acted upon in its own right, independently of (say) society.

This example of medicine suggests that at the core of the professional project is the constitution of disciplinary knowledge as representing or mirroring a 'naturally' isolated and self-contained referent object in the world (for example the body in the case of medicine). The knowledge and expertise of the professions act as a 'centre of translation' (Cooper and Law 1995); it translates a disorderly world made of complex relationships and heterogeneous materials into homogeneous, isolated and ordered patterns; it inscribes complex phenomena into categories and laws allegedly governing their operations and relationships. This process of isolation, categorisation, homogenisation and inscription in natural laws is not 'given' in the order of things but is an achievement contingent upon cultural, historical and economic conditions.

There are two important points to stress about this process of 'making up' the field: first, it serves to constitute rather than merely reflect or mirror the 'reality' it is supposed to 'know' and act upon; and second, the field of professional knowledge thus made up is malleable rather than fixed. The constitutive and malleable nature of the professional field of knowledge is illustrated by drawing upon Hopwood's (1987) discussion of the archaeology of accounting. Hopwood argues that the emergence and development of accounting is not simply the discovery and formalisation of some natural laws of organisational economy, efficiency and effectiveness, it has played a positive role in shaping and constituting managerial roles and actions. Thus 'accounting has emerged in a more positive way than the mere realisation of its essence' (ibid.: 211) and has taken an active part in the construction of the organisational and social order it claims to 'know':

Accounting, when seen in such terms, is not a passive instrument of technical administration, a neutral means for merely revealing the pre-given aspects of organisational functioning. Instead, its origins are seen to reside in the exercising of social power both within and without the organisation. It is seen as being implicated in the forging, indeed the active creation, of a particular regime of economic calculation within the organisation in order to make real and powerful quite particular conceptions of economic and social ends.

(ibid.: 213)

Hopwood draws upon the example of the introduction of accounting in Wedgwood in the eighteenth century to illustrate how the emerging knowledge of 'costing' served to make 'real' and 'endurable' the fact or category of cost that it served to constitute. Although initially Josiah Wedgwood made little use of accounting to inform his prices, things changed in 1772 when a major economic recession pushed Wedgwood to lower his prices in order to boost sales; however, he needed to ensure that prices were still higher than cost, and the problem of costing arose. Hopwood shows that the costing of the products had to be 'laboriously created rather than revealed' (ibid.: 216), costs were not exposed but 'made up'; costing did not reflect some 'true costs' existing independently of the practice of costing, but served to construct the fact or category of cost. The introduction of the 'accounting gaze' in the organisation did not merely create the fact of cost but also provided Wedgwood with new forms of visibility, intervention and surveillance; it provided a basis for 're-appraising the organisation of the manufacturing processes, the advantages of large volume production, and the calculation of piece rates, wages and bonus' (ibid.: 217).

The case of Wedgwood also demonstrates the dynamic and shifting nature of professional knowledge; the field of professional knowledge is extremely malleable and expandable. However, professional knowledge is not expandable in the sense that it is inscribed in a trajectory of becoming 'what it should be' (ibid.), of discovering more about the truth of the object it claims to know about. Rather, the professional field is expandable and malleable in the sense that it is inscribed in a self-perpetuating, self-producing circle of emerging practice (for example costing), constitutive of the object of knowledge (for example the fact of cost), in turn constitutive of new forms of visibility, knowledge and practice. Thus the field of professional knowledge is always in motion, always self-producing and self-expanding; the object that it claims to know about is not independent of the professional gaze, but is constituted by professional practice.

The labour of division and the erection of boundaries

The emergence of the professions as distinctive occupational groups proclaiming exclusive competence over a particular field has often been identified as the product of specialisation, the division of labour characteristic of modern forms of production and knowledge (Weber 1987). Thus the emergence of the professions is seen as an integral part of the process of rationalisation: the increasing complexity and extensiveness of knowledge and information leads to specialisation and the division of labour. However, as Samuel Weber (1987) points out, the division of labour is insufficient in explaining the distinctive status conferred on the professions:

> For all studies of professionalism, even the most descriptive and functionalist, concur in identifying certain characteristics that differentiate the professions from specialised occupations in general. First and foremost, there is a tendency of the professional to present himself [*sic*] as relatively autonomous within his field. Such autonomy, however, does not derive simply from the specialised skills involved; the 'services' rendered by a doctor, a lawyer, a research scientist are not merely specialised (as are those of the auto mechanic), they are, in a crucial sense, incommensurable, and upon this incommensurability the distinctive autonomy and authority of the professional is founded.
>
> (Weber 1987: 26)

This incommensurability characteristic of the professions is described by Weber in terms of the attempt through various 'defensive strategies' to place professional activity apart from, outside of, the sphere of ordinary relationships and activity, and in particular, outside of the market. Incommensurability can be understood in terms of creating boundaries between the sphere of competence of the professions and other spheres of activities. Professions may thus be better seen in terms of the labour of division than as an outcome of the division of labour; in other words, they are not the technical outcomes of the intellectual division of labour but are constituted and maintained through processes of isolation and boundary construction.

An emphasis on the labour of division turns our attention to the work which goes into creating and maintaining boundaries around the professions, into making transient distinctions, categories and structures look stable, certain, and 'in the order of things' (Cooper and Law 1995). The creation of these distinctions and boundaries becomes an achievement, one which is uncertain, reversible, and requires constant effort to be maintained. Such a perspective seeks to identify the strategies and techniques which are deployed to impose order, stability, and fixed boundaries around the professions. The labour of division that goes into the making of the profession is discussed here in relation to three types of divisions and boundaries: the boundaries between different professional groups, the boundaries between the professions and clients/lay persons, and the boundaries between the professions and the market.

The boundaries between professional groups

First, the professions engage in various strategies to erect boundaries between their and other professions or occupations' jurisdictions. This has attracted much attention in the literature; the various strategies and tactics that professions deploy to close their jurisdictions and fields to other occupational groups have been well documented (for example Larson 1977; Witz 1992; Macdonald 1995) and range from credentialism to discursive strategies and legalistic tactics (Larson 1977; Witz 1992). The discussion here does not attempt to provide a comprehensive review of this literature but draws on one example – namely Abbott's (1988) notion of 'cultural work' – to illustrate the type of work which goes into the construction of boundaries. Abbott uses this notion of 'cultural work' to refer to the strategies that the professions deploy to manipulate their systems of knowledge in such a way that they can appropriate various problems as falling under their jurisdiction. Abbott (1988) sees abstraction as the essential quality of professional knowledge which enables a profession to erect and maintain divisions between its own and other occupations' sphere of competence:

> For abstraction is the quality that sets interprofessional competition apart from competition among occupations in general. Any occupation can obtain licensure (e.g. beauticians) or develop a code of ethics (e.g. real estate). But only a knowledge system governed by abstractions can redefine its problems and tasks, defend them from interlopers, and seize new problems – as medicine has recently seized alcoholism, mental illness, hyperactivity in children, obesity and numerous other things. Abstraction enables survival in the competitive system of the professions.
>
> (ibid.: 9)

Abbott's suggestion that the professions engage in 'cultural *work*' to establish their claim to exclusive competence over a particular 'chunk of the world' emphasises the active work that professionals have to put in to maintain the boundaries defining their jurisdiction (and possibly to extend the limits of their jurisdiction), and clearly illustrates the labour of division which goes into the making of the professions.

The boundaries between the professions and clients/lay persons

Second, the authority of the professions relies on the creation of boundaries between themselves and the client or lay person. An indispensable feature of professional autonomy and authority is the corresponding passivity and dependence of the lay person, and in particular the client (Weber 1987). Professional authority needs to be established and reinforced through symbols which make the public conscious of its dependence on the professions. The professions may create this pattern of dependence by playing on the weaknesses of the clients, their vulnerability, helplessness and general anxiety, which in turn are generated, or at least exacerbated, by professionals' cultivation of an atmosphere of crisis or emergency in which they both create work for themselves and reinforce their authority by intimidating clients (ibid.): 'the culture of professionalism drew much of its force, its social credit, credibility, from the cultivation and exploitation of anxiety' (ibid.: 28).

One way in which the professions can cultivate these relationships of dependence and maintain barriers between themselves and the lay public is through the formalisation of their knowledge in ways that make it obscure and unintelligible to those without the appropriate training and credentials. The boundaries between the professions and the lay public are established by maintaining an appropriate level of 'mysteriousness' and esotericism within professional systems of knowledge; such systems of knowledge are then resistant to codification and standardisation, and become inaccessible to the lay person. For example, Larson (1977: 41) observes that 'The leaders of the professional project will define the areas that are not amenable to standardization; they will define the place of unique individual genius and the criteria of talent "that cannot be taught".'

Larson draws on Jamous and Peloille's (1970) claim that professions need to have a high indeterminacy–technicality ratio. This is to counteract the tendency of modern knowledge towards codification that would render it more accessible to the public, thus undermining professionals' privileged position. Professional practice must thus be seen to be based on an element of intuition and talent that cannot be taught or translated into techniques and transmissible rules, that hides professionals' activity behind a screen of 'mysteriousness', and that puts their actions and decisions beyond the scrutiny of the lay public. This use of intuition and talent becomes the boundary marker between the professional and the lay person.

Here again, the work of Abbott (1995) is useful to illustrate the labour of division that goes into the construction of boundaries between the professions and their clients. With the notion of 'professional regression', Abbott suggests that high status in a profession goes with being able to talk purely professional language and to avoid the confusion and complexity that clients' problems present to professional knowledge systems. According to this argument, professionals maintain high status only if they do not compromise the purity of their scientific knowledge, and hence if they spend more time talking to each other (in pure professional terms) than dealing with clients' problems, which may not lend themselves to conceptualisation in pure professional terms. Professional status is achieved by constructing boundaries isolating professionals from clients.

Another important barrier sustaining the status of the profession establishes a division between the professional and the lay person or amateur. Taylor (1995) offers an interesting account of the construction of this division by professional archaeologists. Taylor refutes the evolutionary thesis according to which trained professionals came to replace enthusiastic amateurs in a move towards progress and rationalisation. Instead he suggests that professionals retrospectively construct and define amateurs as part of a strategy to legitimise their positions. He argues that the invention or construction of the amateur, from which the professionals can then distinguish themselves, is crucial to the self-definition of the professions: 'Far from amateurism preceding a supplanting professional class, the notion of "the amateur" as a pre-professional can be considered as part of the professionals' self-justification. The process of professionalization, in this sense, requires the "invention of amateurism"'' (ibid.: 504).

Thus here again, professional status comes with inventing an 'other' (in this case the 'amateur') from which professionals can then 'work' to distinguish themselves.

The boundaries between the professions and the market

Finally, there is a clear distinction between the field of the professions and the market. The professional service is not *sold* but *rendered*. The activities of the professional stand outside the commodity market. The professional service is characterised by its use value rather than exchange value (Weber 1987). The professions profess to be concerned with the public good, which they can deliver through their special access to scientific knowledge. This concern for objective knowledge for the public good, which sets the professional apart from the manager or the politician, can be traced back to the early association of the profession with gentlemanhood (Haber 1991). In the eighteenth century, a profession was seen as an activity that a gentleman could engage in without demeaning *him*self (Freidson 1986; Haber 1991). While there has been a shift in the strategy of demarcation (from building on notions of respectability and gentlemanhood to building on notions of qualifications and scientific knowledge), both strategies serve to distinguish the professions from the ordinary activities and relationships of the market. Professionals' actions are not (allegedly) governed by self-interest but by a body of objective and scientific knowledge which is used to inform decision and intervention carried out for the public good. Thus professionals are not accountable in terms of the laws of the market but in terms defined by their own jurisdiction: i.e. appeal to truth, effective intervention, code of ethics; or in terms of 'ideal-regarding' and internal criteria of the 'practice'[2] (Keat 1991b). The 'objectivity and scientific nature' of professional knowledge places professionals in a special social position that transcends the favouritism of politicians or the self-interest of market relations (Weber 1987); the professional becomes distinguished from the manager or the politician.

In summary, it is argued that the making of the professions can be understood in terms of two key processes related to 'boundary work': first, the constitution of a field of expertise or discipline as a self-contained, autonomous area of knowledge deemed to reflect a natural object which can itself be understood and governed in isolation; this process of the constitution of the professional field of knowledge is historically and culturally contingent (rather than inscribed in 'natural laws'), and it in fact constitutes rather than reflects its object; furthermore, the field of professional knowledge is expandable and malleable rather than fixed by 'the reality of its object'. Second, the making of the professions is contingent upon the labour of division which goes into the establishment and maintenance of the boundaries defining the professions. Both processes are transient and fragile in the sense that they are contingent upon the laborious effort involved in constructing and maintaining boundaries and assemblages out of disorder and movement. Both processes suggest that the construction of boundaries (boundary work) and their malleable rather than fixed nature are crucial to the making, and understanding, of the professions.

These constructed fields and boundaries have proved quite robust to various challenges in the past (Ackroyd 1996); however, their ability to resist the attacks of the market has been questioned. The next section analyses the extent to which the logic of the market does constitute a threat to the professions, by exploring the effects of its discursive and material practices upon the two mechanisms central to the establishment of the professions.

The spreading logic of the market and the unmaking of the professions

As argued above, the professions have sought to situate themselves outside the commercial logic of the market by appealing to notions of gentlemanhood in the seventeenth and early eighteenth century (Haber 1991), and later, to ideas of scientific knowledge and truth. However, this distinction between the professions and the market is being challenged by new organisational discourses and practices articulated around concepts of enterprise, excellence and market liberalism. Several writers (for example Sommerlad 1995; Reed 1996) are suggesting that current economic, political, technological and cultural trends of change are threatening the foundations and legitimacy of the professions.

The early 1980s saw the coming together of various trends of change – technological, economic, ideological and political – which facilitated and legitimised the intensification and spreading of the logic of the market to new domains (Keat 1991a,b). The effects of these trends of change upon organisational practices have been indexed under various labels, such as the culture of excellence or enterprise (du Gay 1996), flexible accumulation (Reed 1996), commercialism (Hanlon 1996) and managerialism (Dent 1993; Sommerlad 1995; Parker and Dent 1996). The problem in trying to capture changes in organisational practices under one label is that there is a danger of portraying change as a coherent and unidimensional force, and of invoking some dualism between the 'old way' (for example bureaucracy) and the 'new way' (for example enterprise). However, for the sake of convenience, I will use the notion of 'the logic of the market' to refer to these changes; this term has the advantage over (for example) 'the culture of enterprise' of avoiding a dualistic account of a move away from bureaucracies towards entrepreneurial forms.

The term 'the logic of the market' is used here to refer to a broad range of discursive and material practices closely aligned with market liberalism and articulated around notions of flexibility, individual freedom and responsibility. The logic of the market appeals to notions of globalisation, intensification of competition and turbulence in the organisational environment to introduce various programmes of economic and institutional reforms. These programmes of reforms can be articulated around three core themes of particular relevance for the present purpose. First, politicians or managerialist writers celebrating the logic of the market (for example Peters 1987, 1992; Kanter 1990) promote the extension of the domain of activities governed by the market (Keat 1991b); for example, the Conservative government, and it seems the New Labour government, have taken steps to introduce quasi-markets in the provision of state-financed professional services such as health and education (see Crompton 1990; Macdonald 1995). Second, the logic of the market involves a reification of the 'sovereign consumer' who displaces the dependent patient, client or student; meeting the demands of the sovereign consumer becomes an imperative (Keat 1991a; Heelas 1991). Third, the discourse of the market challenges occupational, functional and professional monopoly and division; instead it celebrates integration and flexibility. This third dimension entails on the one hand the deregulation of the professions and the breakdown of monopolies of competence; and on the other hand, the collapse of barriers between occupations and functions within organisations, so that members of different occupational groups are now required to work in multi-functional teams (Kanter 1990; Drucker 1993; Casey 1995).

If the erection and maintenance of boundaries, the segmentation of the world into independent fields of disciplinary jurisdiction, are as central to the professional project as was argued in the first section of the chapter, one could anticipate the spreading of the logic of the market (stressing the value of the free market, transparency and flexibility) to have some profound effects on the (un-)making of the professions. The market is likely to distort, disturb and counter the labour of division which goes into building boundaries around the professions. Some of these effects are explored below in terms of the dismantling of three of the boundaries essential to the making of the professions: the dismantling of the independent and self-contained field of knowledge, the dismantling of the barriers between the professions and the market, and the dismantling of the boundaries between the professions and clients/lay persons.

The dismantling of the independent field of professional knowledge

The constitution of the 'independent field of professional knowledge', deemed to reflect some natural division and an isolated object of analysis, is challenged by the logic of the market at several levels. First, professional knowledge rests upon the fragmentation of the world into isolated fields of analysis and intervention, and a corresponding demarcation between areas of single disciplinary jurisdiction. However, the logic of the market challenges the legitimacy of such fragmented knowledge; the 'turbulent and global' world of the market (Peters 1987, 1992; Kanter 1990) does not lend itself to segmentation and demarcation between areas of exclusive and single professional jurisdiction. The discourse of the market portrays the world as being too complex and dynamic to be divided up into autonomous and fragmented fields of knowledge. This supposedly increased complexity and turbulence serves to undermine the validity and usefulness of the independent field of knowledge which formed the foundations of the professions, and to legitimise the breakdown of barriers between disciplinary areas. If the world itself is becoming interwoven into more complex and dynamic relationships, any valid and useful knowledge about the world will need to reflect this growing interdependency, and any form of knowledge based on a single discipline will find it more difficult to make claims which are regarded as credible or useful. For example, Casey (1995), in an analysis of change in a large US company, argues that computer technologies have displaced the need for individuals holding specialist knowledge and expertise, and have facilitated the integration of different functions previously held by professionals or highly skilled technologists. Employees with specialist training and knowledge are now required to participate in functions and to acquire knowledge formerly reserved to other specialists. Specialisation and demarcation are giving way to generalisation, flexibility and the erosion of professional power and privilege (Casey 1995).

Second, the logic of the market, which rests on the idea of market liberalism, stands against the erection of barriers in the labour market and seeks to dismantle professional monopoly over certain areas of practice. This attack on professional monopoly has itself taken several forms; one of which has been the reconceptualisation of problems normally falling under a certain professional jurisdiction in terms which make them open to different forms of understanding and intervention. For example, a strategy used by the government has been to reinterpret many of the problems normally dealt with by the 'caring professions' as 'community problems', thus leaving them open to treatment by lay persons or other occupations and placing them outside the field of competence and expertise of the caring professions. This strategy of reconceptualisation was also illustrated in the proposals concerning the reorganisation of the legal profession; what was regarded as a 'legal problem' requiring the intervention of the legal profession can now be conceptualised in terms falling outside the jurisdiction of the legal profession, allowing a range of non-legal forums to deal with the disputes (Matthews 1989); some legal problems are also being reinterpreted as community problems (Stanley 1991). Another form of attack on professional monopoly has been the opening of the professional fields to other occupational groups. Thus even when the professional field of knowledge is deemed to be a legitimate and valid way of conceptualising a problem, the monopoly of a particular professional group over that field (acquired through state licensure and credentialism) has been challenged.

In summary, the attack of the logic of the market on the legitimacy of professional knowledge works through two processes: a process of diffusion or dispersal of professional knowledge beyond the confines of the professional group, and a process of integration of different systems of knowledge to deal with an allegedly increasingly intricate and complex world.

The dismantling of the boundary between professionals and clients/lay persons

The logic of the market and enterprise gives the 'sovereign consumer' a privileged position (du Gay and Salaman 1992). Customers are no longer passive, simply accepting the authority of the professional and consuming what is on offer. Consuming is transformed into an enterprising project through which people assemble their chosen lifestyle by taking responsibility for, and making informed choice about, the acquisition of appropriate goods and services (Heelas 1991). The so constituted consumer shares very little with the passive, philistine and dependent client. This newly found independence of the customer is a challenge to the relationship of dependence between client and practitioner central to the establishment of the professions. The sovereign consumers question the authority of the professions and the value and cost of their services, they shop around for alternatives within and outside the profession. This constitutes another pressure on professionals to locate their activities in the market: they have to sell their product or services. Professionals competing for customers have to satisfy the preferences of their potential consumers. In the world of enterprises and markets, the consumer supposedly rules; what counts as a 'good product or service' is judged by reference to the consumer's wishes and preferences, whether or not these are consistent with professional practice. In order to make better-informed choice, the customers are demanding and accessing information previously guarded by the professionals; there is a proliferation of 'DIY' manuals, software packages and media programmes diffusing professional knowledge (from medicine to accounting) to the public. For example, information technology has allowed clients of accounting firms to gain access to specialised knowledge previously held exclusively by accountants; as a result, clients are in a better position to assess the services offered by accounting firms and are becoming more demanding, challenging professional firms to justify their services and fees (Greenwood and Lachman 1996). Thus one of the boundary markers between professionals and clients – namely the screen of mysteriousness of professional knowledge which served to maintain the relationship of dependency between professional and client – is being eroded by the diffusion of professional knowledge to the 'sovereign consumer'.

The dismantling of the boundaries between the professions and the market

While the professions have always depended on outside funding (through fee-paying clients or public funding), they have sought to establish independent and internal criteria and standards to judge the quality of their service, rather than rely on the market. The professions have located their activities outside the market by using 'ideal-regarding' criteria (internal to their practice and field) rather than instrumental or 'want-regarding' criteria (such as customer satisfaction or financial success) (Keat 1991b). However, with the extension of the market into professional domains, professionals are increasingly required to compete for public funding or for customers seeking 'value for money'. In this endeavour, the professions become subjected to the laws of the market, and their activities become governed by external rather than internal criteria; professional practice becomes vulnerable to various forms of 'corruption' of their internal practice (Keat 1991b). By having to operate and compete on the market, professionals have to reorientate their activities towards meeting 'external criteria' such as customer satisfaction, and to view their services less in terms of ideal-regarding criteria of the practice than in terms of marketability or commercial success.[3] For example, Stanley (1991) argues that lawyers no longer earn respect by providing justice, but through their success in the market place; the provision of legal services is increasingly seen in terms of its marketability rather than the negotiation of justice (Stanley 1991; Sommerlad 1995). Similarly, Hanlon (1996) argues that accountants have rearticulated their professional services along more commercial lines by shifting the emphasis of accounting away from the policing role of the audit aiming to protect public interest by fighting fraudulent practice, and towards providing advice that enables clients to become more profitable. This shift towards profitability and client satisfaction has involved a rearticulation of 'the good accountant' around notions of commercial awareness at the expense of technical knowledge (Hanlon 1996).

The discussion above shows that the logic of the market seems clearly inimical to the reproduction of the modern professions, at least in the ways they have sought to establish and define themselves in the past. The discourse of the market undoes much of the labour of division which went into the erection of the boundaries defining the professions, and undermines the foundation of the modern professional project. However, the discussion, as it stands, provides a too deterministic and unidimensional analysis of the logic of the market and its consequences for the professions. The final section of the chapter qualifies this vision of doom and argues that the logic of the market may not have such a pervasive and destructive effect.

Discussion: possibilities for the re-making of the professions

The aim of this tentative discussion is to counter an over-deterministic analysis of the effect of market logic on the professions which could be implied by closing the chapter at the end of the previous section. The discussion explores the space that is left, or even created, by the logic of the market and focuses on two points: first, it suggests that the logic of the market shifts rather than eliminates boundaries and thus may create new divisions upon which the professions can (re)construct themselves. Second, drawing upon the arguments presented in the first part of the chapter, it is suggested that professional knowledge is malleable and constitutive of, rather than bound by, its 'field'; thus it can be reinvented to map onto market considerations.

But before exploring these two points, it is worth questioning the pervasiveness of market logic. The anticipated demise of the professions is based on the assumption of the inevitable and pervasive spread of the logic of the market, with its emphasis on competition, flexibility and the sovereign consumer. However,

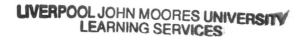

several critical writers (for example Whitaker 1992) have questioned the validity of this thesis and have provided evidence of continuing bureaucratic practice and control. Thus the extent to which the logic of the market is spreading and eroding the professions is disputable.

Shifting rather than eliminating boundaries

The rhetoric of the market may celebrate flexibility and boundarylessness, and it may challenge some of the established boundaries defining the professions; but this is not to say that it operates without boundaries, or that it does not shift and re-create boundaries. The process of erosion of the traditional boundaries protecting the special status of the professions can reconstitute boundaries along which the professions can build new strategies of legitimisation.

For example, the diffusion of professional knowledge to the public through various 'DIY' manuals, the media or software packages is, I would argue, in some cases increasing rather than decreasing clients' dependence upon professionals' knowledge. This works in two ways: first, the circulation of professional knowledge and vocabulary across the public increases the chance of the public conceptualising their problems in professional terms, and hence calling upon professional expertise. It serves to socialise the public into problematising their lives in terms that open them up to professional scrutiny. Second, the circulation of professional knowledge among the lay public serves to cultivate the public's anxiety that Weber (1987) identified as central to the authority of the professions. The little knowledge that the lay public acquires is likely to increase the sense of complexity and indeterminacy of their problems, and make their reliance upon the judgement of the professional more necessary (Gadrey 1994). For example, a 1996 article in *The Guardian* commented on the growing dependence on doctors created by the mass circulation of medical knowledge:

> Paradoxically, as patients have become more willing to challenge doctors' expertise, they have also become less able to look after themselves. Says Dr Rice: 'Patients are better informed now and more health aware but it certainly isn't leading to an ability to cope with things better . . .' The boom in media coverage of health issues is giving patients just enough information to worry them, according to Dr Tony Mathie of the Royal College of General Practitioners. Every day he sees anxious parents who fear that their child has meningitis: they've read that a rash or headache are symptoms of the disease.
>
> (Agnew 1996: 61)

Similarly, the introduction of the market into professional domains is in some cases providing professional groups opportunities to reaffirm their separation from the market. Thus the introduction of market principles in organisations dominated by professionals, such as the NHS, provides new strategies of legitimisation to professional groups. Far from being slavishly entrapped into the new market culture, doctors can point to the 'greediness' and 'immorality' of the market (represented by managers) and realign themselves with the clients; the introduction of market principles increases the demarcation between professional practice and the market, and provides professionals with the moral high ground to differentiate themselves from the market logic (Parker and Dent 1996).

The malleable and constitutive nature of professional knowledge and boundaries

As was argued earlier, the anticipation of the erosion of professional knowledge by the logic of the market is based upon two arguments. First, it is argued that the introduction of market principles will serve to diffuse professional knowledge; second, the professional field of knowledge, based on a compartmentalisation of the world into areas of single jurisdiction, is said to be no longer a valid way of representing an increasingly complex and turbulent world.

However, both arguments are based on the assumption that professional knowledge is fixed by the essence or reality of the object it professes to know; these arguments see the independent and self-contained nature of the professional field as the essence of professional knowledge rather than as a contingent achievement itself sustained by professional practice and knowledge. The vision of the erosion of professional knowledge attributes too much 'fixity', 'reality' and 'endurance' to both the object of professional knowledge and professional knowledge itself, by assuming a correspondence between the two. There is the assumption that in the past, the 'reality of the world' did lend itself to division into independent and isolated fields of knowledge, but that now this 'reality' is too complex. However, this image of the 'reality of the past' was itself partly constructed by professional knowledge rather than independent of its development.

Seeing professional knowledge and the constitution of its field as performative and malleable, as an achievement (as proposed earlier in this chapter), rather than as a discovery and reflection of the 'true nature' of some independent reality, suggests the possibility for the professions to reconstitute their field and knowledge in line with the version(s) of reality popularised by recent discourses celebrating the value of the market and enterprise. As mentioned in the previous section, the discourse of the market, far from eroding all boundaries, is rearticulating them, and in this process is giving rise to two privileged entities: the market and the customer. Some professions have already and successfully reconstituted their field and knowledge around these two categories: accountants, lawyers, business consultants, advertising agencies are all 'professing' about the market and the customer (Ackroyd 1996; Reed 1996). Professional knowledge is malleable and expandable, it is constitutive of its field of knowledge rather than bound by it, it may contain the possibility of being reconstituted to claim broader, newer expertise which map onto concerns of enterprise and the market.

Conclusion

The logic of the market, with its celebration of flexibility, transparency and 'boundarylessness', certainly seems inimical to the boundary work central to the making of the professions, and hence threatens the foundations of the professions. However, such a vision of doom is based on a perspective of professional boundaries and knowledge as fixed, immutable and determined by the essence of the object or field of professional knowledge, rather than as malleable, expandable and self-constituted. Thus the prediction of the demise of the professions underestimates the power of professional knowledge to remake itself, to reconstruct its boundaries. Furthermore, this vision of doom is based on an over-deterministic view of the logic of the market. Finally, the introduction of market principles does not so much eliminate as shift boundaries, creating new divisions along which (at least some) professions can seek to rearticulate and reconstitute their fields of knowledge.

This is not to say that the breakdown of professional boundaries by the logic of the market should not be taken seriously, nor that all professions will be able to reconstitute themselves. The celebration and introduction of market principles is certainly challenging the strategies of legitimisation the professions can deploy to build and maintain their privileged status. Furthermore, some professions may be better equipped than others (in terms of discursive and material resources) to remake themselves and to realign their field of knowledge with the logic of the market. However, the analysis of the threat that market principles constitute for the professions should be balanced by a consideration of the possibilities that remain, or that are created, for the professions to remake themselves.

Notes

1 Here we should note the possible exception of Larson (1977), who sees as one of the key dimensions of the professional project the creation and control of the professional market, i.e. the creation of a distinctive service which has to be standardised to be recognised as such.
2 Although the 'aura of independence' is central to the professions' self-definitions (Sikka and Willmott 1995), it is important to note that this independence is only possible to the extent that the professions have established the legitimacy of the 'internal criteria' governing their practice (such as the validity and usefulness of their 'scientific truth', or code of ethics) in the eyes of their constituency or of other relevant party (such as the state). Thus the independence and autonomy of the professions are themselves fragile and contingent achievements (Sikka and Willmott 1995; Fournier 1999).
3 It should be noted that the pursuit of commercial success and the creation of a market for professional services is by no means new to professional practice (see Larson 1977). What is argued in this chapter is not that the logic of the market is imposing a commercial orientation on professionals previously only governed by altruistic concerns, but that it is contributing to a shift in the strategies of legitimisation the professions can use to justify and maintain their privileged position.

References

Abbott, A. (1988) *The System of the Professions*, London: University of Chicago Press.
—— (1995) 'Boundaries of social work or social work of boundaries?', *Social Service Review* December: 547–62.
Ackroyd, S. (1996) 'Organization contra organizations: professions and organizational change in the United Kingdom', *Organization Studies* 17(4): 599–621.
Agnew, T. (1996) 'Mind and body: doctor impatience', *The Observer*, 2 June: 61.
Armstrong, P. (1993) 'Professional knowledge and social mobility: post war changes in the knowledge base of management accounting', *Work, Employment and Society* 7(1): 1–21.
Casey, C. (1995) *Work, Self and Society after Industrialism*, London: Routledge.
Cooper, R. and Law, J. (1995) 'Organization: distal and proximal views', *Research in the Sociology of Organizations*, 13: 237–74.
Crompton, R. (1990) 'Professions in the current context', *Work, Employment and Society*, Special issue: 147–66.
Davies, C. (1996) 'The sociology of professions and the profession of gender', *Sociology* 30(4): 661–78.
Dent, M. (1993) 'Professionalism, educated labour and the state: hospital medicine and the new managerialism', *The Sociological Review* 41: 244–73.
Drucker, P. (1993) *The Post-capitalist Society*, New York: HarperCollins.
du Gay, P. (1996) *Consumption and Identity at Work*, London: Sage.
du Gay, P. and Salaman, G. (1992) 'The cult[ure] of the customer', *Journal of Management Studies* 29(5): 615–33.
Foucault, M. (1975) *The Birth of the Clinic: An Archaeology of Medical Perception*, New York: Vintage Books.
—— (1977) *Discipline and Punish: The Birth of the Prison*, Harmondsworth: Penguin.
—— (1980) *Power/Knowledge: Selected Interviews with Michel Foucault 1971–1977*, ed. C. Gordon, Brighton: Harvester Press.
Fournier, V. (1999) 'The appeal to professionalism as a disciplinary mechanism', *The Sociological Review* 47(2): 280–307.
Freidson, E. (1986) *Professional Powers: A Study of the Institutionalization of Formal Knowledge*, Chicago: University of Chicago Press.
Gadrey, J. (1994) 'La modernisation des services professionnels: rationalisation industrielle ou rationalisation professionnelle?', *Revue Française de Sociologie* 35: 163–95.
Gouldner, A.A. (1957) 'Cosmopolitans and locals', *Administrative Science Quarterly* 2: 281–302.
Greenwood, R. and Lachman, R. (1996) 'Change as an underlying theme in professional service organizations: an introduction', *Organization Studies* 17(4): 563–72.
Haber, S. (1991) *The Quest for Authority and Honor in the American Professions, 1750–1900*, Chicago: University of Chicago Press.
Hanlon, G. (1996) ' "Casino capitalism" and the rise of the "commercialised" service class: an examination of the accountant', *Critical Perspectives on Accounting* 7: 339–63.
Hattersley, R. (1996) 'Restoring the teachers' historic status', *The Guardian*, 10 June: 10.
Heelas, P. (1991) 'Reforming the self: enterprise and the characters of Thatcherism', in R. Keat and N. Abercrombie (eds) *Enterprise Culture*, London: Routledge, pp. 72–92.
Hopwood, A. (1987) 'The archaeology of accounting systems', *Accounting, Organizations and Society* 12(3): 207–34.
Jamous, H. and Peloille, B. (1970) 'Changes in the French university hospital system', in J.A. Jackson (ed.) *Professions and Professionalization*, Cambridge: Cambridge University Press, pp. 111–52.
Johnson, T. (1972) *Professions and Power*, London: Macmillan.
Kanter, R.M. (1990) *When Giants Learn to Dance*, London: Unwyn Hyman.

Keat, R. (1991a) 'Introduction: starship Britain or universal enterprise?', in R. Keat and N. Abercrombie (eds) *Enterprise Culture*, London: Routledge, pp. 1–17.

—— (1991b) 'Consumer sovereignty and the integrity of practices', in R. Keat and N. Abercrombie (eds) *Enterprise Culture*, London: Routledge, pp. 216–30.

Larson, M. (1977) *The Rise of Professionalism: A Sociological Analysis*, London: University of California Press.

Macdonald, K. (1995) *The Sociology of the Professions*, London: Sage.

Matthews, R. (1989) 'Green paper recipes for a second class service', *The Guardian*, 24 February.

Mihill, C. (1996) 'GP exodus threatens NHS disaster', *The Guardian*, 26 June: 8.

Parker, M. and Dent, M. (1996) 'Managers, doctors and culture: changing an English health district', *Administration and Society* 28(3): 335–61.

Peters, T. (1987) *Thriving on Chaos*, Basingstoke: Macmillan.

—— (1992) *Liberation Management*, Basingstoke: Macmillan.

Randle, K. (1996) 'The white-coated worker: professional autonomy in a period of change', *Work, Employment and Society* 10(4): 737–53.

Reed, M. (1996) 'Expert power and control in late modernity: an empirical review and theoretical synthesis', *Organization Studies* 17(4): 573–97.

Sikka, P. and Willmott, H. (1995) 'The power of "independence": defending and extending the jurisdiction of accounting in the United Kingdom', *Accounting, Organizations and Society* 20(6): 547–81.

Smith, C., Knights, D. and Willmott, H. (eds) (1991) *White-Collar Work: The Non-Manual Labour Process*, Basingstoke: Macmillan.

Sommerlad, H. (1995) 'Managerialism and the legal profession: a new professional paradigm', *International Journal of the Legal Profession* 2(2): 159–85.

Stanley, C. (1991) 'Justice enters the marketplace: Enterprise culture and the provision of legal services', in R. Keat and N. Abercrombie (eds) *Enterprise Culture*, London: Routledge, pp. 206–15.

Taylor, B. (1995) 'Amateurs, professionals and the knowledge of archaeology', *British Journal of Sociology* 46(3): 499–508.

Weber, S. (1987) 'The limits of professionalism', in S. Weber, *Institution and Interpretation. Theory and History of Literature* 31: 19–32, Minneapolis: University of Minneapolis Press.

Whitaker, A. (1992) 'The transformation of work: post-fordism revisited', in M. Reed and M. Hughes (eds) *Rethinking Organization*, London: Sage.

Witz, A. (1992) *Professions and Patriarchy*, London: Routledge.

5 Personal business advice, professionalism and the limits to 'customer satisfaction'

Matthew Gorton

Introduction

Since the 1980s, successive British governments have developed a plethora of support services aimed at assisting small and medium-sized enterprises (SMEs). The flagship of government policy for aiding SMEs is the Business Link (BL) network. Three concepts were central to the development of the BL network:

1   the role of personal business advisers (PBAs) as providers of advice on a one-to-one basis with small business managers,
2   the network acting as a gateway for other support services and
3   a drive to improve the quality and 'professionalism' of small business support.

This chapter draws on survey work conducted by the author into SME – support provider relationships in the south-west and south-east of England. The first section details the evolution of small business support in the UK. This is followed by a discussion of the attempts of central government and many practitioners to improve the standards and professional basis of small business support. The degree to which this has been achieved is investigated through interview analysis of the interactions between small businesses and support agencies. The methodology and results of this process are presented in the 'Research design' and 'Results' sections respectively.

The evolution of small business support in the UK

The overriding strategy for post-war development in disadvantaged areas was the attraction of in-migrant branch manufacturing firms from core regions or abroad (Drudy 1989). However, by the 1980s, dissatisfaction with this approach was manifest. Such strategies had not delivered the employment boosts envisaged, either because of the low linkage between plants and the wider local economy or the transient 'footloose' nature of such production units. With large firms downsizing their workforces attention turned to the potential role of small businesses in economic development strategies. This was stimulated by the turnaround in the number of small businesses in Western economies by the

mid-1970s; employment analysis by Birch (1979) prepared convenient if somewhat uncritical findings in support of the dynamic nature of new and micro-
enterprises. Moreover, successive Conservative governments saw small business
ownership correlating well with their ontological view of human beings as
individualistic, goal oriented and aspirational.

This change in approach led to a whole raft of local, regional and national
schemes to increase new business formation and the growth of SMEs. Local
Enterprise Agencies (LEAs) were initially stimulated by the precedent of US
Community Development Co-operations. Set up with government grants detailed in the 1982 Finance Act, they were designed to bring together the best
leadership qualities from local businesses and public authorities. Most LEAs
concentrate on the delivery of advice and counselling to start-up businesses,
with follow-up aftercare and more specialised one- and two-day training courses
for established businesses. Training and Enterprise Councils (TECs) took over
from the Training Agency, which in turn succeeded the Training Commission.
The functions of the TECs were specified as: analysing local labour markets and
key skill needs, the management of youth and adult training programmes, and
providing selected small business support (Hodgson 1993). In rural areas these
new bodies joined traditional actors such as the Agricultural Development
Advisory Service (ADAS), which provides scientific, technical and business
advice to farmers, and the Rural Development Commission (RDC), the objective of which was to stimulate job creation and provision of essential services in
the countryside. In urban areas a parallel development occurred with the formation of Urban Development Councils (UDCs), Enterprise Zones and City Challenge Initiatives. All of these urban development schemes saw the stimulation of
new and existing small businesses as central to local regeneration, and an array of
support services were funded as a result. However, the growth in small business
support provision was *ad hoc*, with a considerable degree of duplication and
fragmentation. For example, Ritchie *et al.* (1984) identified 125 agencies offering some form of assistance to SMEs within the single county of Humberside.
Taken together, national spending on these support services is significant: over
£2 billion during the course of the 1980s (Curran and Downing 1993). By the
mid-1990s spending in real terms had increased further and institutional proliferation was still apparent. Table 5.1 details 20 agencies operating in rural areas
alone.

However, it was apparent by the early 1990s that considerable confusion
existed about what help and advice was available to individual businesses. Moreover, more detailed longitudinal research highlighted that while some SMEs do
grow extremely rapidly this is not a characteristic of the sector as a whole.
Considerable anecdotal evidence existed that much of the support provision
was of poor quality. There thus appeared a rationale for streamlining support, not just in terms of the number of initiatives but also with regard to
potential recipients of support, with more uniform and higher standards of
provision. These aims formed the central rationale for the establishment of
Business Link.

Table 5.1 Sources of public assistance for SMEs in rural areas (1996)

	Premises	Finance (loans/grants)	Advice	Marketing	Training
ADAS	1	1	1	1	1
Agricultural Training Board–Landbase				1	1
Business Link	3	3	3	3	3
Countryside Commission				3	3
County councils	3	3	3	3	3
Department of Trade and Industry	3	2	3	3	3
District councils	3	3	3	3	
English Nature			3		
English Partnerships	3				
English Tourist Board			3	3	
Farm Retail Association			1		
Local Enterprise Agency	3	3	3	3	3
Ministry of Agriculture, Fisheries and Food		1	1	1	
National Farmers Union	1	1	1	1	1
Prince's Youth Trust★		3	3	3	3
Regional tourist boards			3	3	3
Rural Development Commission†	3	3	3	3	3
Sports Council	3		3		
Training and Enterprise Councils		3	3	3	3

1 agricultural businesses only;
2 non-agricultural-based businesses only;
3 both agricultural and non-agricultural-based businesses.
★ Prince's Youth Business Trust assistance is only available to individuals between 18 and 29 years old.
† RDC services are normally only available in Rural Development Areas (RDAs).

Source: RDC (1995: 33); personal communications

The first Business Link (BL) was opened in Leicester on 27 September 1993, followed by Birmingham in October of that year (*Business Link Bulletin* [*BLB*], no. 1). By the end of May 1995, 100 Business Links were open (*BLB* 17). The central objective of BL is to provide small and medium-sized businesses with high quality support services from a single local contact point. It aims to provide a gateway to, and deliverer of, business support information and services. The key resources to be delivered are specified as:

- an information service, ranging from answering common queries to providing in-depth research;
- a professional advisory service, using independent personal business advisers;
- local business promotion to raise awareness and skills among the local business population via events, seminars and conferences.

The introduction of BL was prompted by a widespread belief that the fragmented and highly diverse nature of support provision in the UK was counter-productive, with uneven quality and poor integration of methods and message. The introduction of BL was designed to rationalise and unify support under a national and clearly identifiable 'banner'. While open to all businesses, the target group was specified as businesses employing between five and two hundred individuals, with special attention paid to those with significant growth potential. The charges for these services vary considerably but many are either free or subsidised by the Department of Trade and Industry (DTI).

In each area (based on existing TEC boundaries) the lead partners were intended to be the TEC and the Chamber of Commerce (wherever there was one of any substance) the relevant local authority and other business organisations and local providers where appropriate. Despite the key partners being based in the public sector, the BLs were intended to be led by the private sector. The funds for BLs should stem from four sources:

1   TEC Enterprise Funds,
2   DTI and other government support,
3   resources provided by partners, and
4   income from commercial activities.

It was intended that public funding would only form a small part of the resources of a fully operational Business Link.

The drive for professionalism

It is a stated aim of public policy that support services should be better co-ordinated and professionally managed, with local Business Links acting as the chief gateway and co-ordinator of an array of complementary but specialised agencies. Local Business Links have to be accredited, holding an Agreed Branding Licence, certification to BS EN ISO 9001:1994, and be recognised as an Investor in People. Many Business Links and TECs insist that their PBAs are members or associate members of the Institute of Business Advisors (IBA). IBA membership is dependent on advisory experience, education and the satisfactory completion of continuing professional development (CPD) courses. This is likely to become a mandatory requirement for PBAs: 'We will discuss with the appropriate professional bodies the introduction of a comprehensive range of national standards of professional competence for all those delivering Business Link branded services, with the aim of introducing them in six months' (Roche 1997: 3).

> Continuing Professional Development (CPD) within Business Links is probably the single most effective strategy for developing and maintaining a world class service. It constantly updates professional knowledge and skills by looking ahead, preparing for change and responding to immediate challenges. For effective performance, commitment to CPD is essential and a recommended practice for Business Link advisers.
>
> (BLB 46: 4)

A national PBA Assessment Centre has been proposed to establish minimum core standards, applicable on both a pre-recruitment basis and on a regular annual/biannual review basis for all existing PBAs (Agar and Moran 1995). The BL literature consistently refers to advising small businesses as a profession.

The rationale for professionalisation has been made on two principal grounds: enhancing customer satisfaction and as a form of competitive advantage. It has been argued that by becoming more customer driven, service provision and quality will improve. The latter is seen as important for improving the productivity and profitability of small business clients, which contribute to Britain's performance in the world economy. This provides the justification for the small business field becoming a legitimate area of knowledge and intervention. The small business has become an object of knowledge and a valid target of control and intervention. In this way it is interesting to draw a parallel with Fournier's arguments (pp. 67–86) on the erection of professional boundaries, which draws on Foucault's (1975) reading of the development of medicine as a profession.

Exactly the same arguments have been made by those that wish to see small business advisers as professionals. According to their logic, small businesses can be turned from 'idle bodies' into more productive, internationally competitive units by the application of best practice administered by 'qualified advisers'. As with medicine, the techniques of 'observation, documentation and constitution of files on individual cases' have been applied to produce training courses and a syllabus for new professional examinations and CPD programmes. The degree to which this drive for professionalism in small business advice is accepted will, however, depend on clients accepting these boundaries, acquiescing to being patients and recognising the legitimacy of this self-contained field of knowledge.

Research design

To understand the nature and degree of acceptance of boundaries between small business support providers and potential clients, interviews with agencies and a random selection of non-agricultural SMEs (taken from the Dun and Bradstreet directory) and agricultural businesses (from Yellow Pages) were conducted. The Dun and Bradstreet database was used because it gave a list of enterprises and detailed their age and size information based on credit references. This meant that the sample was not biased in terms of whether the business had used external sources of advice or training. Businesses were sampled from two distinct geographical areas to avoid a localisation bias: (1) economic core localities in Surrey, Hertfordshire and Berkshire and (2) the economically peripheral area of Devon and Cornwall. The core–periphery divide is based on Webber and Craig's (1976) index of local authority districts, a cluster analysis of like authorities based on 23 socio-economic indicators. Within this classification, core regions can be defined as 'those which have achieved a high level of economic activity per capita relative to others' (MacMillian 1990: 95). As the study areas are predominantly rural, both agricultural and non-agricultural small

Table 5.2 Structure of interviews conducted

	Farmers	Non-agricultural SMEs	Support agencies	Total
Rural core	4	5	4	13
Rural peripheral	7	6	8	21
Total	11	11	12	34

businesses were sampled. As well as interviewing consultants and managers from Business Link, the opinions of other support providers were elicited. The number and type of interviews conducted is shown in Table 5.2.

These interviews were conducted in parallel with quantitative analysis of spatial variations in small business performance, the results of which are presented elsewhere (Gorton 1999). In some cases the interview material presented below is supplemented by answers to open-ended questions taken from the postal questionnaire phase of the research.

Results

Agricultural businesses

The majority of farmers interviewed stated that their main desire was that they 'just wanted to be farmers' and had a marked degree of antagonism towards the development of alternative enterprises. This meant that the agenda of support providers, geared up to new enterprise creation and diversification, was in stark conflict to the desires of most farmers interviewed, reinforcing the divide and boundaries between the two groups. Two responses from medium-sized, family farmers in Devon and Cornwall respectively, present this view most eloquently:

> In a world in which millions starve, the job of a farmer is to grow food, not run zoos, circuses, shops, golf courses, hotels or places of entertainment. If politicians do not wish food to be grown they should pension off farmers in the same way as steel, coal and ship building workers and take land out of production, allowing it to revert to nature. Starting with so-called less favoured areas. So-called diversification is a political stunt and not viable in more than the short term. If at all.
>
> (Interview, dairy farmer, Cornwall)

> We are ruled by too many administrators and criticised by too many un-appreciative, ignorant members of the general public who currently have the luxury of complaining with full bellies. This is forcing farmers into searching for alternative, but basically unwanted, ways of supplementing eroding agricultural incomes. I, personally, despite my love for what I do,

am becoming increasingly despondent about the future for both me, and more importantly, my little boy and girl. I hope she marries well!

(Interview, mixed farmer, Devon)

The main complaint against external agencies was that they failed to understand the 'farming way of life' and the motivations of farmers, producing unrealistic schemes:

> There has to be financial help available other than to partly fund ADAS feasibility studies – which in our case was money, ours, thrown down the drain. The expensive plans and estimated cost fell light-years outside our capabilities. Our bank manager could not believe such hare-brained schemes could be put forward. It was converting buildings for light industry in an area with empty units in abundance.
>
> (Interview, medium-sized farmer, Surrey)

The gap between advisers and advised would seem to be greatest for small and tenant farmers. Most felt disenfranchised from support agencies:

> Most small tenanted holdings have limited capital, so we just plod along I'm afraid, with not too much headway made. Most diversification needs lots of money, time and thought.
>
> (Interview, tenant farmer, Devon)

This gap can lead to a feeling of betrayal, particularly where different agencies appear to give conflicting advice, with a lack of co-ordination or consistency:

> We started a business on this farm repairing and servicing farm machinery and Land Rovers. Caradon Council, who we come under, would only give us two years temporary planning permission to see if the business was a success. The business grew, employing two local men and one part-time man on the farm, as I didn't have the time for all the farm work owing to increased demands in the workshop. When we applied for permanent permission for the workshop, which was an existing farm building, we were given two more years temporary, and told we would then have to move out to an industrial estate, because it was unsuitable to stay on the farm. The business was 400 yards off road, and was not visible from any other property. We appealed against the decision and lost. In April 1994, we moved to an industrial estate. This was completely impractical, having the farm one and a half miles from the business, especially with cows calving and Christ knows what, also because of the cost of renting a unit, and the insecurity of the premises, and also the size of the building, which was much smaller: one employee lost his job, and the part-time man on the farm had to go. We have since disposed of the business, and I am now back where I was six years ago. Diversification has left a very bitter taste in my mouth . . . We

received no help whatsoever from Caradon District Council, who were always most unhelpful and two-faced.

(Interview, dairy farmer, Cornwall/Devon border)

There tends to be poor linkages between farmers and agriculturally based agencies and non-agricultural small business agencies. Two comments from a TEC business adviser and a Business Link information manager illustrate these fissures:

I don't have much contact with farms – the numbers who take up [support] services I could count on one hand. From experience many have buried their heads in the sand and the point of contact is desperation when it's too late. Unless you build up a relationship you will be used as a last resort. One farmer had just let the overdraft go up and up and was going to be repossessed the week after he got in touch. If he had been in touch six months before we probably could have done something about it but as it was it was too late and he lost the lot.

(Interview, TEC business adviser)

To tell the truth we haven't had much contact with them in the past. However, with the 5b money [an EU rural development initiative] coming on stream we had several meetings and it is an area we are looking closely at.

(Interview, Business Link information manager)

Farmers' reluctance to use non-agricultural-based agencies stems from both supply- and demand-side factors. Ignorance of the services available (supply side) and the feeling that these agencies 'don't understand farming' and so 'could be of no use' (demand side) were particularly pertinent. In the small number of successful relationships, advisers worked in sympathy with the aims and prior beliefs of farmers, so that the latter felt 'less out of control' in the relationship. However, the overall take-up of training schemes by farmers is low (Gorton 1999).

The main fears surrounding business development, as perceived by farmers, were concerns about planning and bureaucracy, especially the anxiety of 'falling foul of government regulations'. This is a major barrier to the use of external agencies as they were perceived as 'being all on the same side', 'bureaucrats' or 'not knowing about each other let alone us'. Particular concern was raised about the lack of co-ordination between the economic development and planning departments of district councils. Farmers felt there was a lack of consistency and ambiguities in the advice given. This has not been helped by changes in central government guidance towards development in rural areas and the reluctance of some planning authorities fully to accept these guidelines (Evans 1989).

We have been applying for planning permission for a golf driving range in this area. One of the main stumbling blocks from planners is that it is taking away grade II agricultural land. MAFF [Ministry of Agriculture, Fisheries and Food] have really been no help at all and we feel no one is really there to help you. In fact our farm shop is under threat because of an Asda superstore opening on the same road.

(Interview, mixed farm, north Cornwall)

Farmers are encouraged by the government to diversify but when planning goes into local councils it is turned down. Not worth the effort most times.

(Interview, estate farmer, Berkshire)

The majority of farmers are unsure of the planning process, as most agricultural development has been exempt from planning permission requirements under the General Development Order (Evans 1989).

The majority of farmers wish to earn their living purely through agricultural activities, have strong attachments to the way of life and view enterprises outside of agriculture as very risky. The plethora of agencies to assist small businesses is not well understood by farmers and there is little use of any agency outside of the agricultural community (ADAS, National Farmers Union (NFU) and Agricultural Training Board (ATB)). Business Link is virtually unknown – given the fact that diversification often involves markets well outside of agriculture (for example tourism and retailing), it should be a more appropriate gateway to services than the traditional agricultural agencies. A similar argument can also be made with regard to local authorities, in that while local authorities are part of the Business Link network, the main point of contact is via economic development officers, with planners not directly involved. Yet it would appear that of all the functions of local authorities, it is planning regulations that most concern farmers.

For those farmers which do use training and advisory services, their two principal requirements are: (1) information on how planning systems operate and how government legislation will impact on their proposed or already operating enterprise, and (2) practical suggestions for the implementation of strategy. This subset of farmers are also clear that they still firmly want the relationship with external parties to be 'hands off' and for themselves to remain fully in control of decision making. Maintaining a clear boundary and 'having the final say' in decision making was perceived as being essential.

Non-agricultural SMEs

Before conducting these interviews it was expected that questioning would mainly concern the range of support services offered. However, it emerged that while reviews of public policy have focused on evaluating support services, SMEs were more concerned not with the spending *for them*, but the costs *imposed on* them, by government. As the quotations below indicate, particular anger was expressed about the Uniform Business Rate (UBR):

First, we need better understanding from councils regarding business rates and the importance of cash flow. Second it's Customs and Excise, again same problem.

(Interview, wholesaler, Cornwall)

> If tax was not as high we could reinvest our own money. Grants and loans would not be required and I'm too busy to apply.
>
> > (Interview, specialist manufacturer, Devon)

The majority of respondents felt that a banded system that was tied more to firm size and ability to pay was required. As with farmers, there is a divide between the agenda of support advisers and issues deemed most important by small business owners.

The second biggest area of concern surrounded sectoral and payment legislation. Comments fitted into two categories: those who wanted additional legislation (consisting overwhelmingly of calls for tighter laws surrounding late payment of debts) and second, demand for the reduction of 'red tape':

> Main problem is getting paid on time.
>
> > (Interview, machine tool manufacturer Devon [repeated in similar form by five other respondents, with calls for legislation by three])

> A major problem is having to collect government taxes [PAYE/VAT] free of charge – companies should be reimbursed for this work.
>
> > (Interview, haulier, Surrey)

> Efforts should be made to eliminate, or at least simplify, many of the regulations concerning employment law which combine to make the duties, responsibilities and risks of employing people progressively more onerous. One faces health and safety, Employer's Liability (insurance premiums have rocketed since the employer always seems to be presumed to be 'responsible'), PAYE, enforcement of court orders, SSP [statutory sick pay], SMP [statutory maternity pay], statutory holidays, dismissal procedures and redundancy rights, which are unfair.
>
> > (Interview, machine tool manufacturer, Devon)

For medium-sized firms and exporters it was not just British legislation which was perceived as a barrier to growth, but European directives as well. In the same way as farmers felt frightened by planning regulations, the EU was seen as a similar labyrinth of restrictions with the sheer weight of legislation leaving 'traps' for the unaware small business.

On the issue of grants and incentives the interviews highlighted four fairly common themes:

1   a belief that grant aid assistance should be locally focused,
2   that there is a lack of focus for development (particularly in the south-west study area),
3   a better relationship with planners should be established, and
4   there is general ambivalence towards Business Link.

The idea that assistance needs to be targeted locally was expressed in terms of both large employers establishing better linkages with local small firms and that 'outsiders' often abused inward investment aid:

> The main problem I have faced is that national and local organisations i.e. South West Gas, South West Water, Caradon, Plymouth councils, etc. do not want to employ small local companies and use London or out-of-county-based (hence expensive) companies. My work is almost all overseas.
>
> (Written response, business consultant, Devon)

> More grant aid for *genuine* small businesses attempting to grow – generating *real* employment. Tighter control of the 'big boys' who relocate to Corn-wall for the grants and then asset strip the new site.
>
> (Written response, builders' merchant Devon, emphasis in the original)

The perception of a lack of focus for development stems from the confusion as to precisely what assistance is available and a belief, particularly strong in the south-west, of being ignored by central government. In the south-east study area, by contrast, there was no perception of a need for a regional focus or separate spatial focus. The latter may reflect its greater economic prosperity and lack of past regional assistance. While Business Link has been designed to reduce the confusion surrounding agency proliferation and assistance, there is little evidence of this actually occurring:

> Investment grants should be made available for business to start investing in capital again. There appear to be so many schemes but no single source of information.
>
> (Interview, steel fabricators, Cornwall)

> It would be nice to see some real development and investment in the Ply-mouth area to employ the wealth of skills which are wasting away through age and neglect by our government . . . start trying to identify land the other side of Bristol.
>
> (Interview, industrial property manager, West Devon)

> Business rates, Corporation tax, employers' NIC [National Insurance con-tributions] and bank interest rates should be lowered to give an incentive to companies to employ. Why do we keep getting offers from the Welsh Development Agency? Do we have a similar agency? If so what do they do for a living?
>
> (Interview, manufacturer, mid-Devon)

There is a need for local authorities and the Government Office for the South West to invest in real jobs for twelve months of the year instead of promoting tourism, which is for only twelve weeks of the year. Investment in infrastructure is essential.

> (Interview, timber merchant and panel manufacturer, Cornwall)

The process of applying for grants has become so complicated, one county council now offers SMEs a grant to obtain grants:

> We have also found problems of attracting grants from the DTI. This was often due to applications being unprofessional. So we are now offering a grant to get professional advice to get other grants. Are you with me?
>
> (Interview, county council economic development officer, south-west)

The Business Link network has not reduced these complications as much as initially envisaged, as the partner agencies only include a small selection of the key relationships maintained by SMEs. In rural areas the planning process can be particularly controversial and, like farmers, non-agricultural owner managing-directors (OMDs) felt the advice they received was poor. Yet the Business Link network has no direct links with planning departments:

> Problems encountered with highways authority in signing our business on the public highway particularly as we are 60 per cent tourist reliant. This does not appear to be a problem in other EEC countries, especially France.
>
> (Interview, craft centre, Cornwall)

> Our main problem has been the complete obstruction and delays to development at district and county council by bureaucrats. They pay lip service to industrial requirements.
>
> (Interview, timber merchant, Cornwall)

The criticisms of Business Link cited by SME respondents ranged from views that it was unnecessary to disappointing personal experiences:

> As a small and successful business we went to Business Link for help with business planning. They said they had no experience with such a successful company and could offer very little help. We welcomed their honesty and good service. However, it would have been advantageous to have something more tangible.
>
> (Written response, service sector firm employing under ten people, Surrey)

A gripe cited by one OMD and several of the other public sector agencies was the size of the initial capital investment involved in establishing the BL network and the level of ongoing fixed costs:

> If Business Link spent as much on small firms as feathering their own offices I might have some time for them.
>
> (Interview, medium-sized manufacturer, Devon)

When these complaints were put to Business Link representatives they stressed that individuals were not always going to be happy with the advice they receive. When asked how blunt this advice was, one respondent replied:

> Very blunt – it's futile not to be honest. They will tell people not to waste their time. On each review [PBAs] file a report, currently on paper, to individual offices but we hope to have all reports on a computerised database which can be accessed centrally . . . Many businesses who come to us say they are interested in growth but really it's much more a question of survival than growth.
>
> (Interview, information manager, Business Link)

This highlights the difficulty of services being entirely 'market driven', where service quality is measured in terms of customer satisfaction. Professionalism with regard to business advice often involves the delivery of 'hard truths', where the principal receiver of advice may be part of the problem. The delivery of customer satisfaction within the adviser–advised relationship may not always be commensurate with assisting business survival and growth, as 'hard truths' may not always be palatable. On the issue of the costs of establishing the network, respondents were more conciliatory:

> It wasn't thought out. But we have to be self-funding in three years, that has concentrated people's minds.
>
> (Interview, marketing manager, Business Link)

The information most desired by SMEs related to planning, legislation, finance and market contacts. However, these are not the strengths of the Business Link partners. There are currently no direct linkages with planning departments, accountants and banks. It would appear difficult for Business Links to reduce institutional proliferation and confusion if its own internal relationships do not include those areas that SMEs themselves perceive as being most important.

Inter-agency professional relationships

Nearly all agencies criticised the small business policy in the 1980s, with its focus on start-ups and, in particular, the emphasis placed on 'getting people off the dole'. With institutional proliferation and very frequent changes in assistance (both in terms of regulations and the actual names of schemes) confusion was heightened. As one TEC business adviser describes:

> With the fragmented provision . . . there is great reluctance and many are unaware. The quality has not been there in the past. Training providers were generally low quality, focusing on bums on seats and geared up to business start-ups. This has changed with the end of the Business Start-up Programme in March 1995 with the quality of start-ups hit.
>
> (Interview, TEC business adviser, south-west)

A Local Enterprise Agency trainer who specialises in start-ups also questioned the usefulness of policies to encourage the unemployed to set up their own businesses in his rural locality. The nature of start-up businesses reflected the skills and background of the clients; very few have higher qualifications or employment experience that they could utilise. Most of the businesses launched under such schemes are thus into already developed, often saturated markets. Though there have been some notable successes, very few businesses grow to employ more than the founder:

> Most of the businesses created involve basic skills: mobile hairdressers, plumbers, odd jobs, child minding services, cleaning, you name it . . . You get a few. There is — and — [names of a parcel delivery firm and pasty maker]. They were mine. But for every one of them you get the rest. It's getting worse, they've changed it again so that now you have to be unemployed six months before getting on TFW [Training for Work] Enterprise.[1] In some areas it's stopped altogether. We are only keeping going with Euro cash.
>
> (Interview, LEA business counsellor, south-east)

The long-term unemployed on the scheme face key problems, in addition to saturated basic markets, concerning access to resources and markets. Bank managers are unwilling to fund new business proposals without the provision of collateral and/or matching funding by the prospective client. Yet the vast majority of participants are simply incapable of meeting this criterion, with little or no personal savings after long-term unemployment. Moreover, these groups are, to a certain degree, disconnected from the local business community. Few have connections or ready access to markets, and even less have the confidence to undertake business negotiations. As outsiders, many find it difficult to enter new markets. As the LEA respondent describes:

> They haven't got a lot going for them. It's really a question of inputs and outputs. You cannot expect them to be big deal entrepreneurs. They've got no money and no experience. I'd say about 10 per cent of the people I see cannot fill in the forms. You're not going to get Richard Branson. Let's face it, you can't make chicken soup out of chicken shit.
>
> (Interview, LEA business counsellor, south-east)

Support agencies were also asked about the design of their initiatives and whether there was consideration of two potential pitfalls (displacement and additionality) of external funding. Additionality refers to the extent to which public sector initiatives stimulate net increases in activity, as opposed to activities which would have occurred anyway within the market. Measures of displacement seek to quantify the extent to which supporting some firms leads to the decline or death of others which have not been helped. On both issues there appeared to be little quantitative monitoring or synergy between agencies. To give an example, one district council in the south-west offers a business loan of £1000 to SMEs based within its boundaries. For this it receives 'about one application a month' (according to the local economic development officer). Past users were not monitored as to whether the service was beneficial to performance, and a Business Link information manager, when questioned, did not know of its existence. This would appear to be still symptomatic; the aims of integration and co-ordination are for the large part, so far, not being met. This is a widespread view, not just from small businesses and farmers but – crucially – of those employed by the agencies themselves:

> MAFF are based in Exeter, the Government Office for the South West in Bristol and Plymouth and never the twain shall meet. It's a real problem.
> (Interview, NFU regional director, south-west)

> There are 72 different agencies in Devon and Cornwall alone offering some form of support to small businesses. With 72 bodies including banks, small business advisers, accountants and local authorities (there are six in Cornwall alone) all operating there is enormous duplication and fragmentation. Business Link will pull this together.
> (Interview, Enterprise Agency workspace manager, west Devon)

> No. They very much do their own thing.
> (Interview, TEC business adviser on contact with MAFF,
> ADAS and NFU, Devon)

> We have a good reputation and our main aim is carrying that forward.
> (Interview, RDC business adviser, south-west)

These findings are echoed in two other reports. KPMG Peat Marwick (1994), analysing the performance of the first wave of BLs, discovered that although partners may have worked together previously, bringing all the partners together for Business Link was far more difficult, with the integration of partner staff taking considerable time. Deakins and Philpott (1995) highlight how networking between financial institutions and external support agencies was higher in Baden-Württemberg, Germany than in the UK, where there was general low-level integration. In fact as Table 5.1 indicates, little appears to have changed in terms of institutional proliferation since the early 1980s, when Ritchie *et al.* (1984) identified 125 agencies operating in Humberside.

The reasons for this lack of integration and maintenance of strong organisational boundaries between small business support providers can be divided, albeit not cleanly, into questions concerning internal and external agency relations. The implicit, and not surprising, chief priority of each agency interviewed was to continue their own existence. Agencies tended to begin by searching for new sources of funding to prop up diminishing or soon to be withdrawn existing revenues rather than devising innovative co-operative solutions.

For all the talk of responding to local needs, the most striking point about support agencies is their reliance on external funding, usually from central government and/or the EU. Agencies overseeing SME support projects are not independent, but rely on higher patronage. The key relationship for each agency is thus with central government, not other agencies, as it is the former which decides their level of future funding or whether they continue to exist. The imperative for agencies is to justify their own existence and maintain external funding. Even schemes funded by local government are still heavily dependent on central government policy, given the dominance of the executive in the British constitutional system. Moreover, government funding for small business support has been subject to much chopping and changing in the annual spending round conducted with the Treasury. The environment for local agencies is thus unstable, with the interviews conducted highlighting how each agency felt an acute need for self-justification. Future funding was often felt to be contingent on successful initial phases, where success would be measured by national government and Whitehall. Many agencies interviewed therefore believed they had 'responsibility without power'. Agencies had pre-set targets and objectives to reach, but with minimal influence on the local economy within which these targets were to be met. As the LEA representative (south-east) remarked: 'At the end of the day you do your best but don't expect too much.'

The requirement of agencies to justify their existence, and the way consequent funding is contingent on 'success', often leads to a dilemma for agencies surrounding the trade-off between meeting most pressing needs and, on the other hand, dealing with those most willing to participate or who are cost-effective for the agency. Empirical studies have detailed how those living in the poorest conditions, with the most constrained opportunity sets, are also the least accessible community for agencies to reach (Shaw 1979). With the instability of funding and a treadmill of self-justification, this stratum in many cases is ignored in the quest for short-term results, which can be generated from more accessible, 'cost-effective' and less constrained groups.

This conflict is apparent in TEC funding, as their finances are increasingly subject to payment by results and output related. There has been a backdrop of cuts in real payments per trainee from Whitehall but TECs now have the freedom to allocate any surpluses generated to activities they consider to be of strategic importance (Jones 1995). An Employment Department report (ED 1994) investigated the surpluses of nine TECs, which amounted to £43.5 million. In building up these surpluses, the report found training was skewed towards producing clerical officers and hairdressers, the training of which was quick, cheap and easily assessable. Those TECs which placed greater effort in higher cost, skilled training (such as engineering and the provision of special needs) were less able to achieve surpluses (ibid.). Cost effectiveness and results for the TEC may have very little correlation with the needs of the local community. There is a kind of 'Tom and Jerry' politics between the TECs and central government in terms of obtaining autonomy in spending budgets. Those TECs which place greater emphasis on meeting the needs of more disconnected groups or dealing with sophisticated skill shortages are penalised by the funding system. This system of funding also means that individual SMEs are really the *secondary customer*, after the government, as it is the latter, in most instances, which pays the (initial) bill.

The lack of historical integration of support services is also inimical to contemporary drives aimed at sustaining co-ordinated action. One cannot expect meaningful collective representations or mutual awareness between institutions to develop overnight. Trust and co-operation, if it has any depth, is not by its very nature instantly produced. Moreover, integration in the study areas is not merely restricted within the public sector, but also extends to relationships between firms. Stimulating co-operation between firms appears to try to 'work against the grain' of the motivations and desires of most SME OMDs in the UK. Very few want active involvement with other firms, let alone support agencies. Only if the government has something to offer which is desired by SMEs will OMDs be interested. With the slimming down of direct grants and a greater emphasis towards expertise and training provision, which most do not believe they require, only a small subset of SMEs will want active relationships with support agencies.

Finally, professional co-operation should not be perceived as an end in itself; in fact, closely integrated but closed systems of professionals can become isolated from the very sectors they are supposed to be aiding. A precedent for this problem is highlighted in Dintenfass's (1993) review of co-operation and integration of coal owners in the first half of this century. Coal-mine owners shared very similar educational backgrounds that set stability and institutional loyalty as a high priority, a tendency also noted by Church (1993) within ICI. With strong networks embodying trust and information, established and reinforced at school, university and in various clubs, the information gained from these networks was often used to resist innovation in production techniques and marketing strategies. The efficiency of the network may have contributed to a wider inefficiency in the use of resources (Chick 1995). Integration is only desirable to the extent that it aids the performance of SMEs, and one should not confuse *institutional* efficiency with *policy* efficiency. Co-ordination and professionalisation may lead to a more efficient delivery of services but this does not answer the question as to whether such services are actually necessary or currently delivered in the most appropriate manner.

Conclusions

The number of small business support agencies has burgeoned since the 1970s in an *ad hoc* manner. This fragmented growth has led to considerable confusion with potential clients. The structural environment inhabited by support agencies has limited the much heralded desire for co-ordination in activities. The dependence of agencies on funding from Westminster, frequent changes of policy and the setting of targets linked to funding at the organisational level are all factors inimical to the co-operation and integration of support provision.

Organisational rather than professional boundaries still take precedence in the decision making of support agencies.

The government has argued that the development of support services should be market driven, with a linkage between the delivery of high quality services and customer satisfaction. However, professionalism with regard to business advice often involves the delivery of 'hard truths' where the owner manager of the business (and principal receiver of advice) may be part of the problem. The delivery of customer satisfaction (measured in the short term) within the adviser–advised relationship may not always be commensurate with serving the long-term interests of the business. Hard truths may not always be palatable or met with instant approval. Customer satisfaction as a driver of service quality is, in this regard, problematic.

While the logic for small business advisers to be seen as professionals has been strongly promoted, transformation has foundered on an unwillingness of potential clients to accept the proffered professional boundaries or recognise small business advice as a self-contained, external field of knowledge. The agenda of small business advisory agencies has, in the main, not been accepted by either the agricultural or non-agricultural business communities. While advisory agencies promote government spending *for* small businesses, when enterprise managers are asked to detail their priorities they are far more concerned with *costs imposed on* SMEs. These costs (such as local Uniform Business Rates) lie outside the remit and influence of small business support agencies so that their service cannot be fully driven by the predominant concerns of clients.

Note

1 There are some notable exceptions to the six-month rule: ex-armed forces personnel, ex-prison offenders and certain disabled groups.

References

Agar, J. and Moran, P. (1995) 'Developing excellence in Business Link services: a continuing professional development process for personal business advisers', paper presented to the 18th ISBA National Small Firms Conference, University of Paisley, Scotland, 15–17 November.
Birch, J. (1979) *The Job Generation Process*, Cambridge, MA: MIT Press.
Chick, M. (1995) 'British business history: a review of the periodic literature for 1993', *Business History* 37(1): 1–16.
Church, R. (1993) 'The family firm in industrial capitalism: international perspectives on hypotheses and history', *Business History* 35(4): 17–43.
Curran, J. and Downing, S. (1993) 'The state and small business owners: an empirical assessment of consultation strategies', in R. Atkin, E. Chell and C. Mason (eds) *New Directions in Small Business Research*, Aldershot: Avebury, pp. 139–54.
Deakins, D. and Philpott, T. (1995) 'Networking by external support agencies and financial institutions', *International Small Business Journal* 13(2): 47–58.
Dintenfass, M. (1993) 'Family, training and career in the British coal industry in the era of decline', *Business and Economic History* 22(1): 273–84.

Drudy, P.J. (1989) 'Problems and priorities in the development of rural regions', in L. Albrechts and F. Moulaert (eds) *Regional Policy and the Crossroads: European Perspectives*, London: Jessica Kingsley, pp. 125–41.

Employment Department [ED] (1994) *TEED/TEC Funding Arrangements*, Sheffield: Employment Department.

Evans, J.M. (1989) 'Diversification – the planning issues', *Farm Buildings and Engineering* 6(1): 34–5.

Foucault, M. (1975) *The Birth of the Clinic: An Archaeology of Medical Perception*, New York: Vintage Books.

Gorton, M. (1999) 'Spatial variations in markets served by UK based small and medium sized enterprises', *Entrepreneurship and Regional Development* 11(1): 39–55.

Hodgson, D. (1993) 'UK training policy and the role of TECs', *International Journal of Manpower* 14(8): 3–16.

Jones, M.R. (1995) 'Training and enterprise councils: a continued search for local flexibility', *Regional Studies* 29(6): 577–80.

KPMG Peat Marwick (1994) *Process Evaluation Report on Early Business Links*, London: KPMG Peat Marwick.

MacMillian, M.J. (1990) 'The core–periphery concept in economic terms: with special reference to Brittany and Cornwall and Devon', in M. Havinden, A. Queniart and J. Stanyer (eds) *Centre and Periphery: A Comparative Study of Brittany and Cornwall and Devon*, Exeter: Exeter University Press, pp. 95–107.

RDC (1995) *Action for Rural Enterprise: 1995/1996 Edition*, Salisbury: RDC.

Ritchie, D., Asch, D. and Weir, A. (1984) 'Research note: the provision of assistance to small firms', *International Small Business Journal* 3(1): 62–5.

Roche, B. (1997) *Enhanced Business Links – A Vision for the 21st Century*, London: DTI.

Shaw, J.M. (1979) 'Editorial introduction', in J.M. Shaw (ed.) *Rural Deprivation and Planning*, Norwich: Geo Books, pp. 1–9.

Webber, R. and Craig, J. (1976) 'Which local authorities are alike?', *Population Trends* no. 5, London: HMSO, pp. 13–19.

6   Colleagues or clients?

The relationship between clergy and church members

Helen Cameron

Introduction

One aspect of enterprise culture has been a challenge to the professions as a means of organising work (Ferlie *et al.* 1996) and a questioning of the power differential inherent in professional–client relationships (Crompton 1990). This chapter explores the challenge posed by enterprise culture by looking at the work of a profession already on the margins of society to see what workplace practices its members use to sustain their professional modes of interacting with their clients, church members. The data discussed are drawn from a larger study of the social action of the local church. The disciplinary base of the study is organisational theory, but the chapter seeks to make some connections with the sociology of the professions. The chapter assumes that clergy can be regarded as professionals, and focuses on the workplace practices of a sample of clergy, rather than looking at the clerical profession as an entity.

The rest of the chapter is divided into five parts. The first introduces the relationship between clergy and church members, then the second reviews the literature that was used to frame the study and makes some reference to the literature on professionals. The next part presents the data, followed by a discussion of the data which seeks to interpret the workplace practices of the clergy studied. The final part summarises the argument and makes connections between the experiences of clergy and those of other professions affected by enterprise culture.

The relationships between clergy and church members

Clergy work in a range of organisational settings, for example as denominational executives (Harrison 1959), workers in church-related agencies (Jeavons 1994), or as chaplains to public institutions (Abercrombie 1977; Prison Service Chaplaincy 1984; Hospital Chaplaincies Council 1987). By far the most common setting for clergy is in the local church (Jarvis 1975). This chapter deals with the local church and the ways in which clergy interact with church members.

Three modes of interaction seem to dominate the clergy–church member relationship. The first mode is as a pastor relating to church members as clients.

The client approaches the pastor with personal problems seeking guidance and spiritual direction. An extensive literature exists advising clergy how to undertake this role, much of it drawing upon psychological concepts (Wright 1980; Taylor 1983; Jacobs 1987; Foskett and Lyall 1988; Leech 1990; Blair and Sharpe 1992). Only rarely is the social context of the client addressed (Bradbury 1989; Furniss 1994). The literature suggests that the role of pastor is distinctive and central to the working life of congregational clergy. For example, Greenwood in Nelson (1996: 101) notes: 'the expectation [is] that clergy are chiefly pastors, that they are in sole charge, with lay help carefully controlled'.

The second mode of interaction between clergy and church members is as worship leader and worshipper. The context of worship may not seem particularly interactive in the sense normally understood in professional–client relationships, but in the context of studying religious organisations, the rituals of worship can symbolise the relationships in the church (Cameron 1996; Francis 1996).

The third mode of interaction between clergy and church members is as colleagues working together to run the congregation and undertake its work. Clergy normally have a leadership role but church members also have leadership as well as operational functions. There is little literature on this aspect of clergy's work. As Rudge (1968: 5) has noted,

> The administrative side [of the church's work] has been seen as in opposition to the pastoral; the one is despised, the other regarded as the essence of the ministry. In the training of clergy, only the latter has been taken seriously.

Before looking at the data gathered on these three modes of interacting, it seems appropriate to review the literature used to guide the data collection, and to make some initial connections with the literature on professionals which will be used to help interpret the data.

Concepts of power and conflict

This part of the chapter briefly reviews three types of literature. First, the literature on religious organisations; second, the organisational theory literature which addresses the issue of power; and third, ideas on power relations in the sociology of professions.

Within the sociology of religion, the literature on religious organisations plays a significant, if minor, role (Beckford 1975). Only a few writers address the issue of clergy–church member relationships, but those that do, suggest that conflict is inevitable. Dempsey (1969, 1983), in his ethnographic study of an Australian congregation, suggests that, for clergy, there is an inevitable conflict between their pastoral role and their desire to issue a prophetic challenge to their members. Clergy who challenge the beliefs and practices of their members will experience conflict. Jarvis (1976) is equally clear that conflict between clergy and church members is inevitable, but attributes it to a clash between clerical and lay religious subcultures. The former is based upon an educated and highly rational exposition of Christian doctrine, the latter is heavily influenced by folk religion. Herman's (1984) study of a Canadian church uncovered a split in the congregation between conservative and liberal outlooks. The clergyman was seen as having sympathies with the liberal faction, which led to conflict. Finally, Spencer's observations of clergy in Hull led her to conclude:

> The part played by the laity is important in enabling the minister to per-form his role, but without clearly defined clergy and laity roles, there is a risk that the layman's involvement can become an intrusion into the cler-gyman's professional sphere, and the clergyman can feel his authority is threatened.
>
> (Spencer 1995: 55)

This literature led the researcher to expect conflict between clergy and laity in the case studies undertaken. This pointed to the need to use organisational theory which dealt with the issue of power in framing the study. Power has long been a theme in scholarly work on organisations (Weber 1947; Michels 1949), but from the 1960s onwards, sustained attempts have been made to develop theories which view organisations as political institutions (Emerson 1962; Cyert and March 1963; Crozier 1964). These theories have been attacked, for exam-ple by Donaldson (1995), because they challenge the dominant view of organ-isations as institutions which seek to achieve goals by rational means. Burrell and Morgan (1979) argue that to take a political perspective on organisations is to question the unitary view of power that underlies the field of organisational studies and requires a shift to a pluralist perspective that views society as the outcome of conflicts between parties serving their own interests.

Unsurprisingly, power theory contains differing views as to how its central concept is to be defined. From the 1960s scholars moved from seeing power as an attribute of individual actors to seeing it as the property of social relationships (Emerson 1962). A commonly cited definition is that of Dahl (1957: 202): 'A has power over B to the extent that he can get B to do something that he would not otherwise do.' Bacharach and Lawler (1980) argue that power is too broad a term to be defined meaningfully and that it needs to be broken down into more clearly definable concepts which can be operationalised for empirical investigation.

Many writers on power start by outlining the work of Weber, who defined the concept of authority as power legitimated by a means acceptable to those subject to it (Weber 1947). Some writers have taken Weber's emphasis on authority and concluded that it is the only form of power in organisations. This leads to a unitary and often managerial view of organisations which Burrell and Morgan (1979) diagnose in much of the organisational literature. Some studies of bureaucracies have shown another form of power at work, namely influence. Crozier's (1964) study of public and private sector bureaucracies in France shows how groups within these organisations use informal means to shape the impact of authority on their working lives.

The ability of groups within organisations to frustrate the aims of those with authority has led to explorations of the bases from which power is exercised. Etzioni (1969) identified coercion, remuneration and normative ideas as means of enforcing power. The possession of knowledge, whether in the form of expertise drawn from outside the organisation, or knowledge about the internal workings of the organisation, has been added by subsequent writers (Mintzberg 1976; Bacharach and Lawler 1980) as an important power base, which is of particular relevance to professionals.

If authority is power that is accepted by organisational participants, how is it that the occasion for exerting influence arises? Some scholars have argued that it is an inevitable outcome of the division of labour in work organisations. Pfeffer (1981) goes so far as to describe power as a structural phenomenon. Others would argue that the main reason for exerting influence is to secure scarce resources (Pettigrew 1973).

To summarise, following Bacharach and Lawler's (1980) suggestion, power has been broken down into a number of concepts: authority that is formally legitimised, and influence that is informally available to all organisational members. A further concept has been the bases of power, from which enforcement takes place, with knowledge being particularly relevant.

Methodologically the study of power in organisations is difficult. The structure of authority may be fully described in an organisation's documents, but influence is often felt to be illegitimate and its exercise carefully disguised. Pfeffer (1981) suggests that power can be elusive and that a number of indicators should be sought before concluding how power is distributed in an organisation. He proposes power bases, outcomes of decisions, symbols of power, reputation and position in the organisations as possible indicators.

Finally, this part of the chapter turns to the literature on professionals and notes that ideas about power and power relations have formed one strand of enquiry within the literature (MacDonald and Ritzer 1988). Hugman (1991), in particular, reviews ideas on the power of professionals and distinguishes between overt, covert and latent conflict. He suggests that the relationship between professional and client is an arena for power relationships and that any apparent consensus between professionals and clients must be explored rather than accepted at face value. He also signals that communication between professionals and clients can be an avenue for the exercise of power. These suggestions will be used later in the chapter to examine the data gathered in the study.

To summarise, the literature on religious organisations suggested that clergy–church member relationships were likely to be conflictual. The literature on organisational theory warned that power was difficult to study empirically and suggested a distinction between authority and influence and an investigation of the different bases from which power is exercised. The literature on professionals suggested that power relations is one model for studying professional–client relationships.

Conflict avoided: the data on clergy–church member relationships

As was explained at the outset, the data presented here are drawn from a larger organisational study of the social action of the local church. Case studies were conducted in five congregations in an English city, each of which ran a social action project providing a small-scale welfare service for local residents. Running the projects involved a substantial commitment of resources for each congregation and meant that, as membership-based organisations, they were under some pressure. The initial supposition was that examples of conflict would be likely in such churches.

This section briefly describes the five case study congregations and presents data on three topics: first, the way in which clergy and members regarded the three modes of interacting; second, data on overt, covert and latent conflict; third, workplace practices which clergy seemed to be using to minimise conflict. Pseudonyms are used throughout, and some details have been changed to protect the anonymity of the research subjects. The case studies involved semi-structured interviews, informal discussions with participants, participant observation and analysis of documents.

The five congregations represented four different denominations. Three were located in an inner city area and the other two in a prosperous suburb. The three congregations in Underhill are on a road that runs through what was once the industrial heartland of the city. All Saints Anglican Church has about 200 people on its roll, an equal mix of whites, Afro-Caribbeans and Asians. A former church hall houses a community project that serves around forty families, with a playgroup and after-school club. Barton New Testament Church of God is an Afro-Caribbean congregation with affiliation to the New Testament Church of God in the USA. It has 250 members. The congregation bought a former Methodist chapel in the early 1960s, a Victorian building with extensive ancillary rooms. There is a substantial commitment to social action including a nursery, a day centre for Afro-Caribbean elders and a supplementary school. The Christian Centre, Underhill, belongs to the United Reformed Church and has 75 members, one-third of whom are Afro-Caribbean. The building was erected in the early 1970s, at the same time as the estate that surrounds it. As well as the worship area, there is a large ancillary hall and several side rooms. These facilities are used for a day centre for elders that has mainly white clients, although one afternoon a week it attracts mainly Afro-Caribbeans. The final two congregations are in Parktown, an affluent suburb on the edge of the city. Divinity Road United Reformed Church is in the shopping centre in Parktown. Its worship area is an elegant Victorian building, but a substantial extension was built on in the early 1970s. This provides ancillary halls that are widely used by the community, and houses a drop-in centre and a family contact centre. The church has 300 members, all of whom are white. The contact centre provides a place where divorced parents who have been unable to agree access to their children can, subject to a court order, meet their children in a secure and supervised environment. Eastgate Methodists is a short walk from the Parktown shopping centre. It has a large suite of buildings erected in the 1930s when the membership of the church was at its greatest. There are 350 members, who are all white. The extensive ancillary rooms are used on a Wednesday morning for a toddler group that attracts 50 children under the age of four, with their carers.

First, data are presented which attempt to assess the way clergy and members regarded their three modes of interacting: as pastor–client; as worship leader–worshipper and as colleagues engaged in running the congregation. It was apparent in all five churches that members placed a high value on their clergy's role as pastor. In all congregations unprompted comments were received about how clergy had been available to members at times of personal crisis. At All Saints, one member described how the priest had given practical and emotional support as well as religious guidance during a difficult bereavement. Members seemed to agree that this aspect of clergy work should receive a high priority. At Eastgate Methodists, a member compared the present minister unfavourably with his predecessor, because he placed less emphasis on visiting members in their homes. At the Christian Centre, there had been considerable debate when the minister had said that he didn't need a car. Older members had raised the concern that the minister might not be able to reach them 'in an emergency'. In the larger churches, lay people were involved in visiting members who were unwell, but clergy recognised that most members did not regard a visit from another member as being as valuable as a visit from themselves.

A high value was also placed on clergy's role in leading worship. Clergy saw this role as the place where their theological and ministerial training was most significant. Church members took a strong interest in the quality of the worship. Favourable comments were made about clergy whose preaching was seen as stimulating. Of particular interest were the differences in the ritual of communion. For example, at All Saints, the celebration of communion emphasised the dependence of the members on the priest. At the Christian Centre, the emphasis was on equality between all participants. These rituals could be interpreted as symbolic of the organisational relationships between clergy and members in the different congregations (Cameron 1996).

Finally, the role of clergy as colleagues of church members was assessed. Clergy who were competent organisational leaders and administrators were highly valued by the core activist members (Fichter 1953), although this role seemed to go largely unnoticed by the majority of members. Clergy seemed highly ambivalent towards this role. On the one hand, they saw it as entirely secular and a distraction from their more sacred duties. On the other hand, they recognised that they could not undertake the work of the church single handed and that time spent on the processes of the organisation was a necessity. Only one of the clergy had had any formal training on organisational issues and that had been instigated on his own initiative in response to the complexities of running a social action project.

Of the three modes of interaction between clergy and church members, the first two seem to be highly valued by both clergy and members and to draw upon the specialist religious knowledge of clergy. The third, colleague relationship, seems to be valued only by core activist members and to be viewed ambivalently by clergy.

The second set of data presents the results of the search for conflict in clergy–member relationships. In all the case study congregations, it was clear that both clergy and members recognised the presence of sensitive issues which had the potential to provoke conflict. Only two examples of overt conflict were presented, and both concerned disagreements over the style and content of worship. When the present priest had arrived at All Saints, he sought to change the style of worship from the purely traditional practices of the past. This resulted in friction with the organist, who eventually resigned and left the church. At Eastgate Methodists there had been disagreement in church meetings about the inclusion of modern hymns and drama in family services. Some members made a point of avoiding services that they knew would contain those elements.

Apart from these two examples, all the references made to conflict referred to issues that were known to be controversial but had not resulted in open disagreement, or issues that were well known to be a source of tension and so rarely dealt with overtly. At All Saints, some of the members resented the rather autocratic way in which the priest behaved. He consulted widely, but it was felt that ultimately he made all the key decisions. Several members mentioned this issue to the researcher but it was clear that they did not want it to become a matter of conflict because of their admiration for the way in which the priest had prevented the church from being closed. Brante (1988) speaks of the 'myth of the hero' as being a feature of some professionals' images, and this seemed to be the case in this church. At Barton New Testament Church of God, all key decisions were checked informally with the pastor. He was seen as the final arbiter where differences of opinion arose. Authority was clearly delegated to officers and committees within the church, but that authority was seen to come from the pastor. Open conflict was avoided by informal consultations with him. The minister at the Christian Centre was quite clear that his role included avoiding open conflict. He used the following analogy to describe his role:

> It's like crossing the graveyard in the dark. The first time you do it, you trip over all the gravestones, but you soon learn and can make your way without bumping into difficulties. Now, I kick myself if I don't spot difficulties coming.

He had sensed a developing tension between older members, who wished to control the workings of the day centre, and the organiser, who wanted reasonable autonomy in day-to-day operations. The minister reorganised the committee structure of the church to create a committee that acted as a buffer between the day centre and the decision-making committees of the church. At both the Christian Centre and Divinity Road churches there was a stress on all members being involved in decision making. Nevertheless, the clergy were expected to chair key committees, which gave them an opportunity to shape agendas and control the way difficult issues were discussed. A member at Divinity Road observed: 'Although we all have a vote, there are some older members who won't vote until they know what the minister thinks.' The tensions between traditional and modern worship at Eastgate Methodists have already been mentioned. Although not universally the case, older members tended to be more traditional, and younger ones more modern in their preferences. The church had decided to employ a lay worker on a two-year contract to work with young people in the church. He was seen as carrying the modernising agenda within the church, enabling the minister to distance himself from the resulting tensions.

Contrary to expectations raised by the literature, there seemed to be few open conflicts between clergy and members in the congregations studied. What latent conflicts there were, seemed to be recognised and a variety of tactics employed to prevent open disagreement.

The final set of data attempts to identify the practices used by clergy to minimise conflict. Five examples can be given. First, as full-time paid workers in these churches, clergy were well placed to retain an overview of what was happening across the organisation. Members and paid lay staff would report to them on their responsibilities and consult them over problems. This meant that clergy usually had at their disposal alternative accounts of situations from those presented by members, who, by virtue of their part-time participation, could not be aware of everything.

Second, although the level of leadership expected from clergy varied between the different denominational polities of these churches, the clergy invariably chaired key committees. This gave them a strong influence over the content and ordering of agendas. If issues proved contentious during a meeting they were also in a position to suggest postponement to a future occasion.

Third, although clergy had decision-making authority in some congregations, they were invariably consulted informally about difficult issues prior to their being raised in more formal arenas. This enabled them to have an early warning of difficulties and enter into negotiations with the relevant members to attempt to achieve a compromise. Baum's (1994) case study shows how the power to postpone discussions as chair, together with informal negotiations outside meetings, can give the appearance of spontaneous consensus.

Fourth, clergy had the opportunity to remind members of their preferred values and expectations through preaching in the context of worship. Several of the sermons observed contained exhortations to members to remember the beliefs and values of the congregation when engaged in its work.

Finally, the ritual of communion was observed to contain powerful reminders of the metaphor of the church as a body, suggesting unity of purpose and action. These five workplace practices were seen as enabling clergy to anticipate conflict and minimise its overt expression. The next part seeks to explain why clergy sought to minimise conflict in their interaction with church members.

Safeguarding professional work?

This part of the chapter starts by suggesting reasons why clergy sought to mini-mise conflict with church members. It returns to the religious organisation and organisational theory literature to seek useful concepts. Finally, it looks at the literature on professionals to suggest three interpretations of clergy behaviour.

Why did clergy seek to minimise conflict? Five reasons emerged from discus-sion with clergy and members. First, open conflict was seen as contrary to the values espoused by the church. Clergy had a key role as worship leader in reinforcing values which emphasised the value of unity. Metaphors such as the body and the family were used to make this point (Conrad 1988). Second, clergy were aware of the value placed by members on their pastoral role and may have felt obliged to be on good terms with all members in case they had problems which would require them to relate to each other as pastor and client. Third, clergy were keenly aware that they needed the active involvement of members to undertake the work of the church. Overt conflict might lead to reduced activism by members, or to their leaving the church, thus directly reducing the resources available to the church. This reasoning means that it was particularly important to keep core members (who did most of the work) happy, if the clergy were to have sufficient time to attend to the pastoral needs of more peripheral members. Fourth, in the United Reformed Church and Methodist churches, clergy were appointed for a fixed term which might not be renewed if they were unpopular with core members. Finally, clergy realised that mem-bers held diverse views and yet wished to worship and work together. Minimis-ing conflict was seen as a realistic strategy for sustaining that type of organisation.

Returning to the literature, it can be seen that the initial expectation from the religious organisation literature, that there would be overt conflict between clergy and members, was not sustained. From the organisational theory litera-ture, the distinction between authority and influence seems helpful. Clergy did have authority within their congregations, but their preferred mode of opera-tion seemed to be through influence, negotiating with members outside of formal decision-making arenas. As for the basis of clergy power, their specialist knowledge was important with regard to their pastoral and worship-leading roles. Their worship-leader role gave them opportunity to emphasise the nor-mative expectations of the church. However, their religious knowledge seemed not to have prepared them for their role as organisational leaders, a role they viewed with some ambivalence.

Having reported on the study and suggested reasons for the workplace prac-tices of clergy in minimising conflict, it is worthwhile turning to the sociology of professions literature to see whether it sheds any light on this study of clergy–member interaction. Hugman (1991) emphasises the implicit sources of power open to professionals and how these structure their relationships with clients. He looks at issues of 'race' and gender, but in the case of clergy, issues of class and education can be added. In this study all five clergy were male, middle-class graduates who were highly articulate; four of the five were white. This must have influenced their power in interactions with members, particularly those who were black, female, working class or who had minimal education. This issue was raised as a concern by the clergy at All Saints and the Christian Centre, who were aware of the additional power it gave them to influence situations.

An important component of professional work is having the time and resources to exercise discretion (Billis 1984). Clergy are in the unusual position of having clients who, by their voluntary labour, also influence the amount of resources they have to undertake their work. If church members undertake the work of their congregations, the clergy have more time to exercise their 'professional' role of pastor, which both they and members regard as having high value and status.

Brante's (1988) work suggests that the reasons given for clergy minimising conflict with members could be classified in three ways. First, a naive or functionalist interpretation, which sees clergy attempts to minimise conflict arising purely from the desire to be on good terms with members in case of a pastoral emergency. Second, a cynical or neo-Weberian interpretation, which sees clergy suppressing conflict so as to maximise member activism, thus releasing more time for their preferred pastoral work. Third, a realist or Marxian view, which sees clergy as having little alternative but to minimise conflict if they are to sustain a membership organisation with members holding diverse opinions. All three of Brante's categories seem to have explanatory value. My assessment is that the balance of evidence in this study favours the neo-Weberian interpretation, which sees clergy as having to minimise conflict in order to secure the resources to sustain the church. Those resources in turn enabled them to undertake their 'professional' roles of pastor and worship leader and minimise their role as organisational leader, which they viewed with ambivalence.

Having looked at possible interpretations of clergy behaviour in minimising conflict with church members, it seems helpful to conclude by looking at how clergy might compare with other professionals. Are there any connections between the experience of clergy and other professionals?

First, this study of clergy draws attention to the presence of professionals within the voluntary sector and the fact that, within that sector, they may face particular structural and resource issues. Torstendahl and Burrage (1990: 10) suggest that 'Professionals exist in the form in which society – market or state – finds use for their knowledge.' Like other analysts they ignore the question of whether professionals in the voluntary sector have a distinctive societal role (Brante 1988). Voluntary sector scholars would argue that professionals in the sector are more likely to have a multi-faceted relationship with their clients. As well as being users of services, their clients may also be volunteers in the agency and members of decision-making bodies such as management committees (Harris 1989). This may create particular problems in maintaining the boundaries of professional work.

Second, the welfare reforms of the 1980s and 1990s have increased the number of professionals who would also regard themselves as organisational leaders, and who stretch scarce resources in order to retain space within which to exercise discretion. Ideas about the relative status of client focused and organisationally focused work may have relevance in these settings, as may the notion that active engagement with their organisational role may be necessary if professionals are to sustain the resources with which to carry out their professional role. Workplace practices may need to be developed accordingly.

Finally, clergy can be seen as examples of professionals whose social status is in question. The fortunes of professions may rise and wane. The enterprise culture can be seen as a further contribution to the extensive secularisation of English society (Davie 1994). This means that the religious knowledge which forms the basis of clergy professional status is increasingly regarded as private rather than public knowledge. Furniss has argued:

> According to secular standards, religion does not qualify as public truth (as medical science or legal knowledge do) but only as private belief . . . Yielding to these secular expectations, pastoral care becomes a distinct profession in form but not in content.
>
> (Furniss 1994: 133)

Summary and conclusions

This chapter has explored the relationship between clergy and church members as a way of understanding the workplace practices used by clergy to construct their professional identity. Three modes of interaction between clergy and church members were identified: pastor relating to client, worship leader relating to worshipper and organisational leader relating to colleague. The literature on clergy–lay relations created the expectation that these relationships would be openly conflictual. Organisational literature drew a distinction between authority as the legitimate exercise of power, and influence as informal power available to all organisational participants. The literature on professionals suggested that there is a power differential between professional and client and that this might result in overt, covert or latent conflict. Data were presented from five case study congregations. The pastor–client and worship leader–worshipper relationships were highly valued by both clergy and church members. The organisational leader–colleague relationship was valued only by the core church members involved in running the church and was viewed ambivalently by the clergy themselves. Contrary to expectations, these relationships showed little overt conflict. Each congregation had issues which had the latent potential to create conflict but covert means were used to manage these issues. Data were also presented on the workplace practices used by clergy to minimise conflict. It was argued that clergy use influence rather than their authority to resolve conflict. The power differential of the professional relationship was increased by differences of race, gender, class and education.

In conclusion, I want to argue that although clergy may now seem on the margins of UK professional activity, this study has some relevance to the place of professionals in an enterprise culture. The valuing of the market as a model for society, which became prominent in the 1980s, has had a number of consequences that impact on professional work.

First, the reform of the welfare state along market lines has made voluntary sector organisations attractive as an alternative source of supply of welfare services to the state. There has been increasing delegation of service provision to professionals employed by the voluntary sector (Bagilhole 1996), raising questions about the distinctive challenges of working in this sector. Second, even for those members of the caring professions still working within the public sector, there has been a blurring of the boundaries between the roles of professional practitioner and organisational leader. A balance between these two roles has increasingly to be negotiated if room for professional discretion is to be maintained (Ferlie *et al.* 1996). Finally, a culture which values 'enterprise' has led to challenges to the expertise of a number of professional groups, for example teachers, raising questions about how claims to professional status are sustained when the knowledge base of the profession is under attack (Pollitt 1993).

These three points of comparison between the clergy studied here and the more general fate of professional work in an enterprise culture mean that the working practices of clergy may repay a more detailed examination.

References

Abercrombie, C.L. (1977) *The Military Chaplain*, Beverly Hills, CA: Sage.

Bacharach, S.B. and Lawler, E.J. (1980) *Power and Politics in Organizations*, San Francisco: Jossey-Bass.

Bagilhole, B. (1996) 'Tea and sympathy or teetering on social work? An investigation of the blurring of the boundaries between voluntary and professional care', *Social Policy and Administration* 30(3): 189–205.

Baum, H.S. (1994) 'Community and consensus: reality and fantasy in planning', *Journal of Planning Education and Research* 13(4): 251–62.

Beckford, J.A. (1975) 'Religious organization: a trend report and bibliography', *Current Sociology* 21(2): 1–170.

Billis, D. (1984) *Welfare Bureaucracies*, London: Heinemann.

Blair, J. and Sharpe, R. (eds) (1992) *Pastoral Care before the Parish*, Leicester: Leicester University Press.

Bradbury, N. (1989) *City of God? Pastoral Care in the Inner City*, London: SPCK.

Brante, T. (1988) 'Sociological approaches to the professions', *Acta Sociologica* 31(2): 119–42.

Burrell, G. and Morgan, G. (1979) *Sociological Paradigms and Organizational Analysis*, London: Heinemann Educational Books.

Cameron, H. (1996) 'Culture theory and the local church: Interpreting the organisational significance of worship', Centre for Voluntary Organisation, London School of Economics, paper given at ARNOVA Conference, 1996.

Conrad, C. (1988) 'Identity, structure and communicative action in church decision-making', *Journal for the Scientific Study of Religion* 27(3): 345–61.

Crompton, R. (1990) 'Professions in the current context', *Work, Employment and Society* 4 (Special issue): 147–66.

Crozier, M. (1964) *The Bureaucratic Phenomenon*, Chicago: University of Chicago Press.

Cyert, R.M. and March, J.G. (1963) *A Behavioural Theory of the Firm*, New York: Prentice-Hall.

Dahl, R. (1957) 'The concept of power', *Behavioural Science* 2(3): 201–15.

Davie, G. (1994) *Religion in Britain since 1945*, Oxford: Blackwell.

Dempsey, K.C. (1969) 'Conflict in minister/lay relations', *Sociological Yearbook of Religion in Britain* 2: 58–74.

—— (1983) *Conflict and Decline: Minister–Lay Relations in a Methodist Community*, Sydney, Australia: Methuen.

Donaldson, L. (1995) *American Anti-Management Theories of Organization: A Critique of Paradigm Proliferation*, Cambridge: Cambridge University Press.

Emerson, R.M. (1962) 'Power dependence relations', *American Sociological Review* 27(1): 31–40.

Etzioni, A. (ed.) (1969) *A Sociological Reader in Complex Organizations*, New York: Holt Reinhart and Winston.

Ferlie, E., Ashburner, L., Fitzgerald, L. and Pettigrew, A. (1996) *The New Public Management in Action*, Oxford: Oxford University Press.

Fichter, J.F. (1953) 'The marginal Catholic: an institutional approach', *Social Forces* 32(1): 167–73.

Foskett, J. and Lyall, D. (1988) *Helping the Helpers: Supervision and Pastoral Care*, London: SPCK.

Francis, L.J. (1996) *Church Watch – Christianity in the Countryside*, London: SPCK.

Furniss, G.M. (1994) *The Social Context of Pastoral Care*, Louisville, KY: Westminster John Knox Press.

Harris, M. (1989) 'The governing body role: problems and perceptions in implementation', *Nonprofit and Voluntary Sector Quarterly* 18(4): 317–34.

Harrison, P.M. (1959) *Authority and Power in the Free Church Tradition*, Princeton, NJ: Princeton University Press.

Herman, N.J. (1984) 'Conflict in the Church: a social network analysis of an Anglican congregation', *Journal for the Scientific Study of Religion* 23(1): 60–74.

Hospital Chaplaincies Council (1987) *A Handbook on Hospital Chaplaincy*, London: General Synod of the Church of England.

Hugman, R. (1991) *Power in the Caring Professions*, London: Macmillan.

Jacobs, M. (ed.) (1987) *Faith or Fear? A Reader in Pastoral Care and Counselling*, London: Darton, Longman and Todd.

Jarvis, P. (1975) 'The parish ministry as a semi-profession', *Sociological Review* 23(4): 911–22.

—— (1976) 'The ministry/laity relationship', *Sociological Analysis* 37(1): 74–80.

Jeavons, T.H. (1994) *When the Bottom Line is Faithfulness: Management of Christian Service Organizations*, Indianapolis: Indiana University Press.

Leech, K. (1990) *Care and Conflict: Leaves from a Pastoral Notebook*, London: Darton, Longman and Todd.

MacDonald, K. and Ritzer, G. (1988) 'The sociology of the professions – dead or alive?', *Work and Occupations* 15(3): 251–72.

Michels, R. (1949) *Political Parties*, New York: Free Press.

Mintzberg, H. (1976) 'The structure of unstructured decision processes', *Administrative Science Quarterly* 21(2): 246–75.

Nelson, J. (ed.) (1996) *Management and Ministry: Appreciating Contemporary Issues*, Norwich: Canterbury Press.

Pettigrew, A.M. (1973) *The Politics of Organizational Decision-Making*, Oxford: Blackwells.

Pfeffer, J. (1981) *Power in Organizations*, Marshfield, MA: Pitman.

Pollitt, C. (1993) *Managerialism and the Public Services: Cuts or Cultural Change in the 1990s?* Oxford: Blackwell.

Prison Service Chaplaincy (1984) *The Prison Service Chaplaincy Handbook*, London: Prison Service Chaplaincy.

Rudge, P.F. (1968) *Ministry and Management: The Study of Ecclesiastical Administration*, London: Tavistock.

Spencer, C. (1995) 'The clergy in secular society', in P.G. Forster (ed.) *Contemporary Mainstream Religion: Studies from Humberside and Lincolnshire*, Aldershot: Avebury, pp. 46–77.

Taylor, M.H. (1983) *Learning to Care: Reflections on Pastoral Practice*, London: SPCK.

Torstendahl, R. and Burrage, M. (eds) (1990) *The Formation of Professions*, London: Sage.

Weber, M. (1947) *The Theory of Social and Economic Organization*, London: Oxford University Press.

Wright, F. (1980) *The Pastoral Nature of the Ministry*, London: SCM.

Part III

Professionalism and new managerialism

7 The retreat from professionalism

From social worker to care manager

Mark Lymbery

Introduction

The purpose of this chapter is to examine the implications of the change from social worker to care manager following the implementation of the new community care policies in 1993. In particular, it will address the way this has altered the nature of the relationship between the social worker[1] and the service user. Particular emphasis will be placed on the shift of perspective implied by the changing terminology which is applied to those people who use social services, namely from 'client' in traditional forms of social work discourse to 'consumer' under the influence of market philosophies. The chapter will also consider the extent to which the 'new managerialism' (Pollitt 1993) has affected the context within which social workers operate, and further constrained their autonomy.

The chapter critically analyses a range of literature in order to identify themes that can illuminate the changing nature of social work practice in community care. Particular consideration is given to the way this affects the workplace practices of social workers, specifically the boundaries and interactions between social workers and service users on the one hand, and on the other, social workers and the organisations within which they work. The chapter will argue that the implementation of community care has signalled a substantial setback for the 'professional project' (Larson 1977; Witz 1992) of social work, and has heralded increased managerial control over practice. The pivotal position of social workers in the management of the community care quasi-market (Bartlett and Le Grand 1993) will be addressed, and the consequences of this for the nature of social work practice highlighted. The chapter will conclude by arguing that the general thrust of the changes do not necessarily signal the demise of social work in community care, and will identify a number of factors which could contribute to social workers being able successfully to retain some level of control over their practice.

Characteristics and tasks of social work

In order to assess the extent to which social work practice has been affected by the introduction of care management, it is necessary to establish a view of those characteristics and tasks that have traditionally been held to comprise its nature. To accomplish this, reference is made to a number of 'classic' social work texts, many of which are over twenty years old. Although this endeavour is complicated by the contested nature of definitions of social work, common themes do emerge. For example, the relationship between the social worker and the 'client'[2] has long been held to be central (Biestek 1992). As Shaw (1974: xiii) puts it, 'social work . . . is about understanding the individual'. Even while broadening the definition of social work to include a range of indirect tasks under the general heading of social care planning, the Barclay Report argued that these would still take place within the framework of this relationship (Barclay Report 1982: para. 1.23). Much of social work practice has therefore been focused on the interaction between social worker and 'client'. This appears to be true whether social work is defined in terms of casework (Biestek 1992), the combined tasks of linking people to resources while helping them gain insight into their problems (Brown and Payne 1990), a combination of casework, service provision and relief (Rees 1978), or as a combination of direct and indirect tasks (Barclay Report 1982). These definitions are united by the belief that social work should legitimately address both the internal and external circumstances of service users (Butrym 1976), with a particular emphasis on the interaction between the service user and her/his wider social environment.

This idea has been further explored by both Butrym (1976) and England (1986), who argue that the key role of the social worker is to enable the 'client' to draw upon a range of both internal, social and material resources that will enable her/him to confront her/his difficulties. In their view, the social worker must assess the nature of the tasks confronting the 'client', make a judgement about her/his capacity to cope and the internal or external resources available to her/him, and decide the most appropriate ways to seek to resolve the 'client's' problems. It is argued that this professional judgement has always represented the core of social work, and that the social worker's task can therefore never be one of providing a uniform response to differentiated individual need (England 1986). In such circumstances, England argues, social workers would abandon their social work role and become merely 'agents of a bureaucracy' (ibid.: 15). Butrym has identified a range of factors which militate against the effective practice of social work, citing excessive caseloads, poor preparation for the tasks required and the problems to be confronted, and inadequate supervision and guidance. In common with England, she has argued that in such circumstances social work would turn into 'routine administration . . . a form of residual social service', and would therefore no longer be social work (Butrym 1976: 9).

It should not be assumed that all forms of practice have been considered to be of equal merit within the social work world. Research has indicated that direct casework was seen as the most prestigious form of activity, with indirect tasks assuming much less importance (Rees 1978). Social work with children and families has been perceived as offering most opportunity to engage in high status casework activity, due to the fact that social work with adults has had a greater focus on the indirect tasks concerned with the arrangement of services (ibid.).

This was as true in the 1950s and 1960s, where such services were carried out in welfare departments (Younghusband 1978), as it was in the social services departments (SSDs) created following the Seebohm Report (1963; see DHSS 1978). As more recent writing makes clear, a similar perspective is still current (Hugman 1994; Litwin 1994).

A core problem for the public legitimacy of social work is the extent to which the expertise of social workers is seen as something unique, specialised or 'professional'. Howe (1986: 117) expresses the central dilemma for social work thus: 'to the onlooker, the practices of social workers do not appear markedly different from those of ordinary social intercourse'. This is particularly true in respect of the indirect tasks that have characterised much social work with adults.

In summary, there is a recognition that the tasks of social work include a combination of direct and indirect work. The professional judgement of the social worker is needed to assess what form of intervention would best support and maintain the coping capacity of the 'client'. Where this judgement is not required, or when the social worker becomes governed by the requirement of providing standardised responses to need, then the tasks performed should no longer be characterised as professional social work. Historically speaking, much work with adults has been so classified, and hence allocated to staff without social work qualifications (Younghusband 1978).

Social work as a profession

Much social work literature uncritically assumes the professional status of social work; however, sociological literature on professions questions the right of social work to be so defined. For example, the 'trait' theorists (Greenwood, cited in Wilding 1982) identified a range of attributes which they argued were characteristic of all professions. Following this analysis it has been argued that since social work does not meet all the cited requirements, it should be categorised as a semi-profession rather than a full profession (Etzioni 1969).

Deploying a different analytical frame of reference, Johnson argued that trait theories do not define the attributes of professions so much as the characteristics of those occupations that have secured a measure of 'occupational control'. Through this control their interpretations of contested events become accepted as accurate and unproblematic (Johnson 1972; see also Wilding 1982). Johnson contended that some occupations (including social work) face external conditions which effectively deny them a full measure of occupational control, the fact that social work is located within the hierarchical structures of local government being one such example (Witz 1992). This perspective has given rise to a theory of bureau professionalism, based on the view that 'neither autonomous professionalism nor purely bureaucratic hierarchies' have emerged from the establishment of unified social services departments (Parry and Parry 1979: 43). In the light of this, social work is not able to claim the same status as the established professions.

However, notwithstanding this structural problem, some writers have argued that occupations such as social work have sought to improve their status and maximise their degree of occupational control (Witz 1992; Macdonald 1995). They use Larson's theory (1977) of the 'professional project', which can be defined as an attempt to advance both the actual and perceived status of an occupation, as a means of understanding the development of numerous occupations, including social work. Within this frame of reference, the determined lobbying which was instrumental in the passage of the Local Authority Social Services Act in 1970 (Hill 1993) can be seen as an attempt by the social work profession to increase its power, status and prestige. One of the ways it sought to accomplish this was to present the social work task in such a way as to emphasise its professional nature and intellectual complexity (Butrym 1976; England 1986). Rather more critically, Howe has argued that another mechanism whereby social work has sought to improve its status and prestige is by a process he terms 'ditching the dirty work', downgrading certain forms of less glamorous activity to focus on those activities with most 'occupational potential' (Howe 1986).

Another theory with particular explanatory potential for social work has been advanced by Jamous and Peloille (1970), who argue that a profession must maintain an equilibrium between its 'technical' and its 'indeterminate' elements. This distinction is implicit in the way social work has been characterised by Butrym (1976) and England (1986). 'Technicality' rests in the rules and procedures which social workers have to follow, while 'indeterminacy' can be located in the aspects of professional judgement that a social worker must exercise. Maintenance of the balance between technicality and indeterminacy is critical for an occupation to be able to claim professional status (Sheppard 1995). It can be argued that social work has not been notably successful in conveying the complexity of its professional judgements, leaving it vulnerable to the adoption of more technical 'solutions' to problems. This point will be explicitly explored in a later section in relation to care management.

Social work is unusual among aspirant professions in that it contains a substantial element of its workforce that has actively sought to develop an antiprofessional stance (Simpkin 1983; Macdonald 1995). A desire to close the social distance between social worker and 'client' is at the root of this perspective, along with an inherent mistrust of the way the relationship between the two is conceptualised. A significant problem for the professional claims of social work is that this approach has been based on an assertion of the failure of the more traditional approaches to social work which were an integral part of the post-war professional project (Simpkin 1983). The core limitation of this perspective is that it appears to deny that social work is an activity for which special skills, knowledge and vocabulary is required (Wilensky 1964: 148). Such a perspective could be, and was, appropriated by elements motivated by ideological opposition to social work to justify further assaults on its autonomy and status. As will be explored later in this chapter, this perspective – the product of the radical Left – gained currency with the radical Right, and has helped to contribute to a realignment of the occupation of social work.

Changes in welfare: managerialism ascendant

This section examines the rise of managerialism in social services departments, and links this development to the hold that New Right thinking has had on welfare policy and practice. However, as indicated above, the perceived crisis in social work was not simply the creation of the New Right. From the late 1960s onwards, the Left argued that social work had failed the working class, by becoming aligned with overt mechanisms of social control and coercion, and by pursuing individualist psychological approaches to problems which were overwhelmingly structural and class based (Jones 1983; Simpkin 1983). In addition, feminist and Black writers argued that services were at best inappropriate and at worst oppressive to women and Black people (see, for example, numerous contributions to Langan and Lee 1989). This powerful critique jolted the confidence of the aspirant social work profession, and had a marked impact on the content and structure of social work education and practice.

However, the New Right critique assumed a greater importance, not least because it carried the imprimatur of central government policy. Even though there was a change of government in 1997, the acceptance of financial limits introduced by the outgoing Conservative government has ensured that the effects of New Right policies are still evident. Although there has been a change of rhetoric around welfare, particularly in the prominence given to combating social exclusion, much of the fabric of welfare introduced by successive Conservative governments remains unchanged. In New Right thinking, welfare is characterised as an economic burden. There are three ways in which this is expressed:

- in the high proportion of the nation's wealth which is paid for direct care services, and the large numbers of people who are employed in welfare services who add nothing to the productivity of the nation as a whole;
- in the belief that welfare services are overloaded with bureaucracy and are fundamentally insensitive to the needs of people who require them;
- most significantly for the social work 'professional project', it is argued that state welfare has been dominated by the interests of welfare professionals rather than those who use the services (Hill 1993; Midwinter 1994; Sheppard 1995).

Under New Right theories, competition and market mechanisms were to be introduced into social care, to force all providers of welfare to become more economical, efficient and effective. As a means to this end, managerial techniques borrowed from the private sector were introduced, with the aim both to use scarce resources more efficiently and to curb the autonomy of welfare professionals (Kelly 1991; Lawson 1993; Sheppard 1995).

The increasing influence of the Audit Commission through the 1980s served notice of the government's intentions in relation to the personal social services. However, the collection of changes that have followed the implementation of the National Health Service and Community Care Act in 1990 has provided the clearest evidence of the government's agenda in policy and practice terms.

It has been argued that the primary purpose of community care was financial (Lewis and Glennerster 1996); given this, it is unsurprising that the government wished to ensure that resources were tightly controlled and managed by the local authorities, who were to become the lead agencies for community care. For example, the government required the creation of social care markets or quasi-markets (Bartlett and Le Grand 1993), with the establishment of systems of care management to operate these markets, where services users should be empowered to exercise their rights as consumers in the market place (Means *et al.* 1994). This is made absolutely clear by a telling paragraph in the practice guidance for care management and assessment which was widely circulated:

> The rationale for this reorganisation is the empowerment of users and carers. Instead of users and carers being subordinate to the wishes of service-providers, the roles will be progressively adjusted. *In this way, users and carers will be enabled to exercise the same power as consumers of other services.* This redressing of the balance of power is the best guarantee of a continuing improvement in the quality of service.
>
> (DoH/SSI 1991: 9, emphasis added)

The position of social services departments as monopoly providers of care services has been fundamentally altered by this approach. It has led directly to a reduction in care services provided by local authorities, particularly those services used primarily by older people, such as residential and domiciliary care, combined with a marked growth in the independent sector provision of such services. While the discipline of compulsory competitive tendering has not been used for social care, the indirect means chosen by the Conservative government – for example, the tight control of local authority finance and expenditure – has led to the same end (Kelly 1991).

Linked to this is the promotion of managerialist philosophies within public services. In this context, managerialism can be defined as the assumption that 'better management will prove an effective solvent to a wide range of social and economic ills' (Pollitt 1993: 1). Underpinning the idea of managerialism in the public sector is the belief that previous forms of 'bureau-professional' organisation did not provide an effective form of management, and that the presumed technical rationality of managerialism is to be preferred to the indeterminate processes which were held to characterise professionally dominated decision making.

While the growth of managerialism is clearly connected to the theories of the New Right (Pollitt 1993; Farnham and Horton 1996), its development into a dominant force within SSDs cannot be explained solely by this, as the analysis does not account for the acceptance of managerialist ideologies within such organisations. Clarke (1998) has contributed to this understanding; he accepts that managerialism stemmed from New Right ideas, but also insists that those who have been instrumental in establishing managerialism have also been pursuing their own interests. In his analysis, the carriers of managerialist ideology are motivated, at least in part, by a desire to enhance their own status and power. This helps to explain why managers have been reported as being markedly more enthusiastic about their roles than social workers (Pahl 1994), and why they have accommodated massive changes in policy with remarkably little dissent (Farnham and Horton 1996). It also indicates the extent to which managerialist ideologies have been able successfully to define the terms of social work practice through a process of 'hegemonic control' (Howe 1986). While the preference for managerialist solutions is ideological, given that their efficacy in the context of social welfare is unproven and remains hotly contested (Sheppard 1995), they have been adopted by most social services departments. There are two reasons for this: first, it is clearly what the Tory government wanted! Second, it is managers who have been able to exert most control over the process of defining and meeting community care objectives.

The central problem of community care has therefore been re-ordered – it is not the attempt to meet the needs of individuals and communities but is, rather, the management of budgets and resources. The new responsibilities for assessment of need and the purchasing of care services have greatly increased budgets, even though there is evidence that they remain inadequate (Neate 1996). SSDs have had to construct their arrangements for care management and assessment in the knowledge that these arrangements are intended to be a key mechanism for the rationing of services (Lewis and Glennerster 1996). Simultaneously, they have had to create plans to enable them to purchase care services (initially for residential and nursing home care, with the expectation that these plans would also encompass other forms of care) in the independent sector.

This has had an impact on social workers' practice in various ways. For example, social workers now have to operate within systems of assessment which appear to rely on lengthy forms and procedures, and detailed eligibility criteria, thereby reducing the social worker's capacity to retain a sense of professional judgement as the basis of practice. Arrangements for purchasing and contracting have introduced skill requirements particularly around financial management which have not commonly been held as central to social work.[3] Budgetary constraints have also increased the level of monitoring of social workers' actions and decisions, with a widespread introduction of various means of rationing expenditure. Examples of these include cash limits for care packages and quotas for admissions to independent sector care; they further affect the capacity of the social worker to make independent judgements in response to need. In summary, therefore, the impact on social workers has been that there are 'firmer limits on their professional discretion with a constant nibbling away at the edges of their professional autonomy' (Jones and Joss 1995: 19).

The care manager: administrator or professional?

A key objective for community care was 'to make proper assessment of need and good case management the cornerstone of high quality care' (DoH 1989: 5). It was implied that the process of 'case management' would help shift the balance of care away from institutional care to care in the service user's home, and that this benefit could be achieved for the 'consumer' at no additional cost. However, the precise meaning of the term 'case management' was undefined. In the context of the USA, from which it was appropriated, case management had been developed as a way of co-ordinating a disparate range of services within a context of patchy service provision and a highly developed private care sector (Phillips 1996; Sturges 1996). Case management in the USA had never been intended to function as the cornerstone of a coherent national policy, but as a means of co-ordinating fragmented services to people and groups who made up a very small part of the overall population. The wider applicability of case management in the UK, in the terms which were promoted in the community care White Paper (DoH 1989), was therefore unproven (Sheppard 1995; Phillips 1996).

Matters were further complicated by the shift in terminology from 'case management' to 'care management' part way through the implementation process (DoH/SSI 1991). The justification for this was that it was the care services that were actually managed rather than the individual as 'case'; in addition, it was argued that the term 'care management' was less stigmatising and more acceptable to 'consumers'. Some writers are unconcerned about this shift (Challis 1994), but others have argued that it has a wider significance in terms of the de-professionalisation of this area of social work. For example, Huxley (1993) contrasted the high levels of evaluation which have accompanied the development of 'case management' in the USA with the lack of such research into 'care management' as applied in the UK. He argued that it would be a relatively easy task for care management to be used to meet the managerialist priorities of reducing expenditure on care services. Hughes (1995) contended that the introduction of care management is more related to the introduction of market structures and principles into welfare than it is about the development of effective responses to need. Deploying a similar line of argument, Hugman (1994) stated that care management represents a move away from professionally defined responses to need towards an approach dominated by the priorities of resource management and rationing, and therefore represents a de-professionalising trend for social work. Sheppard (1995) noted that there appears to be a tendency for care management to be interpreted in ways that emphasise the following of rules and procedures rather than the exercise of professional judgement. He suggests that this has created a fundamental shift in the balance between 'indeterminacy' and 'technicality' in the care management task, thereby weakening the claims of care management to a professional role.

A certain amount of evidence is now emerging to support these views. From the viewpoint of an American academic, Sturges (1996) has outlined the central features of an administrative model of care management, while expressing the fear that this type of model is assuming dominance within British practice. Typical of her concerns are the high caseloads of care managers, the separation of assessment from care management leading to fragmentation of tasks, the low priority given to routine reviewing leading to inadequate monitoring of care packages, the move away from in-depth work to more practical tasks, and the overwhelming focus on eligibility criteria and other bureaucratic means of rationing services. In their research, Lewis and Glennerster (1996) find many of these elements in place, and conclude that there has indeed been a shift from professional to managerial control over practice. However, they do not believe that this should be interpreted as meaning that an administrative model of care management is being adopted, pointing to the generally accepted view that care management is based on the sorts of skills which have always been central to social work. In this they appear to be supporting the contention that social work is the most appropriate background for care managers (Sheppard 1995).

However, as I have argued elsewhere (Lymbery 1998), social workers/care managers are required to function more as 'technical operatives' (Jones and Joss 1995) than with any pretence of autonomous professionalism. The key determinant of good practice is defined as being the ability to follow rules and procedures competently, rather than the ability to make individual professional judgements. Given this, there are clear implications for the form of training that is deemed to be appropriate for care managers. If the care manager is a 'technical operative', then the best form of training for that role would be one which focuses on its core technical aspects. (The current structure of social work training, with an emphasis on notions of 'competence', fulfils that role rather precisely.) It has been argued that the Central Council for Education and Training in Social Work (CCETSW), the regulatory body for social work education and training, has uncritically accepted the New Right agenda for education and training, with the result that managerialist principles have been accepted as the dominant world view within that organisation (Brewster 1992). The definitions of competence that characterise the Diploma in Social Work, therefore, are essentially managerial rather than professional. Jones has argued that this accommodation to 'the demands of an increasingly authoritarian state in which the role and nature of social work are being transformed' (Jones 1996: 209) represents a threat to the continued existence of a social work which is marked by a commitment to social justice and the promotion of human welfare.

Changing boundaries: social work in community care

There are a number of ways in which the changes that this chapter has addressed have an effect on the nature of social work. The purpose of this section is to illuminate some of the most significant of these, with a particular focus on their impact on two specific boundaries within social work. The first is concerned with the shifting identity of social workers in community care, and the conflict between managerialist and professional values. The second is concerned with the way in which changing requirements for social work practice impact upon the nature of the relationship between the social worker and service user.

Whether or not social work should be characterised as a profession, there seems little doubt that active professionalising tendencies have been present within the recent history of social work. The significance of the professional–

managerialist conflict for social work cannot be under-estimated; many social services departments are reviewing the qualification requirements for jobs in community care, and re-defining a number of them in ways which render the possession of a social work qualification unnecessary. This is a move to be regarded with suspicion, since it appears to stem more from financial than practice concerns. If successful, it will further erode the professional claims of social workers within community care. The establishment of a social care market in which a concern with the whole person is replaced by a focus on the collected needs of that person is also significant. The core identity of the social worker is affected by this process, which is further exacerbated by the fragmented pattern of service delivery that is likely to follow. The social worker's role is now to assess needs, commission others to meet those needs, and hence to manage the social care market. This challenges the primacy of the relationship between social worker and 'client'; the further implications of this will be considered below.

The process of de-professionalisation may be reinforced by the dominance of technical considerations in the practice of social workers, particularly their ability to operate detailed rules and procedures. The impact of managerialist ideologies is a major factor here; the more a social worker's practice is directly controlled in this way, the less feasible it is for that worker to claim a professional status. The shift in the technicality–indeterminacy ratio is another key factor, moving social work away from a professional to a more administrative mode of practice. If the de-professionalising tendency is accepted, then there are clear consequences for social work in terms of the education and training which is deemed to be appropriate for the role. As noted in the previous section, managerialist dominance within social services departments has been reflected by a preoccupation with 'competence' within CCETSW. It is certainly possible to envisage training for the new occupation of care manager to be handled through the route of vocational qualifications, an approach that would erase any residual commitment to professionalism.

The boundary issue that is of overriding importance, however, concerns the changing nature of the relationship between social worker and service user. One way of approaching the modified relationship between the two is to look at three different paradigms for describing that relationship.

The traditional view of social work was that the relationship was between a *professional* and *client*; this held sway in traditional social work theory for many years. The terms used convey a clear sense of power differentials and disparities in knowledge, and heighten the sense of social distance between the two.

With the introduction of a social care quasi-market, the social worker/service user paradigm has shifted: the social worker has become a *purchaser* and the service user is conceptualised as a *consumer*. The consumer is, in theory, able to define her/his needs and the most appropriate manner of meeting them, while the purchaser arranges for them to be provided and mediates any disparity between the level of needs identified and the resources available to meet them. Care services become commodified, and the relationship between 'purchaser' and 'consumer' approximates to the commercial.

The use of the terms *social worker* and *service user* (as favoured in this chapter) represent a variation on the traditional view. In this version, 'service user' is consciously a more neutral term, which seeks to avoid some of the negative connotations of the term 'client', while 'social worker' represents a form of modified professionalism, where the skills and knowledge of the social worker are used in active partnership with the service user, rather than as the basis for social distance and separation. Larson (1977) has argued that this process of 're-professionalisation' can enable a profession to change the nature of its relationship with those people who need its services. In practice this means breaking down the barriers between professionals and service users, so that they are enabled to express their needs as they define them, as well as ensuring that they actively understand and participate in the plans which are developed to meet need. It also implies that social workers must accept that they have to work to earn the trust of those with whom they work, and that they can no longer assume that this level of trust will be freely given. Finally, it means that social workers accept some role in attempting to ensure that service users are sufficiently empowered to act as their own advocates (see Larson 1977: 188). Hugman (1991 and 1998) has explored the implications of this for social work, arguing that such a reformulation is essential for the continuance of social work as an activity that is more relevant to the needs of those who use its services.

At present, the preferred third paradigm does not have significant purchase, due in part to the history of social work's connection with its 'clients', but also to a range of other factors that mediate the nature of that relationship. These include a constant round of assessments, and extremely high caseloads – both of which restrict the capacity for imaginative responses to need. The primary consideration for the social services department is arguably less that the quality of such work is high, and more that it is completed within tight timescales. This places social workers in a difficult position, where they can acknowledge that the development of a relationship with the service user is a distinguishing factor of their role, but also that there is insufficient time to develop it in a way which is in accordance with social work values. Therefore, the quality and effectiveness of that relationship is likely to suffer, with consequences both for the quality of the assessment itself, and for the nature and appropriateness of any services which depend on its results. It is instructive to recall Butrym's observation that in such circumstances the activity of the worker 'ceases to be social work' (Butrym 1976: 9).

Howe has developed a theoretical perspective that helps to shed some light on this process. He has argued that in traditional social work theories, there has been an assumption 'that there is a deeper order of reality which lies beneath individual behaviour and social life' (Howe 1996: 81). However, in much contemporary social work practice, the chief concern is not with causation, but with the practical consequences of given sets of circumstances. Howe has defined this as a move away from the 'depth' that characterised much traditional social work literature to a concern with the 'surface', based on eligibility criteria, standard service responses, and a concern with the classification of needs.

He states that 'it is the category into which the client's behaviour or condition fits which increasingly determines the response required' (ibid.: 91). It could be argued that, given this priority, it is unnecessary – even distracting – for a social worker to seek to establish a relationship with the service user. The social worker's purpose is defined more simply, as the need to secure sufficient information on which to make the categorisation, on which a subsequent purchase of services within the market is based. As Howe has observed, such an approach 'is antithetical to depth explanations, professional discretion, creative practice, and tolerance of complexity and uncertainty' (ibid.: 92). The relationship between 'purchaser' and 'consumer' is predominantly commercial; in this frame of reference, there is no expectation – on either side – that the relationship should become the central focus of the encounter between the two.

Causes for optimism? Some concluding observations

It is important to note that only a few years have passed since the implementation of community care legislation; while this chapter outlines a series of trends which have adversely affected the social work 'professional project', it should not be thought that these are inevitable consequences of the change. A number of factors are highlighted within this section which could yet signal the continued primacy of social work within community care generally, and care management more specifically. The first point stems from Davies's perception that 'the key to the profession's identity lies in the recognition that what makes something social work is not *what* is done but *how* it is done' (Davies 1983: 155, emphasis in the original). Social work is therefore defined as much as an orientation to people as it is a collection of roles and tasks. If true, this has implications for the care management role, which would be clearly connected with traditional social work if performed in a way which demonstrates the centrality of social work values (Stevenson 1995). This links to an important truth about social work, that most of its practice is 'invisible' to the outsider, including the social work manager (Pithouse 1998). Therefore, to follow Davies's point, a manager may be able to dictate *what* is or is not accomplished, but has little way of controlling *how* it is done. This can potentially create an area of practice within which the social worker has considerable discretion. From a similar starting point, Lipsky (1980) has developed a theory of 'street level bureaucracy'. He argues that managerial control over human services organisations must always be such that 'street level' practitioners will have considerable licence to re-interpret the formal policies of the agency and thus, in effect, create an entirely different policy climate. Again, according to this theory, managers are able to control the formal aspects of work – in particular, the outputs of the work in terms of documents, reports, etc. – but are unable to control either what the practitioner does in face-to-face contact with a service user or how the practitioner does it. One of the key implications of Lipsky's analysis is the doubt it casts on the efficacy of traditional top–down managerial styles, which characterise the managerialist world of community care and social services departments.

The second point stems from Howe's adaptation of Freidson's analysis of the location of power within professions; Freidson argued that there are three types of member of any profession: practitioners, administrators/managers and teachers/researchers, and that power within the profession is shared between these three types (in Howe 1991). Howe has developed this argument in respect of social work and contended that while the nature of these relations should not be regarded as permanently fixed, most power in current social work can be located with administrators and managers (Howe 1991). It is important to recognise that there are alternative sources of power within social work, which could help to combat the impact of managerialism. It is possible to interpret the (belated) attempt to reclaim care management for social work (Sheppard 1995; Stevenson 1995) as an attempt to alter this balance of power.

The third point engages with a central fallacy underpinning market theories in social care. The market assumptions of self-actualising consumers are patent falsehoods when applied to the people who need social care services, since they assume a level of power that has been stripped from many such people, who are, in effect, social casualties. Social work has always been concerned with such people – indeed, their existence is what first created the formal occupation of social work. The early social workers recognised that there was a need to engage with the whole person within their social world in order to provide a proper response to their need (Jordan 1984). A similar vision should inform contemporary social work practice, alongside the commitment to empowering practice noted in the previous section. In other terms, there is still a pressing need for theories and practices which explore 'depth' as opposed to 'surface' issues (Howe 1996). In this respect, it is encouraging that social work knowledge, skills and values have been identified as remaining central to the care management task (Lewis and Glennerster 1996).

However, despite the acknowledgement of various factors that might help to change the direction of care management practice, I remain pessimistic about the direction of care management. The anti-professional, managerialist agenda appears omnipotent within the modern social services department, while voices of opposition have been muted (Hadley and Clough 1996). Community care in general, and the shift from social work to care management in particular, appears to have heralded a simultaneous retreat from professionalism and growth of managerialism. As Hadley and Clough (1996) have recently discovered, the results do not appear to be in the best interests of anybody, except the self-interests of the managerial elite.

Notes

1 The term 'social worker' is used throughout this chapter in a general sense; where the term 'care manager' is used, this refers to the new role largely occupied by qualified social workers which has developed following the implementation of community care.
2 The term 'service user' is employed neutrally to refer to those people who require social services. The term 'client' is used when referring to traditional constructions of

social work; the term 'consumer' is used where discussing the position of the service user in respect of the social care market.
3 Indeed, employers are now keen to ensure that social workers possess skills in financial and budgetary management at the point of qualification.

References

Barclay Report (1982) *Social Workers: Their Role and Tasks*, London: Bedford Square Press/NCVO.
Bartlett, W. and Le Grand, J. (eds) (1993) *Quasi Markets and Social Policy*, Basingstoke: Macmillan.
Biestek, F. (1992) *The Casework Relationship*, London: Routledge.
Brewster, R. (1992) 'The new class? Managerialism and social work education and training', *Social Work Education* 11(2): 81–93.
Brown, M. and Payne, S. (1990) *Introduction to Social Administration in Britain* (7th edn), London: Unwin Hyman.
Butrym, Z. (1976) *The Nature of Social Work*, London: Macmillan.
Challis, D. (1994) 'Care management', in N. Malin (ed.) *Implementing Community Care*, Buckingham: Open University Press, pp. 59–92.
Clarke, J. (1998) 'Managerialisation and social welfare', in J. Carter (ed.) *Postmodernity and the Fragmentation of Welfare*, London: Routledge, pp. 171–86.
Davies, M. (1983) *The Essential Social Worker*, London: Heinemann Educational.
Department of Health [DoH] (1989) *Caring for People: Community Care in the Next Decade and Beyond*, London: HMSO.
Department of Health and Social Security [DHSS] (1978) *Social Services Teams: The Practitioners' View*, London: HMSO.
Department of Health/Social Services Inspectorate [DoH/SSI] (1991) *Care Management and Assessment: Practitioners' Guide*, London: HMSO.
England, H. (1986) *Social Work as Art*, London: Allen and Unwin.
Etzioni, A. (1969) *The Semi Professions and their Organization*, New York: Free Press.
Farnham, D. and Horton, S. (1996) 'Public service managerialism: a review and evaluation', in D. Farnham and S. Horton (eds) *Managing the New Public Services* (2nd edn), Basingstoke: Macmillan, pp. 259–76.
Hadley, R. and Clough, R. (1996) *Care in Chaos*, London: Cassell.
Hill, M. (1993) *The Welfare State in Britain: A Political History since 1945*, Aldershot: Edward Elgar.
Howe, D. (1986) *Social Workers and their Practice in Welfare Bureaucracies*, Aldershot: Gower.
—— (1991) 'Knowledge, power and the shape of social work practice', in M. Davies (ed.) *The Sociology of Social Work*, London: Routledge, pp. 202–20.
—— (1996) 'Surface and depth in social work practice', in N. Parton (ed.) *Social Theory, Social Change and Social Work*, London: Routledge, pp. 77–97.
Hughes, B. (1995) *Older People and Community Care*, Buckingham: Open University Press.
Hugman, R. (1991) *Power in Caring Professions*, Basingstoke: Macmillan.
—— (1994) 'Social work and case management in the UK: models of professionalism and elderly people', *Ageing and Society* 14(2): 237–53.
—— (1998) *Social Welfare and Social Value*, Basingstoke: Macmillan.
Huxley, P. (1993) 'Case management and care management in community care', *British Journal of Social Work* 23(4): 365–81.
Jamous, H. and Peloille, B. (1970) 'Professions or self perpetuating systems? Changes in the French university hospital system', in J.A. Jackson (ed.) *Professions and Professionalization*, Cambridge: Cambridge University Press, pp. 111–52.
Johnson, T. (1972) *Professions and Power*, London: Macmillan Education.

Jones, C. (1983) *State Social Work and the Working Class*, London: Macmillan.
—— (1996) 'Anti-intellectualism and the peculiarities of British social work education', in N. Parton (ed.) *Social Theory, Social Change and Social Work*, London: Routledge, pp. 190–210.
Jones, S. and Joss, R. (1995) 'Models of professionalism', in M. Yelloly and M. Henkel (eds) *Learning and Teaching in Social Work*, London: Jessica Kingsley, pp. 15–33.
Jordan, B. (1984) *Invitation to Social Work*, Oxford: Martin Robertson.
Kelly, A. (1991) 'The "new" managerialism in the social services', in P. Carter, T. Jeffs and M. Smith (eds) *Social Work and Social Welfare Yearbook 3*, Buckingham: Open University Press, pp. 178–93.
Langan, M. and Lee, P. (eds) (1989) *Radical Social Work Today*, London: Unwin Hyman.
Larson, M.S. (1977) *The Rise of Professionalism: A Sociological Analysis*, Berkeley: University of California Press.
Lawson, R. (1993) 'The new technology of management in the personal social services', in P. Taylor-Gooby and R. Lawson (eds) *Markets and Managers: New Issues in the Delivery of Welfare*, Buckingham: Open University Press, pp. 69–84.
Lewis, J. and Glennerster, H. (1996) *Implementing the New Community Care*, London: Open University Press.
Lipsky, M. (1980) *Street Level Bureaucracy: Dilemmas of the Individual in Public Services*, New York: Russell Sage Foundation.
Litwin, H. (1994) 'The professional standing of social work with elderly persons among social work trainees', *British Journal of Social Work* 24(1): 53–69.
Lymbery, M. (1998) 'Care management and professional autonomy: the impact of community care legislation on social work with older people', *British Journal of Social Work* 28(6): 863–78.
Macdonald, K. (1995) *The Sociology of the Professions*, London: Sage.
Means, R., Hoyes, L., Lart, R. and Taylor, M. (1994) 'QuasiMarkets and community care: towards user empowerment', in W. Bartlett *et al.* (eds) *QuasiMarkets and the Welfare State*, Bristol: Policy Press, pp. 158–83.
Midwinter, E. (1994) *The Development of Social Welfare in Britain*, Buckingham: Open University Press.
Neate, P. (1996) 'Strapped for cash', *Community Care*, 17 August 1996.
Pahl, J. (1994) ' "Like the job – but hate the organisation": social workers and managers in social services', in R. Page and J. Baldock (eds) *Social Policy Review 6*, Canterbury: Social Policy Association, University of Kent, pp. 190–211.
Parry, N. and Parry, J. (1979) 'Social work, professionalism and the state', in N. Parry, M. Rustin and C. Satyamurti (eds) *Social Work, Welfare and the State*, London: Edward Arnold, pp. 21–47.
Phillips, J. (1996) 'Reviewing the literature on care management', in J. Phillips and B. Penhale (eds) *Reviewing Care Management for Older People*, London: Jessica Kingsley, pp. 1–13.
Pithouse, A. (1998) *Social Work: The Social Organisation of an Invisible Trade* (2nd edn), Aldershot: Ashgate.
Pollitt, C. (1993) *Managerialism and the Public Services* (2nd edn), Oxford: Basil Blackwell.
Rees, S. (1978) *Social Work Face to Face*, London: Edward Arnold.
Seebohm Report (1968) *Report of the Committee on Local Authority and Allied Personal Social Services*, London, HMSO.
Shaw, J. (1974) *The Use of Self in Social Work*, London: Routledge and Kegan Paul.
Sheppard, M. (1995) *Care Management and the New Social Work: A Critical Analysis*, London: Whiting and Birch.
Simpkin, M. (1983) *Trapped within Welfare* (2nd edn), London: Macmillan.
Stevenson, O. (1995) 'Care management: does social work have a future?', *Issues in Social Work Education* 15(1): 48–59.

Sturges, P. (1996) 'Care management practice: lessons from the USA', in C. Clark and I. Lapsley (eds) *Planning and Costing Care in the Community*, London: Jessica Kingsley, pp. 33–53.

Wilding, P. (1982) *Professional Power and Social Welfare*, London: Routledge and Kegan Paul.

Wilensky, H. (1964) 'The professionalization of everyone?', *American Journal of Sociology* 70: 137–58.

Witz, A. (1992) *Professions and Patriarchy*, London: Routledge.

Younghusband, E. (1978) *Social Work in Britain: 1950–1975* (Volume 1), London: George Allen and Unwin.

8 Social work, professionalism and the rationality of organisational change

Tim May and Mary Buck

Introduction

This chapter examines public sector organisational change in terms of the nature and distribution of professionalism and power within one social services department (SSD) in southern England. It incorporates evidence gathered during a qualitative study to illustrate the predominant effects of such transformations.

The chapter is structured into five sections. The first section outlines the aims and methods of the study. Second, there is an exploration of the nature of organisational changes; this incorporates a brief discussion of quasi-markets and the attendant cultural shifts considered necessary for their functioning. Third, there is a consideration of these changes in terms of the literature on the relations between professionalism and human service organisations as it applies to social workers. This provides a basis upon which to examine, in the next section on research findings, the effects of the organisational changes on the professionalism of social workers, as well as the consequences they engendered. The final section then examines these accounts in terms of the relations between organisational transformation, power and professionalism.

Aims and methods of study

The research itself focused upon the effects of organisational transformations on workplace identities and practices. It thus sought to discover social workers' perceptions of their changing roles and powers, their understandings of policy changes and how these affected their daily working practices.

The SSD under study was a large county-wide organisation comprising approximately 8,000 staff employed in urban conurbations, smaller towns and rural areas. The research participants themselves were employed in a variety of both specialist and generic teams, for example adult services, child and family, mental health and learning disabilities. Thus the range interviewed encompassed differences in geographical location and specialism. The research incorporated a two-stage design, with data collected from the middle-management layer of the organisation between February and September 1993 and the qualified social worker stratum between June 1995 and February 1996. Twenty of each class of respondent were interviewed at length. In addition, observations of management meetings and social work activities were completed, as was an analysis of documentation in relation to changes in policy and organisational structure.

A combination of methods enabled a cross-check of information and an enhancement of understanding through an examination of a variety of contexts, sources and perspectives (Bryman 1988). The data presented here are derived from the second phase of the research and so concentrates on the social workers' responses. More detailed findings from the initial stage have been presented elsewhere (see May and Landells 1994).

Organisational transformation: quasi-markets and cultural shifts

To understand the relationship between organisational transformation and its effects on the professional identity of social workers, a brief discussion of quasi-markets and the 'cultural shift' thought necessary for their functioning at an operational level is required.

Changes in the socio-political climate have had a major impact on the functioning of organisations in general:

> Dramatic changes in the realms of geopolitics, consumer and financial markets, technology, government policy and legislation, macro-economic stability and capital flows, corporate organizational forms and practices, and the politics of the environment are only some of the factors which continue to transform the world.
>
> (Kiernan quoted in Greenwood and Lachman 1997: 564)

Accompanying these changes in advanced capitalism, charges of inefficiency and ineffectiveness have been levelled against public sector human service organisations; a process enabled by the disintegration of a corporatist consensus (see Hay 1996). More specifically, organisational change was then called for through the introduction of 'quasi-markets'. The accompanying rhetoric of 'consumer choice' would, at first glance, seem to provide an enhancement of autonomy for the professional social worker. After all, if there was to be a greater range of both public and private services from which to make a purchase, the social worker would, as the broker between client and service, have more power and discretion to make an expert choice based on the identification of client need. This proposition necessitates examination in the light of the implementation of the quasi-market system. For this purpose a brief description of their aims, as well as introduction into welfare organisations, is required.

The quasi-market

A clear suspicion on the part of the Right towards public monopolies informed the introduction of quasi-markets. Take, for example, the view of Patrick

Minford, who writes in relation to social services: 'The only remedy is for production to be private and, simultaneously, for any residual monopoly power to be broken up, and protection to be removed; in short, simultaneous privatization and competition' (Minford 1991: 73). The quasi-market system was actually introduced as a compromise to those such as Minford who argued that large public sector bureaucracies were unresponsive to client need. Its aim was to provide choice, accompanied by a more efficient use of resources, but not to be directly concerned with profit maximisation (see Le Grand 1990). In the process 'consumers' were not to be the direct purchasers of the services but, in the case of social services, represented by 'care managers'. The term 'quasi' also arose

> because the purchasing power of consumers under these new arrangements is not expressed in terms of cash, but in the form of an ear-marked sum which can only be used for the purchase of a particular service (e.g. the budgets of fund-holding GPs).
>
> (Butcher 1995: 116)

The initial phase of Community Care thus heralded the transposition of a market system of purchasing and providing onto previous service-delivery style SSDs.

The main focus of the White Paper on Community Care (Department of Health 1989) concerned the need for local authorities to develop their lead agency role through the skills of enabling, rather than via direct service delivery. Thus the responsibility of the local authority was to create a market in social care through maximising the service delivery role of both the voluntary and private sectors (Means and Smith 1994). Monopolistic public provision was to be provided alongside private and voluntary sector provision, with the enhancement of the latter being afforded through the ring-fencing of budgets (85 per cent of the social security transfer to local authorities was to be spent in the private and voluntary sectors – see Lewis and Glennerster 1996: ch. 1).

In the process a new ethos was introduced into social services via a separation between purchasers and providers of services. This was accompanied by organisational restructuring and alterations in job specifications. Although there was national variability in the types of structure adopted by SSDs, the overall ethos moved from being providers to designers, organisers and purchasers of services (Pilgrim 1993). SSDs were charged with developing a market in social care and subsequently to 'regulate that market through contracts and service agreements' (Means and Smith 1994: 120). They were also expected to identify gaps in provision and to stimulate the filling of these gaps. In order for this to proceed, the Department of Health pointed out that contracting out services would require 'an improvement in information gathering systems and a more vigorous approach to management which is likely to require a clear distinction to be made between the purchasing and providing functions within a local authority' (quoted in Means and Smith 1994: 126). Furthermore, the White Paper stated that the assessment of need, and the purchasing of services to meet such need, would have to be distinguished from direct service provision and that this separation should be reflected at *all levels* in the organisation. The Department of Health then commissioned Price Waterhouse to identify approaches to developing the purchaser–provider split.

The SSD under study had made a decision to follow the third of three models identified by Price Waterhouse. This was:

> Separation of purchaser/commissioner and provider functions at the local level. This model involves a series of separate purchaser/commissioner and provider teams operating under a combined management structure at the areas level . . . Care management teams would take new referrals, assess need and put together packages of care, taking account of resource limitations. They would purchase appropriate care packages from in-house providers or independent suppliers.
>
> (Means and Smith 1994: 127)

In considering the overall catalyst for such changes on the implementation of Community Care, Lewis and Glennerster note

> that the government's prime concern was to hold public spending and if possible reduce it. That did not feature as such in the guidance, but the need to make the most of the infusion of new money into local authorities' budgets did.
>
> (Lewis and Glennerster 1996: 12)

In addition, of the three 'Es' of the government's Financial Management Initiative – efficiency, effectiveness and economy – it was economy that was consistently 'given priority over "efficiency" and "effectiveness" in the attempt to contain and reduce public spending' (Clarke *et al.* 1994: 226–7).

The overall result was an alteration in job specification in a very short period of time. As noted in the first phase of the research (May and Landells 1994), the potential for the co-operation of employees in these changes was deemed to be dependent upon their acceptance of an accompanying cultural shift in working practices and assumptions.

The cultural shift

The arrival of the quasi-market into the public sector was accompanied by an alteration in public sector management styles, as exemplified in new organisational vocabularies (see Willcocks and Harrow 1992; Farnham and Horton 1993; Pollitt 1993; Taylor-Gooby and Lawson 1993; May 1994). In organisational documents it became common to read of 'performance indicators', 'deliverables', 'targets', 'devolved budgets', 'organisational development teams', 'objectives' and 'evaluation schemes'. This process has been charted with reference to the

National Health Service (Fox 1991), probation service (May 1991a, 1991b) and university sectors (Parker and Jary 1995). The result was a proliferation in planning meetings, consultations and organisational development workshops, during which time objectives, performance indicators and targets were set, budgets drawn and new roles and tasks defined.

Writers on Community Care policy have characterised these changes as inducing a greater overall fragmentation in the delivery of care, alongside a decentralisation in administration, but a centralisation in the control of resources (Walker 1993).[1] The overall aim was

> the replacement of the existing bureaucratic hierarchy with one dedicated to 'process'. Instead of being a comfortable reward for past efforts, management posts and their occupants should be continuously reassessed in terms of fulfilment of targets and achievement of strategic objectives.
> (Langan and Clarke 1994: 79–80)

A shift towards fluid and adaptive organisational structures occurred, alongside the engendering of maximum employee commitment to the goals and practices of the organisation; all of which was accompanied by new procedures and the development of quality standards in order to create what became known as the 'culture of the consumer'. The rationale being that

> the consumer . . . can exert pressure on providers to improve the quality of services . . . Performance indicators monitor the progress and compare the performance of different delivery agencies. League tables enable the users of service to compare the performance of competing delivery agencies.
> (Butcher 1995: 158)

During the first stage of the research Tim Yeo (then Under-Secretary of State with Responsibility for Care in the Community) attended a conference in the area and spelt out the aims of Community Care (9 February 1993). The 'culture of the consumer' was to permeate social services. His message was clear: large public sector bureaucracies had been unresponsive to clients' interests and needs. Government policy was now explicitly designed to make sure that social services 'meet individual needs' and not fit 'individual needs into existing services'. This process, he added, did not allow for the opportunity to embark on 'some huge empire building exercise', but to place 'the interests of clients first and foremost'.

In sum, an alteration in the political economy of organisational functioning was coupled with the introduction of a new culture, the justification for which was underpinned by effective needs provision for clients to be delivered via a quasi-market system. Accompanying this was the rhetoric of greater choice and quality of service, alongside the enhancement of social work skills for the assessment of client need. Yet within a climate of budgetary constraints, there was also the potential for the curtailment of these very factors. Before moving on to the research findings, however, it is first necessary to situate these changes in terms of the literature on professionalism in human service organisations.

Professionalism, human service organisations and social work

The potential of the above changes to enhance the decision-making skills of care managers fits into what is known as the 'trait' approach to professionalism. This holds that professionals have a number of key identifiable traits, one of which is autonomous decision making, underscored by a distinct, theoretical, expert knowledge base (see Greenwood 1957; Etzioni 1969; Witz 1992; Macdonald 1995). Nevertheless, it is commonly held that the autonomy of the professional social worker may be in conflict with administrative systems that possess distinct rationales (Glastonbury *et al.* 1982).

Autonomous decision making, unhindered by pressure from both managers and clients, may well be an ideal closely defended by public sector professionals. In practice, however, it has long been a problematic ideal to attain (Hall 1969; Johnson 1972; Lipsky 1980). As such, it is more accurate to define social workers as 'bureau-professionals':

> Autonomous professionalism was never a serious possibility for social workers, partly because of the drive towards state managerialism, but also because of limited market opportunities. What in fact emerged was a hybrid form of organization for social services which was reflected in the Seebohm report and incorporated in the reform of local government in 1974. This form we have called bureau-professionalism.
>
> (Parry and Parry 1979: 47)

In considering this definition and its applicability to social workers, autonomy may be defined as the ability to make decisions free from either client pressures or an employing organisation (Hall 1969). From this we can say that autonomy will be exhibited in accounts of actions along two distinct dimensions: first, from the client, and second, from the employing organisation (Forsyth and Danisiewicz 1985). Yet the 'bureau' or 'state mediated' professionalism (Johnson 1972) of social workers does not appear to enable them to approximate autonomy in either of these two dimensions. The gaining of autonomy from an accountable, state-held organisation, does not appear to be a realistic prospect. In addition, the practice of social work is directly informed by an ethos which either aims to assist or, in the case of much work with children, protect, the client. The work is thus guided and informed by the needs of the client.

Where close interactions occur between the social work professional and client, the client may be said to co-produce the 'expert' knowledge. A recognition of this induces professional organisations to form 'downstream alliances' with clients so that they can regulate and secure access to this expertise. In turn, this impinges on the professional's control of the knowledge itself and on their subsequent power over clients (Greenwood and Lachman 1997). At the same time there is also the possibility that increased monitoring of professional activities by reflexive institutions, whose aims are to improve strategic effectiveness and operational efficiency, are self-defeating. The gains made in these realms do not necessarily outweigh the loss of power of the expert, around which the organisation is centred. Therefore

> expert power and control is an unstable and contestable outcome of the interaction between social constructions and structural constraints as they respond to the dynamics of economic, technological and cultural changes within advanced capitalist economies.
>
> (Reed 1997: 574)

Given these unstable and con-stable conditions and the nature of social work professionalism, a number of questions are begged. These are: how are traditional roles and forms of organisation changing in the face of new legislation? Are they legitimised as before, or has this process been eroded as a result of new policies? Finally, how are professionals reorganising to cope with changes and what are the processes involved in these transformations? (adapted from Greenwood and Lachman 1997).

Further light can be shed on these questions by focusing upon the accounts of social workers. These can also enable an understanding of how and under what conditions, utilising what resources, such transformations are introduced and managed in everyday practice. This, in turn, permits a consideration of their consequences for the professional status of social workers. It is to these subjects that the chapter now turns.

Perspectives on change from the front-line

As noted above, the SSD under study decided to adopt Price Waterhouse's third model of Community Care implementation. The implementation of this took place through five processes: first, the establishment of 'care management'; second, the setting-up of what became known as the 'Organisational Development Team' (ODTs); third, the drawing up of quality standards by a policy team, which included a process of 'accreditation' for service providers; fourth, the monitoring and evaluation of work performance; and finally, as part of a system of need prioritisation for clients, the introduction of a four-fold classification system.

This final aspect was an important component in altering the focus of social work intervention in terms of meeting the needs of individuals for which the responsibility rested with one person: the care manager. In the process of implementation, management produced policy papers whose colour signified whether they were part of a 'consultative process', or viewed as 'policy': that is, whether they were 'open' to negotiation, or 'fixed' in policy. These were coloured green and white, respectively.

A resulting confusion over the terminology that surrounded the process of organisational transformation led to a 'glossary of definitions' being produced. In this glossary, 'care management' was defined as 'A way of tailoring help to meet individual assessed need by placing the responsibility for co-ordinating and evaluating the services they receive with one person' ('Glossary of definitions' April 1992: 10).

On becoming and practising as a care manager

We asked social workers to reflect upon this new role in terms of their experiences of working at the front-line of the organisation.[2] The following replies were typical of the responses we received: 'I don't see myself as a care manager, I see myself as a social worker. Whenever I write letters I always sign myself as "X, Social Worker", not Care Manager.' Another person related this to changes in organisational structure according to the purchaser–provider split: 'I'm told I'm a purchaser; I resent the term; I also resent the term "care manager" '. When asked why, she replied: 'Because I'm a social worker . . . when they said "you're a care manager", I don't feel it's appropriate because I'm not *managing* care at all' (emphasis in original). Another compared her current situation to past expectations and added: 'I hate the terms "care manager" . . . it sounds like somebody who should be working in Tesco's.'

There appeared to be a disjuncture between occupational self-identification and the formal organisational representation of the role through care management guidelines. In pursuing this during interviews, this person expressed the tension in terms of her interactions with clients:

> you are generally the best person to do the work, because you're the person that's seen the child, done the investigation of the crisis and you're the person that the child's really . . . got a lot of trust in. So the idea of care management, that you do assessment and the care plan and write it up for other people to do the work isn't what happens, and it's a lie really because it's not what goes on.

Here the respondent is clearly identifying with the 'old' role of the social worker, as opposed to the 'new' one of care manager, in terms of the pragmatics of everyday practice. This conflict was manifested in the following exchange about an increase in paperwork that detracted from what it was to be and act as a social worker:

> I do get fed up and I think the paperwork can go hang, the people are more important. And then you get someone coming in and saying 'you haven't done your SS1P and you haven't done your care plan and you haven't done your SS610', you know, and you think *for goodness' sake*.

What you're saying is that you still provide some sort of 'old' social work?

> Yes, yes I do, I go out, I mean I just go out and see the people and talk to the children and get involved with them because that is far more use than just referring them on.

In the following account, a social worker links the role of 'care manager' to general policy issues and their consequences for the de-professionalisation of social work:

> It worries me really because anybody can pick up the phone, I mean I've got colleagues in my office who are unqualified and they can pick up the phone to another professional and say 'I'm so and so's care manager' and obviously the person the other end doesn't know their status and that worries me somewhat. Obviously with the more complex pieces of work, not that my colleagues are . . . unable or what have you, it's just that we're all lumped together and I feel that our qualification as a professional is being undermined by this new care management umbrella.

At the mezzo level, the cultural shift and organisational changes necessitated a transformation epitomised by the SSDs' strategic managers' stated requirements for flexibility, adaptability, commitment and control within the organisation. In terms of social work skills, however, this had a particular effect:

> I feel more de-skilled as each month goes past. The skills that I have is direct work with children and families . . . and I'm really being asked to be a business manager more and more.

These criteria are now considered in terms of the intended 'fit' between the devolving of responsibility for care management and the pursuit of organisational goals. In the implementation of policy the overall purpose was to capture a devolved responsibility for actions within organisational systems and structures which were themselves designed to attain specific goals, and so maximise efficiency and effectiveness.

Devolved responsibility and changing roles and tasks

With regard to changes in structure for the purpose of introducing flexibility, those who were previously called 'social work supervisors' were divided up into either practice supervisors or team managers. The role of the team manager was defined in the following manner:

> To assume the full range of managerial responsibilities to ensure the needs of clients are assessed effectively and that the care of those clients is secured, delivered and maintained in a way which balances the need for

cost effectiveness with care packages most beneficial to clients, within available resources (finance and people).

> ('Establishing care management – Phase 2' 10 March 1993)

The role of the practice supervisor, on the other hand, was to:

> Contribute to professional practice excellence through the provision of casework monitoring, consultation and development.
>
> ('Establishing care management – Phase 2' 10 March 1993)

These alterations in job specification were thought to allow for greater integration between professional and managerial matters, and recall Tim Yeo's call for 'new opportunities for managerial decisions at the sharp end' in health and social service organisations.

In asking about the effects of these changes on working practices, the increase in organisational flexibility and adaptability was not emphasised, but decreases in levels of autonomy were noted, alongside an exacerbation of differences between the ends to which people were working. In the following extract, a social worker compares her current experiences in a team managed according to the new ethos, in relation to her previous appointment:

> I think the newer managers are . . . just better in tune with care management and all the rest of it, but they seem much more on the ball you know, the paperwork has to be, you know, really tight. They are really working to the book, because I suppose I come from a team where things were flexible, you know 'get the people seen' you know, 'catch up on that later'. I think the emphasis has changed and I think a lot of workers have found that quite hard to adjust to.

Another person expressed a similar experience to the above, but in terms of the identity of the team manager in comparison to her own: 'I always felt X [team manager] was one of us, whereas the managers we've got now I feel are up there [points to ceiling] and we're down here [points to floor].' In this context, interviewees spoke of the effects of role changes on organisational communication:

> I think they're [the new team managers] being encouraged to be apart and to get all their information from the practice supervisor as opposed to being a presence . . . it's put a block on communication.

Reported decreases in communication, flexibility and adaptability were compounded by perceptions that social workers were bereft of much of the professional support they had received under the old structure:

> I've very little confidence in consultation or sharing, it's all about 'you will do'. The last example is the cost cutting exercise we've had . . . Senior Management Group [SMG] has seen it as a success because there's been no compulsory redundancies, but it's devastating to us – we've lost a team

manager, we've lost a massive amount of support, we're having to chase around for team managers that are all over the place. They must be run ragged and it makes you quite wary of your own practice 'cos in some cases you need a bit of support now and then and that's not there any more . . . I think for SMG the cost-cutting exercise was seen as an end in itself, but that was a beginning for us . . . all that makes you feel you're not coping with the work any more.

A mental health social worker noted how the new role of practice supervisor could be translated in terms of a new managerial ethos. She then alluded to her own experiences in order to substantiate this observation:

There's a new layer [practice supervisors] and the new layer is personified by X who is business-like in her approach, so the personal support and clinical supervision I felt I benefited by from Y [old supervisor] has been lost.

In the course of applying strategies of performance enhancement through the monitoring and evaluation of work, as well as alterations in job specifications, the organisation was viewed as becoming more formalised. This was regarded as negative in terms of its effects on front-line support systems and its consequences for diverting attention from what were regarded as 'core' elements of practice:

It worries me if I've got lots of visits on a Friday afternoon because I know there's no way I can get the paperwork done till Monday, and then if a crisis happens on Monday, you're looking at Tuesday or Wednesday. So I try to plan my day so that I do all my visits in the morning so that I come back and do all my paperwork in the afternoon. But if you've got more than three or four visits then you're snookered, that's in a day, because you just can't cope with the amount of paperwork you have to do for those visits and the phone calls coming in and crises happening and what have you.

In pursuing this issue during interviews, the relationship between quality and quantity – commonly translated as meeting the needs of a number of clients within the parameters of budgetary constraints – was seen to place a particular onus upon the spheres of discretion in which social workers operated:

We are expected to negotiate [prices] and we are being sent on a negotiating course. It's like going into Marks and Spencer's for something that costs five pounds . . . 'well, I'll give you three!' . . . and of course, what you do, you beat down the price. So, OK, there you are, you're a skilled negotiator, you've been on a course, you've beaten them down. What sort of service are they now offering the clients?

The climate of a 'new realism' was evaluated in terms of its effect on patterns and outcomes of interactions with clients:

I can understand why we've got limited budgets. I mean yes . . . we can't be all things to all people, but it seems to me that if you're setting up procedures which say this is the tack that we should go down, if you know damn well that you're restrained by budgets you're leading people into false aspirations and false hope.

The above account illustrates not only how professional autonomy was increasingly in tension with financial constraints and new procedures for extracting formal accountability, but also how this had consequences for the quality of clients' lives. Indeed, with budgets circumscribed, the type of service a client received depended upon the time in the financial year, rather than the application of social worker expertise to an individual service requirement within given financial parameters: 'It's always hard after Christmas till April, to get money.' Nevertheless, these situations were anticipated by senior management and thought to be alleviated by a system of 'priority categorisation' according to which clients were placed in categories A to D. The following person reflected on this system of categorisation in relation to his recent practices:

We used to sort of manipulate people into a category A position so they can receive a service. A lot of it depends on how you view a category A client. I mean we very much take into account the carer's perspective and the way of looking at it that if you didn't provide respite for this client then the situation would break down and then there wouldn't be a carer and then the client would be a category A. We looked at the thing very broadly to try and get people the services, whereas other districts worked a lot tighter . . . I think that again depends on your team manager.

Some respondents, therefore, felt able to preserve degrees of autonomous working via a manipulation of the system. At the same time, social workers reported having to negotiate for cash for individual cases with their team managers. This process led to unintended consequences in terms of an anticipated component to everyday decision making:

As I say, I've done much more applications to charities and stuff than ever I have done before, because I think nine times out of ten it's not worth bloody asking 'cos you know you won't get it, so let's try another means.

Evaluations of the present situation in terms of the past were routine features of the accounts. Nostalgia for a sphere of discretion was referred to which not only provided social workers with an identity, but a purpose for their occupational activities. The following exchange illustrates this point:

you did sense that you had considerable status in the old days. There were lots of messages around to reinforce that unconsciously. There were bigger offices, you had more space, you were regarded as professional, you could phone up anyone from, er, the police to a solicitor to a GP, and I'd say 'Good afternoon, I'm the social worker for so and so' and you would have the person's attention and you knew that you had some kind of value in society. And now, I just sense that people say 'oh yeah, social worker' and they start looking at their watch and they don't see you as having any real influence, and your professionalism is no longer taken seriously.

Why do you think that they feel that you don't have any real influence now?

Because they seem to sense that your assessments are very constricted by budgets and when you get teams that are forced to stack statutory child protection cases when there is evidence of actual physical abuse and those cases go unallocated because of stacking. I mean your name is mud, really, and I've seen that happen in teams. I've walked into teams with lists of cases unallocated from the previous team meeting and I say 'how old are those lists?' and people say 'three weeks', and I'll look at the blurb on the list and it'll say 'child with non-accidental injury discharged from hospital'.

This points towards a disjuncture between what had been promised by policy and what resulted because of budgetary constraints. Concerns around this issue were epitomised by the following remark:

I think in terms of social work it started to become quite restrictive because initially you could be so creative, do all these wonderful care packages that we were all supposed to be doing, and then suddenly, the reins came in and choice and creativity went out the window.

A fragmentation and questioning of occupational purpose was the result for the following respondent:

You don't talk to your colleagues any more, you communicate through forms. There's a hierarchy that's built up and growing, it feels like there's a massive weight, it's getting harder and harder to get to people, OK, individual departments in here are creating their own boundaries . . . 'this is what we do and what we don't do'. You don't know what the hell they are, so you're having to double guess all the time. You've got agencies out there which are far more governed by grants . . . it's incredibly difficult now to try to tap in and try to refer people on. What's your responsibility then? You just stop your bit and pass it on, it's a minefield, it really is. It's just an absolute mess.

The above accounts are unusual because in the policy process the voices of front-line service delivery personnel are frequently omitted from strategic considerations. Why? Because they are viewed as an impediment to effective policy implementation. However, seen in terms of the situated activities of social work on a daily basis, they are pragmatic responses to difficult and demanding working environments.

Although an expression of loss of autonomy was manifested overall, social workers still reported being able to salvage some spheres of discretion from the 'old' ways of working, while inventing new tactics to circumvent current restrictions. In view of these observations, the final section turns to a theoretical understanding of the consequences of organisational change on working practices and the relations between power, resistance and identity.

Power, professionalism and organisational transformation

The above accounts illustrate that organisational change in the SSD under study had a multiplicity of complex ramifications unforeseen by those who were responsible for implementing the changes. In particular, while devolved budgeting and a purchaser–provider split had clear consequences for working practices and professional boundaries, there were also spheres of discretion in which social workers operated that provided for the persistence of what are regarded as 'old' forms of practice. This was manifested in terms of a concern with the quality of client well-being through frequent contacts and support, to the detriment of a focus upon 'process' as required by new forms of practice. In considering these concerns, writers seeking to understand the de-professionalisation of social work have noted that current changes signify a procedural mentality that constantly alludes to *process* in terms of numbers of persons who go through the system, in contrast to concerns with the quality of the client's *experience* (Dominelli 1996). To this must be added both the speed and nature of the changes. From this point of view, it is not surprising that the Audit Commission referred to managers of the new system as the 'Bolsheviks' of a 'community revolution' (see Harris 1996). After all, it was they who were charged with winning 'the hearts and minds' of staff, implementing policy changes and thereby taking the lead in challenging outdated structures, boundaries and vested interests. Flexibility and adaptability are central to these aims, together with the incorporation of social work staff not only into a new management structure, but a new organisational culture.

In terms of the two dimensions of autonomy (from the client and from the organisation), we find in the above accounts a clear identification with the client. In addition, criticisms of the changes run alongside the attempt to adhere to 'old style' practices within what remain of 'spheres of discretion' (May 1991a). Yet it has been suggested that in terms of professionalism, social workers could never enjoy autonomy from the employing organisation. The question therefore arises: why do respondents allude to past practices in terms of creativity, rather than constraint?

It is not unusual to find, in organisational research, allusions to past working practices as symptomatic of a nostalgia that fosters a sense of value in the face of current discontents: 'The discontents of today . . . find partial but effective consolation in gentle reverie of yesteryear' (Gabriel 1993: 133). This leads to what

Yiannis Gabriel calls the 'nostalgia paradox': people's recollections of a past that is now lost forever. In the above accounts, though, there appears a 'double paradox' because autonomy from the employing organisation was never a realistic prospect for social workers. Despite this, such allusions are clear, as are concerns with de-skilling. What induces this effect and renders current concerns different from those of the past, is the speed and nature of these changes; and this takes place against a background of attacks on the power base of social work professionalism that stem from a number of sources. This, in turn, affects the ability to resist what are perceived to be the more negative consequences of organisational transformation.

Historically, social work sought to construct its professionalism based upon the casework method.[3] This provided for the idea of 'expert' diagnosis for which the practitioner received training. A knowledge base was then developed as a key aspect of the establishment and furtherance of these claims to expertise. However, social work found itself subject to a two-pronged attack to which it was particularly vulnerable. As Shaw (1987: 775) puts it: 'professionals, whilst attending to technological aspects of their work, typically ignore the wider social issues. In this respect they are vulnerable to deskilling and erosion of control over their work.'

The profession was sandwiched between two forms of critique: exogenous and endogenous. First, as we have seen, there have been profound transformations in the purpose and process of organisational functioning stemming from changes in governmental thinking. Second, there arose a series of critiques from within the profession itself. Broadly speaking, these suggested that social workers, through putting to one side the political consequences of their work, functioned as an arm of the state. These were coupled with studies demonstrating that the exercise of their professional discretion led to injustices for clients (for example, see Bean 1976; Corrigan and Leonard 1978; Brake and Bailey 1980; Wilding 1982).

Given the above, a reduction resulted in the 'dispositional power' (May 1998) that social workers can mobilise in defence of their interests. This has been further eroded by those who were once social workers becoming the 'Bolsheviks' of the community revolution. This breaks down simple boundaries between managers and professionals and provides the 'technicians of transformation' (May 1994) with an important cultural tactic in the process of organisational change. Quite simply, operational managers reflect the new order by challenging outdated beliefs in the old by means of, if necessary, allusions to their own past experiences. Speaking of what is in the 'best interests' of the client on the basis of experience at the front line is thereby limited in terms of its ability to affect changes in policy. In addition, by producing new posts (such as the team manager, whose purpose is one of budgetary control with devolution of support for practice being made to the practice supervisor), the form of power employed is seen as productive as well as repressive. New roles and rationales are produced in the process, and with that, the form of power and possibilities for resistance are also transformed:

> What makes power hold good, what makes it accepted, is simply the fact that it doesn't only weigh on us as a force that says no, but that it traverses and produces things, it induces pleasure, forms knowledge, produces discourse.
>
> (Foucault 1980: 119)

These observations do not imply that respondents were engaging in false representations of a bygone era. Instead, these accounts represent narratives that provide not only for occupational identity, but also purpose. These take place in the face of changes whose consequences are seen not only as deleterious to client well-being, but also contradictory in their effects on practice. Therefore they represent the modes through which identity is both organised and unified (Harré 1998).

It is also clear from the accounts that these social workers are not 'capitulated selves' for whom the new culture is a 'totalising culture' that influences all aspects of their identity and practice (Casey 1995). Within remaining spheres of discretion, provided for in the ambiguity of policy and the resultant inability fully to determine the 'how' or actual day-to-day performance of tasks, the narratives constituted a sense of purpose that was recognised to be in tension, if not outright opposition, to administrative edicts. In the above sense, these accounts are symptomatic of episodic power. This is defined as referring to protests, or conflicts over the content of ideas, which may or may not be generally normatively oriented, to what are seen as undue encroachments upon the purpose, nature and conduct of work (May 1998). Thus they are rationales for resistance. These cannot be read as generalised struggles that are informed by interests that span time and place, but may be thought of as fights against power in general. To this extent they too have transformative potential. As Foucault (1989: 81) puts it: 'if the fight is directed against power, then all those on whom power is exercised to their detriment, all who find it intolerable, can begin to struggle on their own terrain and on the basis of their proper activity (or passivity)'.

The overall effect of the implementation of these changes is to re-politicise areas of work that were formerly regarded as being amenable to intervention by supposedly neutral and technical expertise. Social workers are implicated in the reconstitution of objects of political intervention because the means for their solution can never be fully determined by formal transformations in organisational functioning. Because of unintended consequences and resultant conflicts, to be a professional social worker is never fixed, but always in the process of *becoming* (Johnson 1993).

Summary

As movements in power occur at every level in reaction to all aspects of the new policies and processes charted in this chapter, there exists the possibility for unintended consequences at every twist and turn. The changes had the effect of de-professionalising social work, despite the rhetoric of providing for 'managerial decisions at the sharp end'. At the same time, these transformations produced new opportunities and identities for those who were prepared to embrace the new ethos.

These transformations produced specific forms of resistance. These were manifested in accounts of action that served to constitute identities and practices that, in turn, existed at various levels of tension with managerial and governmental intentions. This was enabled through the inability of administrative edicts fully to determine the actual performance of work in what are complex, human service organisations. This is not to say that the introduction of quasi-markets, devolved budgeting and performance measures did not affect working practices, produce conflicts and frustrations and even lead to redundancies. It does, however, suggest that there are limits to what Foucault (1991) has termed the 'appropriation of discourse', or Ritzer (1996) the McDonaldisation of society. Therefore, we say that resistance is the direct result of the exercise of power, while the rationality that informs organisational change may find itself questioned by new sets of practices and rationales that were never envisaged by its technicians of transformation. In the process there is the potential for the development of new forms of identity in social work practice.

Acknowledgements

A version of this chapter originally appeared as 'Power, professionalism and organisational transformation', in *Sociological Research Online* 3(2), http://www.socresonline.org.uk/socresonline/3/2/5.html. Our thanks to the editor and publisher for permission to re-reproduce this article. Also our thanks to Mel Landells for the excellent data collection work she undertook during the first phase of the research.

Notes

1 For a more detailed understanding of the legislation and guidelines see Lewis and Glennerster (1996) and Pilgrim (1993).
2 This group will be defined as 'front-line workers' because they are in daily contact with the people for whom the organisation is meant to serve (see Lipsky 1980; May 1991a).
3 For example, Mary Richmond's book *Social Diagnosis*, originally published in 1917, was reprinted 16 times up to 1964.

References

Bean, P. (1976) *Rehabilitation and Deviance*, London: Routledge and Kegan Paul.
Brake, M. and Bailey, R. (eds) (1980) *Radical Social Work and Practice*, London: Edward Arnold.
Bryman, A. (1988) *Quantity and Quality in Social Research*, London: Unwin Hyman.
Butcher, T. (1995) *Delivering Welfare: The Governance of the Social Services in the 1990s*, Buckingham: Open University Press.

Casey, C. (1995) *Work, Self and Society: After Industrialism*, London: Routledge.

Clarke, J., Cochrane, A. and McLaughlin, E. (eds) (1994) *Managing Social Policy*, London: Sage.

Corrigan, P. and Leonard, P. (1978) *Social Work Practice under Capitalism*, London: Macmillan.

Department of Health (1989) *Caring for People – Community Care in the Next Decade and Beyond*, London: HMSO.

Dominelli, L. (1996) 'Deprofessionalizing social work: anti-oppressive practice, competencies and postmodernism', *British Journal of Social Work* 26: 153–75.

Etzioni, A. (ed.) (1969) *The Semi-Professions and Their Organisation: Teachers, Nurses and Social Workers*, New York: The Free Press.

Farnham, D. and Horton, S. (eds) (1993) *Managing the New Public Services*, London: Macmillan.

Fineman, S. (ed.) (1993) *Emotion in Organizations*, London: Sage.

Foucault, M. (1980) *Power/Knowledge, Selected Interviews and Other Writings 1972–1977*, ed. C. Gordon, Brighton: Harvester Press.

—— (1989) *Foucault Live: Collected Interviews 1961–1984*, ed. E. Lotringer, trans. J. Johnston, New York: Semiotext(e).

—— (1991) 'Questions of method', in G. Burchell, C. Gordon and P. Miller (eds) *The Foucault Effect: Studies in Governmentality*, London: Harvester Wheatsheaf.

Forsyth, P. and Danisiewicz, T. (1985) 'Towards a theory of professionalization', *The Sociology of Work and Occupations* 12(1): 59–76.

Fox, N. (1991) 'Postmodernism, rationality and the evaluation of health care', *Sociological Review* 39(4): 709–44.

Gabriel, Y. (1993) 'Organizational nostalgia – reflection on the 'golden age', in S. Fineman (ed.) *Emotion in Organizations*, London: Sage.

Glastonbury, B., Cooper, D. and Hawkins, P. (1982) *Social Work in Conflict: The Practitioner and the Bureaucrat*, Birmingham: British Association of Social Workers.

Greenwood, E. (1957) 'Attributes of a profession', *Social Work* 2: 45–55.

Greenwood, R. and Lachman, R. (1997) 'Change as an underlying theme in professional service organizations: an introduction', *Organization Studies* 17(4): 563–72.

Hall, R. (1969) *Occupations and the Social Structure*, Englewood Cliffs, NJ: Prentice-Hall.

Harré, R. (1998) *The Singular Self*, London: Sage.

Harris, J. (1996) 'Hard labour in a cold climate: developments in the social work labour process', paper presented to the Department of Applied Social Science, University of Plymouth, Devon.

Hay, C. (1996) *Re-Stating Social and Political Change*, Buckingham: Open University Press.

Johnson, T.J. (1972) *Professions and Power*, London: Macmillan.

Johnson, T. (1993) 'Expertise and the state', in M. Gane and T. Johnson (eds) *Foucault's New Domains*, London: Routledge.

Langan, M. and Clarke, J. (1994) 'Managing in the mixed economy of care', in J. Clarke, A. Cochrane and E. McLaughlin (eds) *Managing Social Policy*, London: Sage.

Le Grand, J. (1990) 'The state of welfare', in J. Hills (ed.) *The State of Welfare: The Welfare State in Britain since 1974*, Oxford: Clarendon Press.

Lewis, J. and Glennerster, H. (1996) *Implementing the New Community Care*, Buckingham: Open University Press.

Lipsky, M. (1980) *Street Level Bureaucracy*, New York: Russell Sage Foundation.

MacDonald, K.M. (1995) *The Sociology of the Professions*, London: Sage.

May, T. (1991a) *Probation: Politics, Policy and Practice*, Buckingham: Open University Press.

—— (1991b) 'Under siege: the probation service in a changing environment', in R. Reiner and M. Cross (eds) *Beyond Law and Order: Criminal Justice Policy and Politics into the 1990s*, London: Macmillan.

—— (1994) 'Transformative power: a study in a human service organisation', *Sociological Review* 42(4): 618–38.

—— (1998) 'Forging the docile body? Power and resistance at work', paper presented at the British Sociological Association Annual Conference, Edinburgh, April.

May, T. and Landells, M. (1994) 'Administrative rationality and the delivery of social services: an organisation in flux', paper delivered to the International Conference on Children, Family Life and Society, University of Plymouth, Devon, July.

Means, R. and Smith, R. (1994) *Community Care: Policy and Practice*, London: Macmillan.

Minford, P. (1991) 'The role of the social services: a view from the new right', in M. Loney, R. Bocock, J. Clarke, A. Cochrane, P. Graham and M. Wilson (eds) *The State or the Market: Politics and Welfare in Contemporary Britain*, 2nd edn, London: Sage.

Parker, M. and Jary, D. (1995) 'The McUniversity: organization, management and academic subjectivity', *Organization* 2(2): 319–38.

Parry, N. and Parry, J. (1979) 'Social work, professionalism and the state', in N. Parry, M. Rustin and C. Satyamurti (eds) *Social Work, Welfare and the State*, London: Edward Arnold.

Pilgrim, D. (1993) 'Anthology: policy', in P. Bornat, C. Pereira, D. Pilgrim and F. Williams (eds) *Community Care: A Reader*, Basingstoke: Macmillan.

Pollitt, C. (1993) *Managerialism and the Public Services: Cuts or Cultural Change in the 1990s?* 2nd edn, Oxford: Basil Blackwell.

Richmond, M. (1917) *Social Diagnosis*, New York: Russell Sage.

Ritzer, G. (1996) 'The McDonaldization thesis: is expansion inevitable?', *International Sociology* 11(3): 291–308.

Taylor-Gooby, P. and Lawson, R. (eds) (1993) *Markets and Managers: New Issues in the Delivery of Welfare*, Buckingham: Open University Press.

Wilding, P. (1982) *Professional Power and Social Welfare*, London: Routledge and Kegan Paul.

Willcocks, L. and Harrow, J. (eds) (1992) *Rediscovering Public Services Management*, London: McGraw-Hill.

Witz, A. (1992) *Professions and Patriarchy*, London: Routledge.

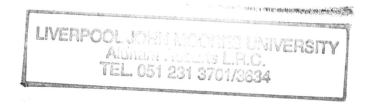

Part IV

Professionalism and credentialism

9 From befriending to punishing

Changing boundaries in the probation service

Tina Eadie

Introduction

PO: So I thought we'd have a look and see . . . how you feel it's going. Did you think that being on probation was going to be like this?

Carol: Um, no, not really.

PO: Did you have any ideas as to what it was going to be like?

Carol: No.

PO: You hadn't thought about it?

Carol: I didn't think it would be like this really . . . I thought it would be more, um, not so, you know what I mean? It's difficult to explain . . . I didn't think it would be so down to earth. I thought it would be more . . . more punishment, do you know what I mean? More harder, like you'd be looked at like you were a piece of shit. Do you know what I mean? Treated like . . . not me and you one-to-one, thought you'd be spoken down to just 'cause you'd done something wrong . . . I thought it would be like a school teacher and a child.

(Edmonds 1996: 36–7)

This conversation between Carol (not her real name), a young woman on a probation order, and her probation officer (PO), a student in training, took place in summer 1996. Asked to share her thoughts about what 'being on probation' might be like, Carol indicated that she expected the order to feel more like a punishment, and equated that punishment with being 'spoken down to', not treated with respect. Historically, although always maintaining a balance between care and control, probation officers have never been regarded as 'agents of punishment'. While the explicit use of the word 'punishment' increased in Home Office documents from the late 1980s onwards (Home Office 1988, 1990a, 1991, 1995a), this chapter argues that there needs to be a tension between this and the way individual probation officers interact with those they supervise. It questions the extent to which Home Office directives and changes in service terminology will transform the nature of probation officer–offender relationships, and considers the impact of this on the professionalism of officers, and of the service as a whole.

The chapter is in four sections: the first outlines the current requirement of the service to combine effective punishment with success in reducing reoffending, and considers the extent to which the relationship this requires between probation officer and offender has changed during the history of the service. The second draws on Freidson's (1994) framework of expertise, credentialism and autonomy to consider changing boundaries in relation to probation officer professionalism. The third explores conflicts arising from different understandings of professionalism, and the fourth addresses future challenges for the service arising from changing boundaries. The chapter concludes that the service still has a way to go in successfully combining a law enforcement role with that of the effective rehabilitation of offenders.

The changing nature of the probation officer–offender relationship

Carol's view, that the order should be a punishment, was reflected in the Home Office's priorities for the service set out in the *Three Year Plan for the Probation Service 1996–1999* (Home Office 1996). The 'Statement of purpose' at the beginning of the Plan stated (Home Office 1996: 1):

> 1.2 The goals of the service are to:
> - reduce crime and supervise offenders effectively;
> - provide high quality information, assessment and related services to the courts and other users;
> - improve value for money and maintain high standards of equity.

The priorities included (Home Office 1996: 8, emphasis added):

> - to ensure that community sentences and supervision after release from custody are effective as *punishments*, through the implementation of the 1995 National Standards and improved enforcement.

Also addressed in the 'Statement of purpose' were values (Home Office 1996: 1):

> 1.3 The service is committed to:
> - treating all people fairly, openly and with respect;
> - challenging attitudes and behaviour which result in crime and cause distress to victims;
> - working at all times to bring out the best in people;
> - reconciling offenders and communities, recognising the obligations of both.

While these had moved some way from the duty of the probation officer enshrined in the Probation of Offenders Act 1907, to 'advise, assist and befriend', they still reflected an essentially humanistic, person-centred approach to work with offenders. There was a certain ambivalence, therefore, between these and an increasing emphasis on punishment.

This ambivalence, currently expressed as combining 'effective punishment with success in reducing reoffending' (Home Office 1998a: 2), requires probation officers to manage the tension between enforcing orders strictly, returning offenders to court for non-compliance if necessary, and, at the same time, building a relationship with them in which their offending, and reasons for it, can be explored and addressed. While this has always been part of the professional task of probation officers, the change in emphasis from a befriending, helping role to one of punishment, reflecting society's increased anger, fear and intolerance of offending, may affect both the way in which probation officers view their role, and the way in which they are perceived by those they supervise.

Reform through the relationship between the probation officer and offender has been a guiding principle throughout the history of the probation service. The Police Court Missionaries of the nineteenth and early twentieth centuries focused their attentions on the reform of the drunk and disorderly, reflecting a particular concern with drunkenness at the time. Theirs was fundamentally a religious philosophy, aimed at 'the saving of souls through divine grace' (McWilliams 1983: 130). They saw their task as influencing magistrates' sentencing decisions by means of persuasion and special pleading (Jarvis 1980). This was gradually overtaken by a more scientific approach: the period from the 1930s to the early 1970s has been called 'the phase of diagnosis' (McWilliams 1986). This reflects the growing professionalism of the service through salaried positions and specific knowledge and skills, acquired through training, 'The gradual movement from the religious, missionary ideal to the scientific, diagnostic ideal, depending, in part, on notions of professionalism, required that probation work should be something for which people were trained to enter rather than called to follow' (McWilliams 1985: 261).

Although the ethos of 'advise, assist and befriend' underpinned the probation officer–offender relationship throughout this period, the relationship also contained an element of control; offenders were released into the care of the probation officer subject to the conditions of their order. The general consensus continued to be that the *rehabilitation* of the offender was the goal, and the relationship a means to that end. The probation officer as 'professional caseworker', having skills in common with social workers, was endorsed in the report of the Morison Committee (Home Office 1962), set up to review the aims of probation. While the report also stressed the regulatory and public protection role of the probation officer, it can be argued that it was the treatment of offenders and a concern with their well-being that was prioritised by practitioners.

The 1960s and 1970s saw the diversification of the service's tasks, including 'welfare' work in prisons, the supervision of parolees on licence from prison, and administration of the community service order. The latter included, for the first time, an explicit punitive element (Pease 1981). At the same time as this expansion, faith in the product – the successful rehabilitation of offenders – was under attack (see Martinson 1974; Brody 1976). Powerful and influential debates concerning probation's role and purpose (see Harris 1977, 1980; Bryant *et al.* 1978; Bottoms and McWilliams 1979; Walker and Beaumont 1981) highlighted the diversity of views surrounding how a clear purpose and direction might be regained. Although the offender remained central in these debates, the probation officer now worked within a framework of policy, no longer being the autonomous practitioner that had for so long been the case (McWilliams 1987: 99). McWilliams (1987) identified three distinct 'schools of thought' emerging in this period – the managerial, the radical and the personalist (ibid.: 105). Briefly, the managerial emphasised the need for the service to be managed as opposed to professionally administered; the radical, often through a 'Marxist analysis' (see Walker and Beaumont 1981), criticised what was regarded as the trend towards greater social control of offenders; and the personalist strove to maintain the humanistic approach within the probation officer–offender relationship. Common to all three in the 1980s was an acknowledgement that the service had moved away from the diagnostic casework model and was, more pragmatically, about providing alternatives to custody, but variations in philosophy and practice did not provide the clarity of purpose sought by the service.

This lack of internal consistency was addressed by the Home Office, which throughout the 1980s began to take increasing interest in the work of the service and to impose its own agenda. The late 1980s witnessed the work of the probation service repackaged as 'Punishment in the community' (Home Office 1988, 1990b), with community sentences no longer 'alternatives' to imprisonment but sentences in their own right. John Patten (then Home Office Minister of State) took a strong line with the service regarding its antipathy towards the word 'punishment', stating: 'The fact is that all probation-based disposals are already in varying degrees forms of punishment . . . It is bizarre to scratch around to find polite euphemisms for what is going on' (Patten 1988: 12).

The punitive element of community orders was to be in the restriction on liberty and in the enforcement of orders, rather than the activities carried out during the order (Home Office 1990b: para. 4.4). The Criminal Justice Act 1991 that followed was the culmination of Home Office initiatives throughout the 1980s to move the probation service centre stage in its criminal justice programme and to ensure that offenders were being supervised rigorously in accordance with the newly introduced *National Standards for the Supervision of Offenders in the Community* (Home Office 1992a, 1995b). The probation service was presented with the challenge of demonstrating to sentencers and the public at large that community sentences contained a penal element as well as a rehabilitative one (Jack 1993). This was made more difficult by the increasingly hostile socio-political climate towards offenders throughout the 1990s – encapsulated in the rhetoric of the Conservative Home Secretary that 'prison works' (Howard 1993) – and the demonisation, albeit in very different ways, of sex offenders and juvenile delinquents (see Worrall 1997: 118–25). Any sentence other than imprisonment was regarded as 'a soft option', putting increased pressure on the service to justify its existence.

Changing boundaries in relation to probation officer professionalism

The question of what impact these changes have had on the professional task of the probation officer depends on the definition of 'professional task'. The work of Freidson (1994) is drawn on here because the three common denominators he suggests are found in professional activities – expertise, credentialism and autonomy – can all be shown to have altered in relation to probation officer–offender interactions in recent years. Assessing the effectiveness of supervision is no longer based on the word of the probation officer supervising the offender – a practice reserved for a time when probation was *assumed* to be a 'good thing' (Harris 1996: 122) – but on scientific and research-based measures which the service has introduced in an attempt to persuade sceptics among sentencers, Home Office officials, and the general public that their 'product' is credible.

Expertise

Until the 1990s, probation officers were trained alongside social workers, developing knowledge and skills in a broad range of areas. Officers were encouraged to develop expertise in any areas of the work that particularly interested them, which might include substance misuse, sexual offending, groupwork, family therapy, and counselling. How an officer worked with offenders on his or her caseload was largely a matter of that officer's professional judgement as to what methods would best contribute to an individual's rehabilitation and thereby prevent re-offending. While the assessment task, particularly risk assessment, remains central to the work, the range of interventions undertaken directly by probation officers has contracted, with expertise being drawn on from organisations outside of the service. These changes have been driven by political, financial and research considerations.

The political climate of the 1980s and early 1990s was heavily influenced by growing managerialism and government attempts to apply free market principles to public services (see Statham and Whitehead 1992; Raine and Willson 1993; Oldfield 1994; Beaumont 1995). While it has been argued that the service was less affected than some by the restructuring experienced in the fields of health, education and the public utilities throughout this period (Harris 1996), the impact of the Home Office's attentions towards the service focused on its *modus operandi* and, implicitly, its professional base. A series of financial audits and inspections (Audit Commission 1989, 1991) forced services to address both internal and external accountability and 'value for money'. A diminishing budget has resulted in a move from the traditional one-to-one approach to working with offenders towards a case management system, whereby responsibility for the assessment and management of cases is separated from the direct provision of services. These might be provided internally by other probation staff (for example groupwork with offenders), or delivered through contract by other agencies (for example drug and alcohol services).

Service provision within the probation service has been dominated by a renewed optimism in the rehabilitative agenda which has arisen from convincing
research evidence into what methods actually do work to prevent re-offending.
The Reasoning and Rehabilitation programme developed in Canada (Ross and
Fabiano 1985; Ross *et al.* 1988) was based on findings which demonstrated that
successful programmes concentrated on offenders' *thinking*. Promising results
from programmes in the UK and research suggesting that less structured approaches such as casework or individual or group counselling are less successful[1]
has resulted in services moving en masse to cognitive-behavioural programmes.
These insist on programme integrity – an assurance that all programmes are
being run according to a clear format. It is acknowledged that this demands the
partial surrender of professional autonomy (Hollin 1995: 206), resulting in a
further attack on practitioners' professionalism. With measures of effectiveness
being so tightly prescribed within the service, broader gauges of success in reducing recidivism are being increasingly located outside of the service.

The 'contract culture' of the 1990s led to services being required to allocate
5 per cent of their recently cash-limited budgets on developing partnerships
with organisations in the voluntary or private sectors (Home Office 1992b)
offering specific expertise to offenders. Examples are employment schemes,
housing projects and community drug and alcohol teams. While formerly, individual officers might have developed personal contacts in such organisations,
and been regarded as the team 'expert', they are now more likely to be sec-
onded to work in those organisations, developing expertise *outside* of the
service.

In relation to expertise therefore, a key change is that the probation officer
or case manager will identify help or treatment appropriate to addressing
criminogenic (directly related to an individual's offending behaviour) and non-
criminogenic need; they will link that person to it rather than provide it. Expertise in assessment will therefore remain, but some probation officers might
undertake an enforcement role only, needing technical as opposed to professional expertise – Ward's 'utilitarian functionary in the justice system' (Ward
1996: 114). Officers involved in running groupwork programmes will develop
expertise in a specific method – that of cognitive-behavioural groupwork – but
will be unable to deviate from this. The impact of all of this on professionalism
will be returned to later.

Credentialism

Freidson's second common denominator of professionalism is credentialism –
evidence of an individual's competence through some form of entry qualification. Entry to the probation service in the UK has, since the Central Council for
Education and Training in Social Work (CCETSW) took over responsibility
for the training of probation officers in 1971, required a Certificate of Qualification in Social Work (CQSW) or, more recently, a Diploma in Social Work
(DipSW). The latter qualification aimed to prepare students for 'employment as

professionally qualified social workers and probation officers and [lay] the foundation for their continuing professional development' (CCETSW 1995: 8) by ensuring that students demonstrate the knowledge, skills and values required for competent practice. In an onslaught which has been described as state-led *de-professionalisation* (Aldridge 1999), the requirement in the 1984 Probation Rules that probation officers had a social work qualification was dispensed with in November 1996.

That the attack on probation training was driven by a political agenda which required a tougher image for the service (see Aldridge and Eadie 1997) is hard to dispute. Despite the 1994 Home Office review of probation officer recruitment and training reporting that 'most people within the Probation Service argued that a social work qualification was appropriate to probation work' (Dews and Watts 1994: 2), a spirited defence by social work academics (Williams 1994; Ford and Sleeman 1996; Ward 1996), and the fact that only 11 out of the 493 responses to the consultation exercise fully endorsed the proposed change (*THES* 1995), the report concluded:

> Although the present system clearly has a number of strengths we have concluded that the shortcomings are too important to be ignored and some fundamental changes are required . . . We think the requirement in the Probation Rules that all probation officers . . . should have a CQSW/DipSW qualification is inappropriate and *we recommend* that it be repealed.
>
> (Dews and Watts 1994: 3)

In its official response to the report (Home Office 1995c), the government proposed direct recruitment into the service with largely 'on-the-job' training to meet core competences set by the Home Office. The proposals rejected the view that professional training should encourage an analytical approach in dealing with offenders and be based in higher education (Willis 1995: 56). In a strongly argued pamphlet written for the Association of University Teachers, Williams (1996) maintained that control of qualifying training had begun to be seen as a way of deterring members of professions from challenging the government's political projects (ibid.: 7), stating that the proposed changes to probation training devalued independent, critical research and showed no appreciation of the concept of reflective practice (ibid.: 8). The government's approach was particularly ironic given that it was taking place at a time when other professions, for example nursing, were moving *into* the universities.

After some considerable delay, a compromise position was announced: the new qualification for probation officers was to be the Diploma in Probation Studies; it was to be service based, but combining a two-year undergraduate degree taught by higher education institutions outside of social work departments with a Community Justice National Vocational Qualification obtained through work-based supervised practice. The relationship between the probation service and higher education was, therefore, not severed entirely, although the separation from social work training had been successfully achieved. It is too soon to say whether and to what extent the change in the training of probation officers will affect their relationships and interaction with those they supervise. The continued contribution of higher education institutions ensures an educative rather than wholly technical approach to the training. The fact that 'values and ethics' appear on the core curriculum gives cause for optimism that trainees will continue to balance the requirement for punishment with that of working in an anti-discriminatory way. Also, while recognising that personal and social factors do not *cause* criminal behaviour, they will be aware that such factors do represent a *constraint* on the exercise of choice and responsibility.

Autonomy

In relation to Freidson's third common denominator of a profession, it can be argued that the autonomy traditionally enjoyed by both the probation service as a whole and individual probation officers began to be curtailed in the 1970s and 1980s; during this time the managerial culture began to take hold in public sector organisations and the Home Office began to dictate the service's agenda. The National Statement of Objectives and Priorities, commonly known as SNOP (Home Office 1984), began this process, defining core tasks as the provision of reports to courts, the supervision of offenders in the community, working with prisoners before and after release from prison, and offering a service to the family courts in advising on residence of and contact to children in disputed divorce cases. SNOP was underlined by the instigation of an annual cycle of objective-setting and Home Office policy papers which outlined the required direction of the service. The introduction of cash limits in 1992 ensured that resourcing was also shaped by central rather than local government agendas. James (1994: 64) notes that 'an outmoded and recalcitrant Probation Service was quickly knocked into shape'.

While feeling the impact of the above changes through Home Office inspections, policy development and internal monitoring, the major impact on probation officers' autonomy has been the introduction of National Standards for the Supervision of Offenders in the Community. First introduced for community service orders in 1987, these were extended to other areas of work in 1992 and revised and further extended in 1995 (Home Office 1992a, 1995b). Their key purpose was to increase the confidence of the courts and general public of the service's ability to supervise offenders in the community effectively through preventing re-offending and protecting the public. The increasing influence of a punitive as opposed to welfare agenda is reflected in the Standards. Those published in 1992 state that supervision in the community can represent both 'a demanding and a constructive sentence of the criminal court', and that for probation and social services staff, supervision is 'challenging and skilful, requiring professional social work in the field of criminal justice' (Home Office 1992a: 1). By the time the revised Standards were published three years later the tone had changed: 'The aims of these National Standards are to strengthen the supervision of offenders in the community, providing punishment and a disciplined programme for offenders, building on the skill and experience of practitioners and service managers' (Home Office 1995b: 2). There was now an explicit reference to punishment, and no mention of social work as a skill. The balance between punishing and helping, however, was still apparent in the statement that supervision in the community was to be an 'effective punishment' while also being a means 'to help offenders become responsible members of the community' (ibid.).

There were two reactions to the introduction of National Standards: one regarded them as a serious threat to the professional discretion of individual probation officers, arguing that the needs and situations of offenders were far too varied and complex to be reduced to a few simple rules. The other took the view that probation officers enjoyed too much discretion and that standards of practice in relation to court reports and supervision should not depend upon the interests and preferences of individual probation officers. There is no doubt that practice in relation to enforcement of orders was inconsistent (see McWilliams 1989), and National Standards have, to a large extent, addressed this. There is a danger, however, that the Standards become minimum standards, and officers do no more than is required by them. They also run the risk of relocating discretion away from professional practice, which ideally offers high discretion while at the same time requiring high accountability from the officer. As was pointed out when the first National Standards for Community Service were introduced, rigid criteria and no discretion will not work in dealing with offenders whose social circumstances are often characterised by instability and chaos (Eadie and Willis 1989).

Conflicts arising from different understandings of professionalism

Reflecting on the service's history throughout the twentieth century, it can be argued that the boundary between practitioners and managers changed, as well as that between practitioners and those they supervised. The power of practitioners to influence the shape and direction of the service shifted to managers. Analysing this from a theoretical perspective, three types of member within any profession have been identified (Freidson 1986): practitioners, administrators (referred to here as managers) and teacher-researchers. Howe (1991) has applied these to the UK context, suggesting that each member holds a different view on the use and interpretation of the profession's formal knowledge (ibid.: 202). These contrasting perspectives lead to alternative ideas about what is to be recognised as good and appropriate practice. While the teacher-researcher will be interested in rigour and consistency of professional performance, the manager will wish to establish practices which are consistent, regular and standardised (ibid.: 207). The practitioner, aware of both perspectives, will use what knowledge and skills she or he requires to deal with any given situation. Howe argues that the service managers 'currently have the lion's share of power' (ibid.: 202).

The power dynamics between all three have been played out over past decades; throughout the first half of the twentieth century probation officers enjoyed a personal relationship with their local magistrates' court, often, it has been suggested (McWilliams 1981), sharing a similar moral position towards the offenders who appeared in court. The attempt to professionalise the service resulted in a more 'objective' stance, reducing the influence of the officer in court. In the 1960s and 1970s it could be argued that teacher-researchers held the power through responsibility for preparing new entrants to the service; Lacey (1992: 7) talks of an age in which 'training was pluralistic, social work based, and was led by academics'. The Training Review (Dews and Watts 1994) noted that the control of the training in the 1990s, despite a new emphasis on partnerships with local probation services, seemed 'to rest with academic institutions rather than the Probation Service' (ibid.: 2). It was clear that one of the agendas of the review was to restore the control of the training to the service. This control has been passed back to managers of the service and, in the current managerialist culture, it is they who now control the direction of the service.

How service managers experience a professional service might be very different from the experience of main grade staff who are actually interacting with offenders on a day-to-day basis. Howe notes (1991: 209) 'they [practitioners] find themselves working in a world which has boundaries and outlooks not of their making'. By increasing rules, routines, and procedures, the manager diminishes the area of professional discretion available to the social worker (Howe 1991: 214). The equilibrium between technicality (the skills and knowledge and their application) and indeterminacy (judgements about how the skills and knowledge should be applied in different circumstances) (Jamous and Peloille in Howe 1991) becomes weighted towards technicality.

There is evidence, however, that practitioners do retain a measure of power, specifically as regards their interaction with the offender; research undertaken by May (1991) highlighted what he called 'the implementation gap' – policies being re-interpreted at practitioner level in relation to what was feasible, which was not always the same as that which was required by service policy. This is reminiscent of Lipsky's (1980) argument that the worker at street level will establish his or her own ways of coping with the uncertainties and day-to-day pressures of the job, which might or might not fit with the bidding of the employer. Ideally, both will retain a sense of professional power within their own spheres of influence, with practitioners able to draw to the attention of managers practice implications of policies which are unworkable or inequitable.

Changing boundaries in the probation service: a challenge for the future

The probation service continues to have little alternative but to engage enthusiastically with the challenges set for it by government – its survival is at stake. Demonstrating its effectiveness in both punishing and rehabilitating offenders through effective supervision continues to be an uphill struggle. Media reports repeatedly describe offenders as 'walking free' after the imposition of a probation or community service order. Respondents in focus groups exploring attitudes towards sentencing (Hough 1996) knew little about the work of the service, and what they *did* know was not perceived as a punishment. The belief in imprisonment as the only effective punishment remains firmly fixed in the public's minds.

One attempt to imply toughness and punishment has been through the changing use of language in the service; since the 1980s, 'punishment' has replaced 'control', 'offender' has replaced 'client'. Even the term 'probation' has itself become 'something of an endangered species' (Leach 1998); a Consultation Document (Home Office 1998b) suggested that the term is associated with tolerance of crime, and proposed seven new names for the service, including the Public Protection Service and the Community Justice Enforcement Agency. It also argues that 'community service' sounds like voluntary activity and 'throughcare' suggests an association with the 'caring' services. It has been argued that when the language used and the conceptual environment it supports undergoes change, those using the language change both the way they think and the way they act (Howe 1996: 93).

There is a view that the service could be doing more to publicise the complexities of its work (Harris 1996: 129), and the expertise with which probation officers undertake their demanding, difficult and, at times, dangerous work. A debate in the House of Lords during the consultation process for the training review demonstrated sophisticated understanding and some sympathy with the work of the service:

> Baroness Seear: 'What is the knowledge and understanding that probation officers require? There can be no doubt that, first and foremost, probation officers deal with human behaviour – in particular, human misbehaviour – in complicated social situations.'
>
> (*Parliamentary Debates* 1995: 194)

'Complicated social situations' characterise the majority of offenders who come to the attention of the probation service: unstable accommodation, unsettled relationships, in poor health, their lifestyle characterised by disorder, chaos and ill-discipline. For many, this state of affairs is utterly normal (Eadie and Willis 1989: 416). To develop a positive relationship with people in this situation, one in which confronting the offending is managed effectively, probation officers need to develop relationship skills of the highest order, not the tough, no-nonsense approach favoured by the Conservatives in the early 1990s.

From the offender's perspective, research evidence suggests it is the relationship which is all-important:

> Lily: Without Probation, well, I'd have gone down the hill. I'd still be on drugs. I'd still be committing offences . . . I realised that he [the probation officer] was the first person I could really open up to about my home, job

worries, being in Care, people that I mixed with, drug abuse and things like that . . . Phil doesn't shout at me, but we sit down and discuss it sensibly.

(Bailey 1995: 129)

You're stood in Woolworths, you're skint and there's something you want on the shelf. Nobody's looking and . . . tsh . . . you can do that. But you're aware that you're letting them [probation] down, and you just don't bother with it. That's when you know it's working.

(Merrington 1996/97: 23)

Not all of the evidence is positive, but the fact that many offenders value the help and support offered to them by their supervising officer, as well as benefiting from the control, accentuates the need for a balance between the two. The service risks losing this balance by playing down the significance of personal relationships between offenders and 'their' probation officers and by moving towards case management systems which de-personalise contact even further (Beaumont and Mistry 1996). Any approach which devalues the relationship between probation officers and offenders is ill-informed. Moreover, if the social context within which the crime is committed is neglected, and probation officers focus solely on offending behaviour, they will have less opportunity to influence social systems which contribute towards the conditions which encourage offending. The role of the probation service will become focused on the offender's compliance rather than on the relationship between the two (Drakeford and Vanstone 1996: 19). There is the danger that technical 'solutions' may be seen as preferable, if only because the decision-making processes are easier both to explain and for the public to understand (Lymbery 1998).

The service needs to reconsider its working baseline; it has been argued that in these new political and cultural contexts, many of social work's theories and practices have become analytically more shallow and increasingly performance-orientated (Howe 1996). In relation to working with offenders, probation officers now ask *what?* rather than *why?*, a switch from causation to counting, from explanation to audit (ibid.: 88). Deep theoretical frameworks, the knowledge base claimed by social work as unique to its professional task, become less important than the visible surface behaviour of clients. While practitioners experience on a daily basis the dire social circumstances of offenders, public rhetoric – and John Major's suggestion that we 'understand less and condemn more' (Major 1994) is a good example – indicates a desire to blame rather than understand. Punishment is far higher up the socio-political agenda than rehabilitation. The emphasis on cognitive-behavioral techniques aimed at changing behaviour begins to fit into place; concern focused on the offender has shifted to concern with the offence and what action is required to prevent a re-occurrence of the offence. While the probation officer has always sought to prevent re-offending, the emphasis has changed.

With changes in tasks, in training, in accountability and in language, the probation officer of tomorrow will address the role differently from the one today. But as Millar and Buchanan have argued (1995: 198), the concept of probation as social work is perfectly compatible with the adoption of a 'challenging' attitude to offending; what is crucial is the manner of the challenge, the attitudes and values of those doing the challenging. This is what will ensure that people already alienated and marginalised from society are not pushed further outside society's boundaries. While the probation service has changed and has, appropriately, become a more publicly accountable agency required to demonstrate its effectiveness, much of its success in doing so relies on the ability of staff to develop positive, professional relationships with offenders – relationships which look to the future with optimism rather than those which focus only on the past. Moreover, the mechanical application of a rigid breach policy to gain compliance will be counter-productive with individuals for whom further punishment holds no threat.

Conclusion

This chapter has explored the role of the probation officer and questioned the extent to which the current changes in that role will impact on probation officer–offender relationships. While intervention to confront a person's offending behaviour is a necessity, a focus on this to the exclusion of the individual in his or her social context is likely to result in that individual's further alienation. Probation officers who lose sight of wider contextual issues will be working with only a part of, rather than the whole, person. Professional practice requires a range of skills and knowledge, and an ability to recognise what is required when.

Returning to Carol, the young woman quoted at the start of the chapter, the following extract shows how the probation officer uses her relationship with Carol to explain the concept of offending behaviour. The probation officer has just told Carol that in addition to monitoring her debts and making a referral to a voluntary sector bereavement counselling service, the two of them need to carry out offence-focused work:

Carol: What does that mean?
PO: Well, offence-focused work is the map that we did last time. I mean, that was offence-focused in the sense that the purpose was . . . to look at how you make decisions and how you make choices . . . that is about the offence because when people commit offences they always say that they just did it, it just happened.
Carol: Mmm
PO: In real terms you do make a choice; you make a choice about what you do and . . . how it came to be that you committed that particular offence. So that's what that means about offence-focused work in supervision sessions.
Carol: Yeah
PO: This is a supervision session; all that means is that we work together and do some exercises that we feel are going to be helpful to you.

Carol: Yeah

PO: I don't want to do exercises or work with you that you're not finding helpful; I mean, the two things we were saying as well was about con-fidence and assertiveness. We can have a go at that. I didn't feel that it was really appropriate to just launch into that without . . . you know, not knowing you that well . . . there has to be an element of trust to work on things like that.

Carol: I'm alright on confidence. I think it's assertiveness . . . I don't like to say no, do you know what I mean?

(Edmonds 1996: 40)

There is no attempt here to mystify the client with jargon or assert the more powerful position of the probation officer. The interview is taken at Carol's pace yet the officer seeks to ensure that Carol recognises her responsibility for her actions, and how they might work to change her behaviour in the future.

The probation service is being required to engage with the rhetoric of pun-ishment in the public and political sphere of its activity but to manage its task with individual offenders in a way that engages their interest and co-operation in a relationship which is, first and foremost, about their lives and their futures. Changing boundaries in relation to the activities of the probation service itself and in the relationships of its officers with offenders continues to be a challenge – one which only those in the service can meet.

Note

1 See McGuire (1995) for a comprehensive overview of the research literature.

References

Aldridge, M. (1999) 'Professions, promotional culture and the public sphere', *Public Administration* 77(1): 73–90.

Aldridge, M. and Eadie, T. (1997) 'Manufacturing an issue: the case of probation train-ing', *Critical Social Policy* 17(1): 111–24.

Audit Commission (1989) *The Probation Service: Promoting Value for Money*, London: HMSO.

—— (1991) *Going Straight: Developing Good Practice in the Probation Service*, Occasional paper, London: HMSO.

Bailey, R. (1995) 'Helping offenders as an element in justice', in D. Ward and M. Lacey (eds) *Probation: Working for Justice*, London: Whiting and Birch, pp. 127–39.

Beaumont, B. (1995) 'Managerialism and the probation service', in B. Williams (ed.) *Probation Values*, Birmingham: Venture Press, pp. 47–74.

Beaumont, B. and Mistry, T. (1996) 'Doing a good job under duress', *Probation Journal* 43(4): 200–4.

Bottoms, A.E. and McWilliams, W. (1979) 'A non-treatment paradigm for probation practice', *British Journal of Social Work* 9(2): 159–202.

Brody, S. (1976) *The Effectiveness of Sentencing*, Home Office research report no. 35, London: HMSO.

Bryant, M., Coker, J., Estlea, B., Himmel, S. and Knapp, T. (1978) 'Sentenced to social work?', *Probation Journal* 25(4): 110–14.

CCETSW (1995) *Assuring Quality in the Diploma in Social Work. Rules and Requirements for the DipSW*, revised 1995, London: CCETSW.

Dews, V. and Watts, J. (1994) *Review of Probation Officer Recruitment and Qualifying Training*, London: Home Office.

Drakeford, M. and Vanstone, M. (1996) 'Rescuing the social', *Probation Journal* 43(1): 16–19.

Eadie, T. and Willis, A. (1989) 'National standards for discipline and breach proceedings in community service: an exercise in penal rhetoric', *The Criminal Law Review* June: 412–19.

Edmonds, C. (1996) 'Final placement project, submitted for the MA/Diploma in Social Work', unpublished, University of Nottingham.

Ford, P. and Sleeman, S. (1996) 'Educating and training probation officers: the announcement of decline', *Vista: Perspectives on Probation* 1(3): 14–22.

Freidson, E. (1986) *Professional Powers*, Chicago: University of Chicago Press.

—— (1994) *Professionalism Reborn. Theory, Prophecy and Policy*, Oxford: Polity Press.

Harris, R.J. (1977) 'The probation officer as social worker', *British Journal of Social Work* 7(4): 433–42.

—— (1980) 'A changing service: the case for separating "care" and "control" in probation practice', *British Journal of Social Work* 10(2): 163–84.

—— (1996) 'Telling tales: probation in the contemporary social formulation', in N. Parton (ed.) *Social Theory, Social Change and Social Work*, London: Routledge, pp. 115–34.

Hollin, C.R. (1995) 'The meaning and implications of "programme integrity"', in J. McGuire (ed.) *What Works: Reducing Reoffending*, Chichester: John Wiley, pp. 195–208.

Home Office (1962) *Report of the Departmental Committee on the Probation Service* (The Morison Committee), Cmnd 1650, London: HMSO.

—— (1984) *Statement of National Objectives and Priorities for the Probation Service*, London: Home Office.

—— (1988) *Punishment, Custody and the Community*, Cm 424, London: HMSO.

—— (1990a) *Supervision and Punishment in the Community: A Framework for Action*, Cm 966, London: HMSO.

—— (1990b) *Crime, Justice and Protecting the Public*, Cm 965, London: HMSO.

—— (1991) *Organising Supervision and Punishment in the Community: A Decision Document*, London: Home Office.

—— (1992a) *National Standards for the Supervision of Offenders in the Community*, London: Home Office.

—— (1992b) *Partnership in Dealing with Offenders in the Community: A Decision Document*, London: Home Office.

—— (1995a) *Strengthening Punishment in the Community: A Consultation Document*, Cm 2780, London: HMSO.

—— (1995b) *National Standards for the Supervision of Offenders in the Community*, London: Home Office.

—— (1995c) *New Arrangements for the Recruitment and Qualifying Training of Probation Officers: A Decision Document*, London: Home Office.

—— (1996) *Three Year Plan for the Probation Service 1996–1999*, London: Home Office Communication Directorate.

—— (1998a) *PC 3/1998: Plan for the Probation Service 1998–1999*, London: Home Office.

—— (1998b) *Joining Forces to Protect the Public Prisons-Probation. A Consultation Document*, London: The Stationery Office, August.

Hough, M. (1996) 'People talking about punishment', *The Howard Journal of Criminal Justice*, 35(3): 191–214.

Howard, M. (1993) Speech by the Rt Hon. Michael Howard QC MP, the Home Secretary, to the 110th Conservative Party Conference, 6 October, London: Conservative Party Central Office.

Howe, D. (1991) 'Knowledge, power and the shape of social work practice', in M. Davies (ed.) *The Sociology of Social Work*, London: Routledge, pp. 147–62.

—— (1996) 'Surface and depth in social-work practice', in N. Parton (ed.) *Social Theory, Social Change and Social Work*, London: Routledge, pp. 77–97.

Jack, M. (1993) Speech to the 10th Annual Conference of the Association of Chief Officers of Probation, 4 March.

James, A. (1994) *Managing to Care: Public Services and the Market*, Harlow: Longman.

Jarvis, F.V. (1980) *Probation Officers' Manual* (3rd edn), London: Butterworth.

Lacey, M. (1992) 'A service for justice', in *Probation Training Issues and CCETSW's Training Continuum*, unpublished conference papers, London: CCETSW.

Leach, T. (1998) 'In defence of traditional terminology', *Vista: Perspectives on Probation* 4(2): 108–12.

Lipsky, M. (1980) *Street-Level Bureaucracy*, New York: Russell Sage.

Lymbery, M. (1998) 'Care management and professional autonomy: the impact of community care legislation on social work with older people', *British Journal of Social Work* 28(6): 863–78.

McGuire, J. (1995) *What Works: Reducing Reoffending. Guidelines from Research and Practice*, Chichester: John Wiley.

McWilliams, W. (1981) 'The probation officer at court: from friend to acquaintance', *The Howard Journal of Criminal Justice* 20(2): 97–116.

—— (1983) 'The mission to the English police courts 1876–1936', *The Howard Journal of Criminal Justice* 22(3): 129–47.

—— (1985) 'The mission transformed: professionalisation of probation between the wars', *The Howard Journal of Criminal Justice* 24(4): 257–74.

—— (1986) 'The English probation system and the diagnostic ideal', *The Howard Journal of Criminal Justice* 25(4): 241–60.

—— (1987) 'Probation, pragmatism and policy', *The Howard Journal of Criminal Justice* 26(2): 97–121.

—— (1989) 'Community service national standards: practice and sentencing', *Probation Journal* 36(3): 121–6.

Major, J. (1994) Speech by the Prime Minister, Rt Hon. John Major, MP, at Church House, London, 9 September, Press notice, PM's Office.

Martinson, R. (1974) 'What works? Questions and answers about prison reform', *The Public Interest* 35: 22–54.

May, T. (1991) *Probation: Politics, Policy and Practice*, Buckingham: Open University Press.

Merrington, S. (1996/97) 'Offenders' views', *Social Action: The Journal for the Centre for Social Action* 3(2): 17–23.

Miller, M. and Buchanan, J. (1995) 'Probation: a crisis of identity and purpose', *Probation Journal* 42(4): 195–8.

Oldfield, M. (1994) 'Talking quality, meaning control: McDonalds, the market and the probation service', *Probation Journal* 41(4): 186–92.

Parliamentary Debates (1995) *House of Lords 5 April 1995 – Probation Officers: Recruitment and Training* (Hansard), 186–242, London: HMSO.

Patten, J. (1988) 'Punishment, the probation service and the community', speech to the Association of Chief Officers of Probation, 15 September, London: Home Office.

Pease, K. (1981) *Community Service Orders: A First Decade of Promise*, London: Howard League.

Raine, J.W. and Willson, M.J. (1993) *Managing Criminal Justice*, Hemel Hempstead: Harvester Wheatsheaf.

Ross, R.R. and Fabiano, E.A. (1985) *Time to Think: A Cognitive Model of Delinquency Prevention and Offender Rehabilitation*, Johnson City: Academy of Arts and Sciences.

Ross, R.R., Fabiano, E.A. and Ewles, C.D. (1988) 'Reasoning and rehabilitation', *International Journal of Offender Therapy and Comparative Criminology* 32: 29–35.

Statham, R. and Whitehead, P. (eds) (1992) *Managing the Probation Service: Issues for the 1990s*, Harlow: Longman.

THES (1995) 'Setback for social work', *Times Higher Education Supplement*, 6 October.

Walker, H. and Beaumont, B. (1981) *Probation Work: Critical Theory and Socialist Practice*, Oxford: Basil Blackwell.

Ward, D. (1996) 'Probation training: celebration or wake?', in M. Preston-Shoot and S. Jackson (eds) *Educating Social Workers in a Changing Policy Context*, London: Whiting and Birch, pp. 103–29.

Williams, B. (1994) 'Probation training in the UK: from charity organisation to jobs for the boys', *Social Work Education* 13(3): 99–108.

—— (1996) *Freedom on Probation*, London: Association of University Teachers.

Willis, A. (1995) 'W(h)ither probation training: a review of the scrutiny report', *Vista: Perspectives on Probation* 1(2): 55–61.

Worrall, A. (1997) *Punishment in the Community: The Future of Criminal Justice*, Harlow: Addison Wesley Longman.

10 Professionalism definitions in 'managing' health services

Perspectives on the differing views of clinicians and general managers in an NHS Trust

Reva Berman Brown and Sean McCartney

Introduction

The professions have been the subject of intellectual interest for most of this century. For instance, around the time of the First World War, there were books and articles by Spencer (1914), the Webbs (1917) and Tawney (1920); the inter-war years saw influential books by Carr-Saunders (1928) and Carr-Saunders and Wilson (1933); and on the eve of the Second World War significant papers by Marshall (1939) and Parsons (1939) were published.

A considerable literature has accumulated since 1945, and especially in the last decade, ranging over a number of connected topics. For example, the work of Goode (1957, 1969), Moore (1970) and Wilensky (1964) was concerned with developing a concept of profession that would distinguish it from other occupations, and discovering the process by which an occupation attains professional status; Auerbach (1976), Platt (1969), and Rothman (1971) analysed how professional activities facilitate control of the poor, the working class and the deviant; Freidson (1970, 1988) considered issues of conflict and power in the medical profession; Larson (1977) viewed professional groups from a Marxist or Weberian perspective.

Research in the sociology of professions has been marked by a shifting and diverse range of theoretical frameworks (Saks 1983: 1). As Meiksins and Watson (1989: 561) state, there is 'no single theory of the professions; rather, there are competing theories, no one of which has become completely hegemonic'.

The two major debates have concerned the process by which particular occupations become professions, and the conceptualising of professions, the professional and professionalism. In this chapter we attempt to contribute to the conceptualising debate, using healthcare as a focus.

In studying the medical profession, writers have rooted their analyses in various contexts, as noted by Ashburner (1996: 211). This may be social context (Abbott 1988; Hafferty 1988; McKinlay 1988); a political, economic, gender and race context (Davies 1983; Navarro 1988; Atkinson and Delamont 1990); a historical context (Larkin 1988; Navarro 1988); how the medical profession impacts on organisational forms (Scott 1985); or how it is linked into the class and labour market systems (Hall 1988). The research reported here was stimulated by a paper by Stewart (undated) which demonstrated the mistrust doctors had of managers and their belief that managers had completely alien values. During previous research (Bell *et al.* 1993; Brown *et al.* 1994), we have corroborated Stewart's findings, uncovering the hostility felt towards general managers by the clinical professionals who work with (or against) them. Comments made to us during this research led to the supposition that such conflict as does arise might have its roots in differing definitions of what it means to be a professional and what 'proper' professional action might be. This chapter reports on the results of our investigation of this assumption.

The next section, therefore, briefly considers various definitions of the concepts of 'profession', 'professional', and 'professionalism' in order to explain the definitions chosen for the research. We then move on to discuss the nature of NHS management and the place of NHS management within the NHS. Next, we describe the research undertaken in an acute hospital to uncover the meanings these concepts have for consultants and general managers working there. The final section discusses the implications of our findings, drawing tentative conclusions.

Definitions and their problems

Profession

The lay and academic meanings of 'profession' are correlated rather than synonymous. To the lay person, a profession is an occupation calling for special knowledge and expertise; to the academic, such as Freidson (1994: 10), it is 'an occupation that controls its own work, organised by a special set of institutions, sustained, in part, by a particular ideology of expertise and service.'

While most definitions overlap in the elements, traits or attributes they include, a continuing lack of consensus persists, and usage of the term still varies substantively, logically and conceptually (Freidson 1977).

One method of solving the problem of definition is to avoid defining the characteristics of professions as 'inherently distinct from other occupations' (Klegon 1978: 268) and to concentrate, instead, on the process by which occupations come to claim, or to gain, professional status. This, of course, leads to the tautology of defining a profession as an occupation that has gained professional status, and defining professional status as the status of a professional occupation, without clear definition of either concept.

Another method is to move from structure, i.e. the static conception of a profession as a distinct type of occupation, to process, uncovering the routes by which occupations are professionalised. But, as Johnson (1972) and Turner and Hodge (1970) have pointed out, an emphasis on process rather than structure – on professionalisation rather than on the elements, traits or attributes of professions – is unhelpful, because one cannot study the process of professionalisation without a definition of the structure (profession) as a guide.

The three original learned professions – medicine, law and the clergy (who then included university teaching in their profession) – originated in the medieval universities of Europe, and Elliott (1972) has termed them 'status professions'. The occupational structure of capitalist industrialism developed what Elliott has called 'occupational professions' out of the middle-class occupations distinct from the three 'gentlemanly', long-established professions.

In the UK and the USA, because the state was relatively passive in this area, these middle-class occupations organised their own training and credentialling institutions, and over time, these became part of the official occupational classification scheme. Each occupation mounted its own movement for recognition and protection, and its members' loyalties and identities were attached to their individual occupation and its institutions. In Europe (which in this instance does not include the UK), the traditional 'status professions' maintained their occupational distinctions, but the new, middle-class occupations did not seek classification as 'professions' – the status and security of professionals were gained by their attendance at state-controlled, elite institutions of higher education which assured them of elite positions in the civil service or other technical-managerial positions. Ben-David (1964) suggests that primary identity was not given by occupation, but by the status gained by elite education, no matter what the particular speciality. This leads Freidson (1994: 19) to assert that 'as an institutional concept, the term 'profession' is intrinsically bound up with a particular period of history, and with only a limited number of nations in that period of history'.

Elliott's distinction covers the two main usages of the term, as suggested by Freidson (1994: 16):

1   The concept of a profession as a limited number of occupations which have particular institutional and ideological traits more or less in common, producing distinctive occupational identities and exclusionary market niches, which set each occupation apart from (and sometimes in opposition to) the others. These are the status professions.
2   The concept of a profession that refers to a broad stratum of relatively prestigious, but quite varied, occupations, whose members have all had some kind of higher education, and who are identified more by their educational status than by their specific occupational skills. These are the occupational professions.

Rather than reinvent the wheel, we have used Elliott's distinction in our empirical research.

Professional

There are two 'opposites' that come to mind when the term 'professional' is used: that of 'professional' and 'amateur', and 'professional' and 'not professional'. In the business sphere, the professional person or activity is easily distinguished from the amateur, because the professional is paid and the amateur is not. In organisational terms, the professional is the person who performs a given set of tasks in a contracted market exchange by which he or she gains a living, and the amateur is the person who performs the tasks without conscious and calculating concern for their exchange value in the market. In this sense, for instance, the voluntary, unpaid worker in a charity shop is an amateur, while the salaried shopworker is a professional.

This particular professional–amateur distinction provides clear boundaries between what is to be defined as work, and what is not, and who is to be defined as a worker, and who is not. It does not, however, discriminate among types of work or occupation, which is where the professional–not professional opposite comes in. Here, the macro-sociological categorisation of the strata of the labour force into a number of 'classes' is relevant. To define the class of 'professional', use is made of either (or both) of two characteristics, both of which are measured by reference to official statistics:

1   The years of formal education required for employment in particular jobs (and here professional workers are those whose work is considered by employers to require four years of post-secondary education). In the context of this chapter, these are the health service managers.
2   Those groups of workers who possess special knowledge (usually distinguished as abstract and theoretical) and skill (usually characterised as requiring the exercise of complex judgement). For the purposes of our research, these are the consultants, but it must be said that the current range of occupations in this broad 'professional' class includes not only physicians, but also engineers, dental technicians, clergymen, schoolteachers, reporters, nurses, airline pilots, social workers, photographers, professors, chemists (Freidson 1994: 113).

We included in the research the usage in lay language of 'professional' as a person who, or activity which, is skilled, proficient, trained or learned, and adept. Here the term 'a professional person' conjures up an individual in a paid occupation so well organised that he or she can realistically envisage a career over most of his or her working years, a career during which he/she can retain a particular occupational identity and continue to practise the same knowledge-based skills, no matter in what institution he/she works (Freidson 1994). (This description would apply to members of the status and the occupational professions, hence its inclusion in the study.) And a professional activity is one which is based on the actor's trained proficiency and ability, expertise and knowledge.

Professionalism

For Freidson (1994), 'professionalism' is the ideology and special set of institutions by which a profession is organised. His description of the ideology carries with it much of the traditional ethos of the professional-as-the-altruistic-servant-of-clients, appropriate for the medical profession which has been the subject of his work, but which can be seen as somewhat outdated in the context of current research. For Freidson,

- The kind of work professionals do is esoteric, complex, and discretionary in character; it requires theoretical knowledge, skill and judgement that ordinary people do not possess, may not wholly comprehend, and cannot readily evaluate.
- Their work is believed to be especially important for the well-being of individuals or of society at large, having a value so special that money cannot serve as its sole measure.
- It is the capacity to perform that special kind of work which distinguishes those who are called professional from most other workers.
- The character of professional work suggests two basic elements of professionalism: commitment to practising a body of knowledge and skill of special value, and to maintaining a fiduciary relationship with clients.
- The course of training required for learning how to do esoteric and complex work well tends to create commitment to knowledge and skill, so that the professional's work becomes a central life-interest which provides its own intrinsic rewards.
- What professionals do is of special value to their clients. But their knowledge is sufficiently complex and esoteric that clients are not able to evaluate it accurately. Therefore clients of professionals must place more trust in them than they do in others. Professionals are expected to honour the trust that clients have no alternative but to place in them.

To come down to earth, it can be said that the concept of professionalism entails commitment to a particular body of knowledge and skill, both for its own sake and for the use to which it is put. In order to do such good work well, and to behave in a professional manner, one must have the nominal freedom to exercise discretionary judgement.

It is here that the clash between consultants and general managers becomes more obvious. The private sector ethos that emphasises the importance of the customer does not fit easily with the public sector professional need to exercise discretion, guided by an independent perspective on what work is appropriate for people who are patients, not customers.

The nature of NHS management and the place of management within the NHS

The characteristics and tasks faced by the managers within the NHS are shared, to a lesser or greater degree, by most other managers in the UK (Leopold *et al.* 1996):

1   UK managers are required to determine and then choose between priorities in order to cut costs or improve efficiency.

2   External forces act upon all managers. In the case of NHS managers, the role of government in bringing about the managerial changes of the last decade have been overt and firm, even though the control of day-to-day local or regional management has been more equivocal.

3   Like other managers in both the public and private sectors, NHS managers tend to be guided by a faith in rationally guided search behaviour, despite the limitations of this approach.

4   As in many organisations, NHS managers emphasise consumption or an end-state or goal over the process of achieving these.

5   NHS managers share a faith in, and place emphasis upon, the value of the general management *of*, rather than specialist management *in*, healthcare.

In a great number of NHS Trusts, one can find evidence of resistance from clinicians to non-specialist, non-expert managerial domination; but one can also find evidence of the existence of the hybrid clinician–manager, operating, perhaps, under the 'If you can't lick them, join them' philosophy. (It is the GP who is an interesting special case – Bennett (1996) showed how some doctors could, by showing entrepreneurial drive, enthusiasm and single-mindedness, use their professional characteristics of autonomy, status and collegiality to enhance, as well as to defend, their positions.)

FitzGerald (1996) portrays a complex and ambiguous situation, with clinicians becoming, over time, both more favourable towards the idea of becoming involved in management, and better educated and trained in order to do so. Harrison and Nutley (1996), however, show how general management had clearly weakened the authority of other professionals in the NHS apart from doctors, especially that of nurses.

Hafferty (1988) suggests five areas of threat to the dominance of the medical profession:

1   A marketplace in healthcare increases competition between professionals, and causes divisions between them.

2   Rifts develop within the profession between the clinical managers and the clinicians who are being managed.

3   External control directly, or indirectly, limits and reduces the autonomy of the professional.

4   Consumer knowledge increases and narrows the gap between the power of the professional and the dependence of the patient.

5   Medicine is unable to control and restrain the right of 'alternative' providers, such as complementary medicine.

We would suggest a sixth threat:

6   Rifts develop among the general managers, the clinical managers, and the clinicians who are being managed.

We have evidence of a rift in perceptions of professionalism, plus some quite strong comments in the responses to our questionnaire.

The research study

It was our suspicion that the professional view of the consultants would be that it is counter-productive to provide whatever customers (patients) desire, when their capacity to evaluate the service or product is seriously limited, and when what they desire contradicts the better judgement of the consultant. We also thought that the professional view of the managers would put more emphasis on the prevailing commercial opinion that the customer is king, and the satisfied customer is evidence of the success of the enterprise.

A questionnaire was devised, piloted and issued to the population of consultants and general managers at an acute hospital in Essex. The questions were phrased in non-academic language but expressed the themes which had emerged from the literature. We assured anonymity and confidentiality and did not ask respondents to identify themselves beyond stating whether they saw themselves as being a clinician, a manager, or both at the same time.

We were concerned to elicit the views of respondents concerning the meaning, to them, of the terms 'profession', 'professional' and 'professionalism'. For 'profession', we used the traditional, dictionary definition, and also Elliott's (1972) division into status and occupational professions. For 'professional', we absorbed the ideas of Abbott (1988), Child and Falk (1982) and Simon (1985). For 'professionalism', we based our statements on Begum (1986) and Freidson (1994).

The questionnaires were distributed under the auspices of the medical audit department of the hospital; responses were returned there in sealed envelopes provided with the questionnaire, and then returned to us in two batches by mail.

We had provided our 'distributor' with 150 questionnaires, which were distributed to managers and senior clinicians. A total of 85 questionnaires were returned, of which 34 were from consultants, 29 from managers, and 22 from respondents who described themselves as consultant-managers – our term for clinical directors and others who have taken on managerial tasks as well as continuing to work as clinicians.

For our analysis, we divided the respondents into three groups, according to self-identification. We present our findings in tabular form (Table 10.1), divided into these three categories, and discuss their implications in the next section. All responses in all tables are expressed in percentage terms.

Table 10.1 Analysis of questionnaire responses

Profession

1 An occupation is only a profession if it has *all four* of the following components: a strong theoretical basis + a specific training process + procedures for professional accreditation + defined ethical codes.

	Consultants	Managers	Consultant-managers
not at all			
to a small extent		7%	
to some extent	18%	16%	17%
to a great extent	78%	70%	83%
have no firm opinion	3%	7%	

2 An occupation is not a profession if it does not have the ability to exclude those without formal qualifications.

	Consultants	Managers	Consultant-managers
not at all	3%		
to a small extent		4%	
to some extent	31%	12%	16%
to a great extent	66%	80%	84%
have no firm opinion		4%	

3 An occupation is not a profession if it does not have the ability to control the supply of practitioners.

	Consultants	Managers	Consultant-managers
not at all	3%		
to a small extent		19%	15%
to some extent	31%	15%	25%
to a great extent	66%	58%	50%
have no firm opinion		8%	10%

4 To what extent do you consider that the two types of profession – status and occupational – are:

(a) of equal value to society

	Consultants	Managers	Consultant-managers
not at all	10%		
to a small extent	14%	8%	
to some extent	41%	20%	55%
to a great extent	21%	56%	35%
have no firm opinion	14%	16%	10%

(b) of equal intellectual standing

	Consultants	Managers	Consultant-managers
not at all	17%		
to a small extent	7%	4%	24%
to some extent	55%	36%	52%
to a great extent	14%	48%	14%
have no firm opinion	7%	12%	10%

(c) capable of co-existing amicably in a health setting

	Consultants	Managers	Consultant-managers
not at all		4%	
to a small extent	14%	8%	14%
to some extent	48%	34%	18%
to a great extent	35%	54%	68%
have no firm opinion	3%		

5 Do you consider that you belong to:

	Consultants	Managers	Consultant-managers
a status profession	100%	19%	44%
an occupational profession		72%	22%
both at the same time		9%	34%

Professionals

1 Professionals are always members of 'colleges' or other registering bodies.

	Consultants	Managers	Consultant-managers
not at all			10%
to a small extent	3%	8%	15%
to some extent		12%	15%
to a great extent	93%	76%	60%
have no firm opinion	3%	4%	

2 Professionals always have a recognised expertise and knowledge.

	Consultants	Managers	Consultant-managers
not at all			
to a small extent	3%		4%
to some extent	93%	12%	41%
to a great extent	3%	88%	55%
have no firm opinion			

3 Professionals serve clients, and are ultimately trying to benefit the community as a whole.

	Consultants	Managers	Consultant-managers
not at all	4%		
to a small extent	4%	8%	
to some extent	21%	62%	38%
to a great extent	68%	15%	52%
have no firm opinion	4%	15%	10%

4 Professionals act in a rational, structured way when solving problems.

	Consultants	Managers	Consultant-managers
not at all	3%		
to a small extent			9%
to some extent	45%	73%	64%
to a great extent	48%	27%	27%
have no firm opinion	3%		

5 Professionals are basically altruistic about their work.

	Consultants	Managers	Consultant-managers
not at all	3%	4%	
to a small extent	7%	48%	16%
to some extent	52%	40%	74%
to a great extent	31%		9%
have no firm opinion	7%	8%	

6 Professionals are committed to an ethic of service to clients.

	Consultants	Managers	Consultant-managers
not at all			
to a small extent	4%	13%	
to some extent	32%	87%	72%
to a great extent	64%		28%
have no firm opinion	%		

7 Professionals define who the client is, what the client needs, and the way in which these needs are to be catered for.

(a) Professionals define who the client is

	Consultants	Managers	Consultant-managers
not at all	11%	21%	24%
to a small extent	19%	26%	19%
to some extent	56%	21%	52%
to a great extent	7%	16%	5%
have no firm opinion	7%	16%	

(b) Professionals define what the client needs

	Consultants	Managers	Consultant-managers
not at all		44%	
to a small extent	14%	26%	16%
to some extent	54%	22%	79%
to a great extent	32%	8%	5%
have no firm opinion			

Professionalism

1 Professionalism can be recognised by the general way the professional behaves.

	Consultants	Managers	Consultant-managers
not at all			
to a small extent	10%	66%	15%
to some extent	28%	14%	45%
to a great extent	59%	10%	40%
have no firm opinion	3%	10%	

2 Professionalism can be recognised by the use of certified techniques of practice.

	Consultants	Managers	Consultant-managers
not at all	7%		
to a small extent	21%	4%	5%
to some extent	51%	48%	42%
to a great extent	21%	48%	53%
have no firm opinion			

3 Professionalism is more a state of mind than specific actions.

	Consultants	Managers	Consultant-managers
not at all	27%	52%	33%
to a small extent	21%	19%	33%
to some extent	27%	19%	19%
to a great extent	21%	5%	15%
have no firm opinion	4%	5%	

The implications of our findings

Overall, our findings confirm FitzGerald's (1996: 196) view that 'Doctors' perceptions of management and what management entails are coloured by their contact with managers in healthcare and by the frequently held view that managers are not well qualified and management is easy to learn.' For 'not well qualified', we suggest, read 'not professionals'.

Turning to the results of our survey, it will be seen that there is a large measure of agreement between all groups in certain respects, but large divergences in others. We had encouraged respondents to add verbal comments at the end of the questionnaire, if they felt so inclined, and we have quoted from them where relevant.

Credentialling the professions

All groups agree about the definition of a profession: that professions must have a strong theoretical basis, a specific training process, procedures for accreditation, defined ethical codes, powers of exclusion, and control over the supply of practitioners. This is perhaps surprising: such features are present in the medical profession, but are lacking in the profession of management (it lacks four of the five defining criteria). Although professional bodies do exist for managers (there is even an Institute of Health Service Management), they do not have the crucial credentialling powers of the status professions. The group who is less committed to this view of 'profession' is the consultant-managers. This may be because, now that they undertake managerial tasks and know from practical experience what general management is 'about', they are willing to accept that there is more than one way of defining, or recognising, a profession. As one consultant-manager commented,

> While the managers here aren't professionals in any way that I'd accept, the good ones behave in what I acknowledge is a highly professional manner.

A manager wrote:

> It's not the closed shop aspect – control over the supply of credentialled practitioners – that makes a profession. It's the existence of theory about

the practice and the existence of an accredited training process. And we've got that, so management is a profession.

Status and occupational professions

Managers are more likely to see the status and occupational professions as of equal value to society and equal intellectual standing, and capable of co-existing in the health service. Consultants are less likely to see the two types of professions as equal or capable of amicable co-existence, while the consultant-managers . . . One consultant commented rather snobbishly:

> Accounting and management are not professions, and it reflects seriously on your credibility that you call them 'occupational professions'.

Professionalism

Turning to other facets of professionalism, both consultant groups agree that professionals must belong to a recognised 'college'. Managers, on the other hand, believe more strongly that the hallmark of a profession is a body of recognised expertise or knowledge. This is corroboration of Elliott's (1972) division of professions into 'status' and 'occupational', and of Freidson's (1994) view that the division is one between those professions with exclusionary market niches and those identified by their members' educational qualifications.

Professional attitudes and knowledge

Managers tend more to the idea that the essence of professionalism is the use of certified techniques. While consultants give more credence to the idea that professionalism is a state of mind, managers lean more towards the idea that the essence of professionalism is the acquisition of a body of defined knowledge/techniques and the ability to apply it/them. To the consultants, it is more than learning and applying rules. As one commented:

> Professionals do not follow set rules – monkeys do that. There is development, modification. Professionals develop – they do not administer.

A manager provided the statement that:

> It's how you apply what you know that marks you out as behaving professionally or not.

Professional ethics and serving the client

Considerable differences emerge over what we might term the ethical side of professionalism. Consultants appear to believe much more strongly than managers that professionals are there to serve clients, or to serve society, and are basically altruistic. Alongside this is a tendency to see the client's needs (and even a decision as to who the client is) as something to be determined by the professional him/herself, who will presumably tell the client what he/she needs to know, and give the treatment the client needs to have. The managers, in contrast, lean more to a 'consumerist' and 'managerialist' view. Whereas the clinician sees him/herself as a professional who does the best possible for the client, focusing on the individual professional–client relationship and his/her own integrity in that relationship, the managers focus on the organisation and its relationship with customers. One consultant commented:

> A professional needs to use imagination, insight and sympathy with the client in the light of past experience and certified techniques, but be able to identify the individual needs of each client.

However, a manager commented:

> A more relevant and useful view of professionalism would emphasise customer service and a greater commitment to achieving organisational goals – this would close the gap between the two professional types [i.e. status and occupational].

Similarly, the consultants lean more to the view that 'professionalism' is an attitude of mind. While the managers view professionalism as determined by behaviour, they tended to be more sceptical of ideas of professional altruism.

Summary and conclusions

Previous research (Bell *et al.* 1993; Brown *et al.* 1994; Stewart, undated) has suggested a considerable degree of friction in the health service between the clinicians (status professions) and managers, who may have no clinical experience at all. Typically, the consultants viewed such managers as useless bureaucrats more concerned with budgets and meetings than patients' needs, who did not care for (or about) the patients.

Managers responded by stressing 'customer satisfaction' and the aims of the organisation rather than the ethics of the profession. This can lead to outright hostility towards the clinicians' view of professionalism, which can be seen as a hypocritical and self-serving cloak for the self-interest of the professionals. One manager commented:

> The health service is predominantly a professional culture preoccupied with status and self-protection. It relies on – and abuses – the traditional view of professionalism to foster the interests of the professional membership.

There appears to be a clash of cultures, one manifestation of which is a radical difference of view as to what constitutes professionalism. It is clear that because of such differences, the interaction between consultants and managers is clouded by different conceptions of what a 'true' professional is, and how he or she acts in a properly professional manner. There are likely to be occasions when clinicians and managers talk past each other, coming from such different starting points that, with all the goodwill in the world, they cannot meet. It is as though, despite their both inhabiting the same material space, in some important way, they are unable to see one another.

The working world in which consultants and managers co-exist is obviously not an uncomplicated one. To understand the differences among occupations in a healthcare setting requires an emphasis on the degree to which they have gained the organised power to control the terms, conditions, and content of their work in the settings where they perform it. For instance, Freidson (1994) draws attention to the difference between the occupations of pharmacist and physician. Both are nominal members of the status professions, both have complex skills, both have a higher education, and both have exclusive licences by which they monopolise certain tasks. But the critical difference between them is that the pharmacist can work only at the order of the physician, and thus may be seen to be in a critically different position in the division of labour, as regards freedom of authority of others over their work. Indeed, a particular kind of work – practice of the tasks of healing, for instance – can be organised as a profession at one point in history and not at another, and in one nation and not another.

One of the ways in which people cope with the complexity and ambiguity of organisational life is to simplify issues which would otherwise be problematic. The research reported here indicates that this is what consultants and managers do about each other. Both constituencies have answered the question, 'Whose "professional" is the real thing?' with 'Mine is'. One encouraging sign, however, is the attitude of the 'hybrids', those who are both consultants and managers, who perhaps can build bridges between the two groups and develop a new consensus on the meaning and role of professionals in the health service.

References

Abbott, A. (1988) *The System of Professions: An Essay on the Division of Expert Labor*, Chicago: University of Chicago Press.

Ashburner, L. (1996) 'The role of clinicians in the management of the NHS', in J. Leopold, I. Glover and M. Hughes (eds) *Beyond Reason? The National Health Service and the Limits of Management*, Aldershot: Avebury, pp. 207–24.

Atkinson, P. and Delamont, S. (1990) 'Professions and powerlessness: female marginality in the learned occupations', *Sociological Review* 38: 90–110.

Auerbach, J.S. (1976) *Unequal Justice: Lawyers and Social Change in Modern America*, New York: Oxford University Press.

Begum, J.W. (1986) 'Economic and sociological approaches to professionalism', *Work and Occupations* 13: 113–29.

Bell, L., Brown, R.B. and McCartney, S. (1993) 'Professionals in health care: perceptions of managers', *Journal of Management in Medicine* 6(5): 49–56.

Ben-David, J. (1964) 'Professions in the class system of present-day societies', *Current Sociology* 12: 247–330.

Bennett, C. (1996) 'The crucial role of professional status in promoting change: the development of services for HIV/AIDS', in J. Leopold, I. Glover and M. Hughes (eds) *Beyond Reason? The National Health Service and the Limits of Management*, Aldershot: Avebury, pp. 103–23.

Brown, R.B., McCartney, S., Bell, L. and Scaggs, S. (1994) 'Who is the NHS for?', *Journal of Management in Medicine* 8(6): 61–9.

Carr-Saunders, A.M. (1928) *Professions: Their Organization and Place in Society*, Oxford: Clarendon Press.

Carr-Saunders, A.M. and Wilson, P.A. (1933) *The Professions*, Oxford: Clarendon Press.

Child, J. and Falk, J. (1982) 'Maintenance of occupational control: the case of professions', *Work and Occupations* 9: 155–92.

Davies, C. (1983) 'Professionals in bureaucracies: the conflict thesis revisited', in R. Dingwall and P. Lewis (eds) *The Sociology of the Professions: Lawyers, Doctors and Others*, Basingstoke: Macmillan.

Elliott, P. (1972) *The Sociology of the Professions*, London: Macmillan.

FitzGerald, L. (1996) 'Clinical management: the impact of a changing context in a changing profession', in J. Leopold, I. Glover and M. Hughes (eds) *Beyond Reason? The National Health Service and the Limits of Management*, Aldershot: Avebury, pp. 189–203.

Freidson, E. (1970) *Professional Dominance: The Social Structure of Medical Care*, New York: Atherton Press.

—— (1977) 'The futures of professionalization', in M. Stacey, M. Reid, C. Heath and R. Dingwall (eds) *Health and the Division of Labour*, London: Croom Helm.

—— (1988) *Profession of Medicine: A Study in the Sociology of Applied Knowledge*, Chicago: University of Chicago Press.

—— (1994) *Professionalism Reborn: Theory, Prophecy and Policy*, Cambridge: Polity Press.

Goode, W.J. (1957) 'Community within a community: the professions', *American Sociological Review* 22(1): 194–200.

—— (1969) 'The theoretical limits of professionalization', in A. Etzioni (ed.) *The Semi-Professions and Their Organization*, New York: Free Press.

Hafferty, F. (1988) 'Theories at the crossroads: a discussion of evolving views on medicine as a profession', *The Milbank Quarterly* 66(2): 202–25.

Hall, R.H. (1988) 'Comment on the sociology of the professions', *Work and Occupations* 15: 273–5.

Harrison, J. and Nutley, S. (1996) 'Professions and management in the public sector: the experience of local government and the NHS in Britain', in J. Leopold, I. Glover and M. Hughes (eds) *Beyond Reason? The National Health Service and the Limits of Management*, Aldershot: Avebury, pp. 227–48.

Johnson, T. (1972) *Professions and Power*, London: Macmillan.

Klegon, D.A. (1978) 'The sociology of professions: an emerging perspective', *Sociology of Work and Occupations* 5: 259–83.

Larkin, G. (1988) 'Medical dominance in Britain: image and historical reality', *The Milbank Quarterly* 66(2): 117–32.

Larson, M.S. (1977) *The Rise of Professionalism: A Sociological Analysis*, Berkeley: University of California Press.

Leopold, J., Glover, I. and Hughes, M. (eds) (1996) *Beyond Reason? The National Health Service and the Limits of Management*, Aldershot: Avebury.

McKinlay, J.B. (1988) 'Introduction', *The Milbank Quarterly* 66(2): 1–9.

Marshall, T.H. (1939) 'The recent history of professionalism in relation to social structure and social policy', *Canadian Journal of Economics and Political Science* 5: 325–40.

Meiksins, P.F. and Watson, J.M. (1989) 'Professional autonomy and organizational constraint: the case of engineers', *The Sociological Quarterly* 30(4): 561–85.

Moore, W.E. (1970) *Professions: Roles and Rules*, New York: Russell Sage Foundation.

Navarro, V. (1988) 'Professional dominance or proletarianisation? Neither', *The Milbank Quarterly* 66(2): 57–75.

Parsons, T. (1939) 'The professions and social structure', *Social Forces* 17: 457–67.

Platt, A.M. (1969) *The Child Savers: The Invention of Delinquency*, Chicago: University of Chicago Press.

Rothman, D.J. (1971) *The Discovery of the Asylum*, Boston, MA: Little, Brown.

Saks, M. (1983) 'Removing the blinkers? A critique of recent contributions to the sociology of professions', *The Sociological Quarterly* 31(1): 1–21.

Scott, W.R. (1985) 'Conflicting levels of rationality: regulators, managers and professionals in the medical care sector', *The Journal of Health Administration Education* 3(2): Pt. II, 113–31.

Simon, W.H. (1985) 'Babbitt v. Brandeis: the decline of the professional ideal', *Stanford Law Review* 37: 565–87.

Spencer, H. (1914) *The Principles of Sociology* Vol. 3, New York: Appleton.

Stewart, R. (undated) 'Involving doctors in general management', Templeton Series, Paper 5, Bristol: National Health Service Training Agency.

Tawney, R.H. (1920) *The Acquisitive Society*, New York: Harcourt Brace.

Turner, C. and Hodge, M.N. (1970) 'Occupations and professions', in J.A. Jackson (ed.) *Professions and Professionalisation*, Cambridge: Cambridge University Press.

Webb, S. and Webb, B. (1917) 'Special supplement on professional associations', *New Statesman*, 211: 9.

Wilensky, H.L. (1964) 'The professionalization of everyone?', *American Journal of Sociology* 70: 137–58.

11 Betwixt and between

Part-time GPs and the flexible working question

Ruth Pinder

Introduction

> I think it would be quite hard for me to go into a practice as a part-time principal or whatever I get. There'll be a part of me that thinks 'hang on, I'm better than that' you know. I'll feel that sense of demotion.
>
> (37-year-old full-time partner)

> I accept that I am part-time, *very* part-time, and as such the practice has accommodated me very well. They've let me know they respect me. I feel happy with the balance I've got right now. If I was to do more, I wouldn't do anything right – rather I'd feel too torn between the two. And that's a problem not only for full-time women, but men as well.
>
> (36-year-old retainer[1])

> There's no comparison between now and before the formation of the NANP [National Association of Non-Principals]. Old attitudes and prejudices are shifting. They're totally irrelevant to modern practice.
>
> (Carter 1998)

In the contemporary era the old adage, 50 hours for 50 weeks for 50 years, is losing its edge as people adapt to the changing demands of the labour force. General practice is no exception to this. Yet as the above quotations show, the question of flexible working for GPs is fraught with contradictions.

As women secure a firmer footing in general practice, the number of GPs wishing to work flexible hours is increasing, and it is estimated that 31 per cent (some 7,000) of all female unrestricted principals[2] now work part-time (Chambers *et al.* 1998). Recent surveys have found a strong groundswell of opinion in favour of more part-time posts in the profession (Allen 1992; *General Practitioner* 1996). During their vocational training, registrars are now asked to think carefully about the importance of personal relationships and the need to strike a balance between work and family (Willows 1997). Moreover, the growing evidence on stress in general practice (Rout and Rout 1993; Chambers and Maxwell 1996; Myerson 1997) is likely to make flexible working for both sexes a more attractive proposition. While the Department of Health and the General

Medical Services Committee may be concerned with notions of justice and equity, they are equally aware of the need to promote a good image, recognising the fact that patients often prefer women doctors. A strong political message underpins the flexibility debate: more family-friendly work policies and practices are seen as an important key to solving the recruitment crisis in general practice. *Pulse* (one of the weekly magazines for GPs) ran a series of features on this theme, and a typical heading read 'Needs of women GPs will be pivotal to solving crisis' (1996).

Some troubling issues are at stake. If flexibility in general practice is 'good for us', why does part-timing still have difficulty establishing its credentials (Gilley 1994; Baker *et al.* 1995; Brooks 1998)? Why is respect for women's choices about the work–family balance still frequently belied in practice? How far is 'getting the balance right' the same balance for women as it is for men? When studies show overwhelmingly that women still shoulder a disproportionate responsibility for domestic and childcare arrangements (Reeves and Gallagher 1990; Segal 1990), is flexibility primarily a women's question? And, more difficult still, what pictures in our heads are being rejected when part-timing is still associated with 'a lack of commitment'? Surveys suggest that significant discrimination against women GPs occurs in general practice (*Doctor* 1996): one in three women GPs (including non-principals) believed they were less likely to have a say in the running of the practice than their male colleagues; and more than one-fifth of women GPs feel that they were less highly regarded than their male colleagues. The NHS Wales Opportunity 2000 project (1996) noted: 'Many women and part-time partners, associates, retainers and locums[3] are treated less favourably in employment terms with regard to salary, allowances and job content.'

While more flexible working options are likely to make it more attractive for women GPs to stay in the profession, Cockburn (1991: 92) argues: 'the more women are permitted various kinds of flexibility in relation to work to enable them to cope with motherhood and other domestic responsibilities, the more they can be dismissed as "different", less serious than male employees'.

Moreover, none of the high profile discourses highlights the tensions between the desirable aspects of flexibility – innovation, creativity, responsiveness to change – and its less attractive features, when flexibility may mean working without opportunity for advancement, paid vacations, paid sick leave or health insurance. The crucial question is: flexibility for whom?

Significant practical questions flow from a consideration of these issues: namely, how can GPs most equitably address the nagging question of 'how much work for how much pay?' When issues of allocation are at stake, as West and Zimmerman (1998: 183) point out, 'significant social categories such as "female" and "male" seem to become pointedly relevant'.

Background: making wider connections

The search for predictability and order is a key to getting by in our lives. We long for clear lines and simple messages, blacks and whites rather than pale shades of grey (Douglas 1966; Perin 1988). Sibley (1995: 32) argues that 'the need to make sense of the world by categorizing things on the basis of crisp sets A, not-A . . . is evident in most cultures'. It reflects the continuing need to define the contours of normality and to eliminate difference.

Thus social categories are loaded with meaning about the kinds and desirability of the behaviours expected of each. To this end every culture establishes boundaries between what is and what is not, who belongs and who does not, and our identities are carved round these definitions. Where people are neither quite one thing nor another we feel uneasy. Ambiguity is unsettling, and intellectually we have a great deal of trouble with something that both is and is not. As Ardener (1993: 19) argues, 'where rules of separation obtain, many difficulties arise at critical points'. As groups have differential power to impose their classifications on others, intolerance often follows in the wake of the drive to 'clean up' anomalies.

The newly formed NANP is raising the profile of part-time GPs in unprecedented ways. Who is to be included, who excluded? Words speak volumes: the 1997 Birmingham Conference of Non-Principals, recognising the potentially divisive effect of a language of special needs and special provision, attempted to abolish the word 'non-principal', but struggled to arrive at a satisfactory alternative. Where is non-principals' main commitment? To home or to work? For GPs who are 'betwixt and between' the public (rational) world of work and the private (feeling) world of the family, the lack of clarity of their status may be unsettling. Belonging simultaneously to two different worlds may be 'a symbolic breaking of that which should be joined or the joining of that which should be separate' (Douglas 1966, cited in Perin 1988: 11).

A moral charge underpins these difficulties. Difference is not merely difference: it involves judgements about 'right' and 'wrong' difference. Some GPs feel that women (and men) should align themselves more clearly on one side of the line or the other. There has been an appropriate reaction against the polarisation of the public–private division (Lopatea 1993): we may have lost sight of the blurred edges between work and family time, the extent to which work rhythms punctuate family time, or the way family and childcare crises often penetrate the workplace (Daly 1996). Simply by virtue of their position, part-timers and non-principals cannot help calling into question some of the values and precepts which those unequivocally 'there' take for granted.

Painting a broader canvas

Polemical writings apart, the empirical writing by GPs themselves on gender in general practice is almost exclusively quantitative (Baker *et al.* 1995; Chambers and Campbell 1996; *Doctor* 1996). While surveys play an important role in mapping the dimensions, they pay comparatively little attention to GPs' 'local moral worlds' (Kleinman 1996). Taking a leaf from the more rounded contributions of social scientists, this chapter offers a different perspective. Drawing on in-depth interviews with a group of 25 women GPs at differing positions within the life course, and some initial interviews currently being conducted with a comparable group of male GPs to provide a counterpoint, it explores not only what people are saying, it also tries to understand why they are saying it: what fuels some of the worries about flexibility? What is at stake?

The chapter argues, first, that at a time when all professions are undergoing radical change, part of the problem lies in a discomfort with people 'on the margins'. The 'comfort of belonging' (Perin 1977, 1988) is a major issue for any social group, and general practice is no exception. The question of where women non-principals belong is integrally related to perceptions about the nature and extent of their commitment to general practice. Second, in suggesting that such questions cannot be understood in isolation from the many other economic, social and political changes which are taking place in and around the profession, it explores some ways in which mapping those invisible structures might pave the way towards a modest agenda for change.

Contested meanings: the 'right' or the 'wrong' side of the line?

Some women GPs who tried to juggle career and family responsibilities experienced no untoward difficulties negotiating part-time status and a position of respect from their partners. One GP, who had taken several non-principal posts while bringing up her family, reflected with some satisfaction:

> When I look back, I feel proud that I have done this and worked hard and done something for myself. I feel more professional because of the experience.

Greater life experience gave women an added edge in contributing to their partnerships later: 'because I mixed with the world, played other games' (course organiser) they were 'more rounded people'. Non-principals had different skills to contribute, 'a broader vision to offer', as one male GP put it. Moreover, flexible working had distinct advantages, both for the practice and for non-principals themselves. One newly established partner had recently appointed a clinical assistant:

> It was a really excellent solution to a gap in the running of a practice. There would be absolutely no way we could offer the sort of salary which would attract a new partner, and we had quite a lot of work that we just weren't able to do adequately, and we needed more manpower. Having somone who could be there on a permanent basis who we and the patients could get to know, is much more satisfactory than having people coming in and out . . . I actually admire our assistant hugely for the way she does set her boundaries, she just doesn't let general practice overwhelm any other aspects of her life. I can really identify with that . . . But it is different from the way the rest of us work. She does what we need her to be there for exceedingly well, and she's happy with the arrangement.

Combining familiar things in an unfamiliar way seemed to pose no undue threat here: difference could be accommodated without upsetting the social fabric of the practice. It also had important financial advantages: extending the bound-aries of the 'normal' working day allows a practice to claim more money for additional staff and resources.

Yet, offering flexibility simultaneously involved signalling to one's partners a reduced career ambition. With the exception of two informants, most women in the study did not want high-powered careers, and often pointedly avoided the 'masculine' activities, such as the finances, in their practice. (The term 'femin-ist' was generally considered a pejorative label.) For those who did, one of the ways to keep a part-time schedule without violating the unspoken rules of the practice was to work more like a full-timer. Hayden (1991: 733) notes that 'Although many women nominally work part-time, their rates of consultation and the time they spend with patients are almost identical with those of their male partners.' Evidence from this study goes further: it suggests that women spend *more* time with their patients than do their male colleagues, as 'women invariably pick up the emotional problems' (full-time female partner). More-over, it raised provocative questions about the opposition of 'emotional' woman to 'unemotional man' (Lupton 1998), and the negative connotations with which vulnerability is still regarded in medicine. However, the question of how part-time was part-time work aroused scepticism in some male GPs: 'women part-timers say they work more like full-time GPs, but they don't really' (GP tutor).

Moreover, being on the 'wrong' side of the line – working less than full-time – still evoked some unfavourable reactions, such as the fear of 'not being taken seriously', or 'using the system for your own ends'. 'You're seen as quirky, different, not going with the flow' (female locum GP). The constant worry was, as one non-principal put it, that 'I'm not doing enough, whatever "enough" is'. The symbolic significance of working even fractionally less than full-time was confirmed by this course organiser:

> Dropping one session, that little bit makes all the difference in terms of status. You become three-quarters time with three-quarters pay and three-quarters say in the running of the practice. You're much more likely to meet charges of 'not pulling your weight' then.

Such comments reflect the unease with new working patterns which might compromise high standards of professionalism and dedication to patients, an intense source of pride and identity to GPs. Worries about ensuring part-timers' standards of clinical competence following maternity leave frequently surfaced. Although some GPs argued: 'it's rather like riding a bicycle, it's always there once you have it', lack of confidence was a major concern, and retraining schemes are currently addressing this question. It has been proposed that the body of knowledge required for professional practice is too vast to accommodate a part-time commitment only.

Crucially, notions of flexibility were often at variance with the increasing standardisation inherent in contemporary healthcare delivery which requires GPs to be at their desk for large tracts of their time, a trend likely to continue with the formation of primary care groups. As this course organiser commented:

> Flexibility doesn't work round here. A lot of doctors still think women should be looking after their children at home. Flexibility is one of those things that are good in theory but don't work very well in practice, well not round here anyway. The *system* is inflexible, you can't negotiate in and out of more hours or less.

'Lack of commitment' and a loss of 'specialness'?

Ensuring appropriate standards of clinical competence was only part of the problem. When boundaries are no longer clear-cut, what are the dangers to those safely ensconced? Most of the anxieties about part-timing centred around the question of 'commitment', or the perceived lack of it, to the practice. One GP, with a young family, now working full-time in a go-ahead practice, knew the difficulties of working part-time all too well. Nevertheless, competing imperatives guided her thinking:

> Part-timing is a bit marginal. Part-timers are saying by their actions: 'There's something as important as medicine in my life', and that's quite a strong statement to make. We chose medicine. If you're part-timing, you're not quite one of us . . . You're not seen as committed by other women, as well as by other men. I was asked recently: 'how would you feel about having a part-time partner?' I wouldn't want it. When you know how much work is involved around the practice, the lifestyle. Logistically it's harder to provide continuity of care. You're not *there*. It's a fact.

> RP: Like renting a house rather than being an owner-occupier?

> That's it exactly. And clinical assistants are out of the equation completely. They've made statements about themselves, not wanting the responsibility.

The desire for peer group approval and the sense of belonging to a profession this GP loved often outweighed other considerations. Like tenants renting a property, non-principals had made the choice of not having the 'bother' of a house: commitment and shorter hours were mutually exclusive. In a profession traditionally organised around continuous care for patients, lack of permanence and fragmentation of care raised the possibility of different motivations, different levels of responsibility to the practice. With partnership (or ownership), on the other hand, came prestige, stability, security and predictability.

GPs routinely worried about covering the workload and overloading their colleagues when they were unavailable. A potentially de-stabilising trend had emerged, as this course organiser reflected:

'Part-timers' not only want to work part-time, but to work *selected* part-time, normal working day hours, rather than weekends or evenings.

She recalled interviewing one of her 'girls', who said

'I'm doing far too much work and not getting a fair share of the income.' She'd wound herself up. I suggested we'd have a look and see exactly what was going on in her practice and we went through exactly what each part-ner did, how many surgeries, how many weekends, who's the trainer, who does the fundholding, who's on the LMC [local medical committee]. When we got the list completed, she was actually doing less than half the work her full-time partners were doing. She was quite stunned and in fact rang me up about six months later and said she'd decided to become a trainer! She'd decided to do some extra as well.

Drawn into the pressure to 'be like us', she narrated this incident to me entirely without irony: implicit norms about what was an appropriate investment of time were taken for granted. Other partners (male and female) stressed the obvious aspects of a full-time contribution to the practice:

What worries me is the commitment, and that's the practice and the run-ning of the practice. I want the commitment because I don't want to have to do all the work. If everyone's committed, they're all sharing out work equally, that's how I have it impacting on me . . . I'm not too worried about the medicine side of it, I don't see why part-timing should lower standards, it's the nitty-gritty of the practice running, keeping the staff happy and making sure that the notes are in order, things like that.

Underpinning the material 'facts' of her concerns were idealised notions about equality in a situation where equal workloads are notoriously difficult to define and quantify.

Commitment was presented almost exclusively as a reification: you either have 'it' or you don't. One male senior partner now encourages his female partners 'not to stint on childcare in case there's an emergency and you haven't got the back-up'. Yet his own commitment was not entirely foolproof: he, too, was obliged to take time out to respond to a crisis with his ageing parents. As one academic male GP, planning to return to general practice on a one day per week basis, put it insightfully:

There's still the sense that *either* you're committed *or* you're not. There's an absolutist sense to the word . . . It's partly linguistic, nobody would say 'I'm partly committed!' It's absolutist in the word, but in terms of its meaning, no. You can be completely committed doing one session a week, as long as you deal with what that half day a week means in terms of your responsibil-ity to your colleagues and to your patients.

As the recent increase in the number of sessions which retainers are allowed to work also indicates, notions of appropriateness were constantly shifting. What constituted the minimum acceptable amount of sessions necessary to maintain a viable presence was fluid and arbitrary: there were as many 'bottom lines' as there were practitioners who sought to justify their own particular working balances.

Underpinning worries about part-timers' lack of commitment lay apprehensions about the growth of a salaried service undermining the independent contractor status – and hence earning power – of GPs, as well as a fear that general practice was becoming less personal, more instrumental. It is the import as much as the actuality which is at stake here: what it might imply by way of a practitioner's ability to predict and order the world. GPs sometimes felt that they were reduced to being mere technicians. The following full-time female partner reflected this awareness:

> I suppose it's the cliché, particularly for GPs who've been in general practice for a long time, they've always thought of it as being a real vocation, the lynchpin of their lives. So people are coming along now and saying 'no thanks' – and they're just not doing that. Maybe it's going to have some knock-on effects on all sorts of things. Maybe the respect that GPs are held in if it's just becoming a nine to five job, then how can it be something more than just a normal job? Most people do feel that what they're doing is much more valuable.

> RP: Medicine's a bit special?

> That's right.

Working more routine hours might mean a loss of specialness in a profession which has traditionally been associated with charisma, the sacred rather than the mundane (Horobin 1983), a speculation confirmed by a part-time female GP at a gender workshop with registrars run by the author. However, other factors were already eroding the moral boundaries of the profession (Armstrong 1988; Ehrlich 1998). The curtailment of doctors' out-of-hours commitment and the growth of co-operatives are merely the newest contenders in a changing ethos which is reducing GPs' traditional 24-hour availability to their patients.

The part-time partner: a very real anomaly?

The blurring of boundaries was more evident in some positions in general practice than in others. Being a part-time partner, for example, smudged the lines in complex ways.

The following GP had invested considerable energy in re-locating her practice in central London. However, the strain involved was exacerbated by her additional responsibilities as a part-time partner. At interview she had reached a crisis point in her life, and was seriously depressed:

> You see my life would have been absolutely fine if I could have been a smaller cog in a big wheel. At the start, I'd always been ambitious and I knew I could be a senior partner quite quickly, but if I'd known what I know now, I'd have gone into a more established practice with more part-ners where I could have taken a quieter role.

> RP: So the issue was being part-time and being a senior partner at the same time?

> That's right. Having to make decisions and be the one to carry the can and having a family on top of that . . . I'm a perfectionist and I think it's been my downfall, I've been trying to juggle too many balls in the air at one time and I can't do it any more.

The demands were not compatible: she could not comfortably shuttle between the two worlds.

More routine difficulties arose for other GPs in maintaining a clear separation between work and home, as this part-time partner, with four sessions a week, explained:

> There has been this problem about meetings from time to time. The full-time partners say 'you weren't there'. Then I say 'It's my time off', other-wise I'd be going in all the time and not getting paid for what I'm doing. But again I'm saying 'Anything urgent, I'm quite happy to be contacted at home.' I don't grumble.

Despite a strong professional commitment, her limits were not always suffi-ciently respected. Time with her family was poachable in a way that for those with two part-time *paid* jobs it was not. Was she on duty when, strictly speak-ing, this was private family time? Where were the boundaries drawn?

Others had more positive views about mixing categories, as this part-time partner, working in a more rural practice with her (part-time GP) husband, explained:

> I can only say that it's worked for me, and I suspect it works round here, there are quite a lot of women who are part-time partners. It's more diffi-cult to do the administrative stuff if you're part-time, and it's very easy to feel that you don't participate in the decisions that are taken . . . So it's quite easy to feel that things are happening without you, well then, what's the point. But I certainly wouldn't go as far as saying you shouldn't have partners who are part-time, because that's the thin end of the wedge, isn't it. If you only have clinical assistants, then you don't get the balance right

with organising the practice, they don't have any input with anything, just number-crunching the patients. No, I don't think part-time partners should be relegated to being assistants.

Despite some anxieties, crossing boundaries was a viable compromise, particularly in an area where the maintenance of general practice coverage relied heavily on a pool of women working flexible hours. A balanced practice needed to be attentive to difference: it required alternative kinds of contributions.

Some room for manoeuvre in practice organisation had allowed two female part-time partners to tailor their practice exactly to fit their childcare requirements, as this female GP, now winding down her hours, remembered:

> My current partner had two young children and we both saw eye to eye. We had a room set aside with a telly in it and games, and if any child was on holiday or ill, we'd bring the child to work. We decided to make the practice so that we could cope, being two married women with children who wanted also to be mothers. Very often there'd be children loitering around, hers and mine, *and* the practice paid for a colour TV licence! This, I think, is a very good model for women for the future . . . When I came in as a part-time partner, we shaped the practice so there was never more than one doctor on in the evening. *We* decided we would do the bulk of the work in the morning so that we were home when the children came home. And this has been the philosophy of the practice.

Tilting at the margins was always possible. Women were able to devise creative solutions to the problem of childcare, challenging the notion of public space as uncontaminated by the feeling (and feeding) work of children. However, with the streamlining implicit in the formation of new primary care groups, women will need to search out other crevices when combining work and childcare.

A correct chronology of life

GPs are still expected to have negotiated life's competitive hazards, medical school, vocational training, membership of the Royal College of General Practitioners, passing through its mundane stages to the final social category, that of full-time partnership. A minutely differentiated hierarchy (or pecking order – Allen 1992) was observable, with the (senior) partner at the apex. Despite the fact that full-time work is losing its edge, the full-time partner still carries a distinct aura. To 'arrive' in general practice, there is a 'natural' progression for GPs to follow, and being a locum was the first step on the ladder. As Perin (1977: 44) notes, 'The life cycle is believed to consist of moving from a less safe to a more safe status.' Those considered most safe are those who are settled, who have not changed categories for some time.

Locums were, by definition, in transition. However, those on the move found being 'neither quite in nor quite out' unsettling. Although locums felt there were important advantages to 'biding their time so that they might pick and choose the best practice', GPs were also relieved when the ambiguities of locum status were finally resolved and they became partners. Two GP locums had negotiated this transition during interviews, as this full-time GP, after a trying time feeling herself 'neither fish nor fowl', explained:

> Now I feel totally that I'm part of the team, absolutely 100 per cent along-side everyone else, and I really don't feel any uncertainty about that. That's a very different feeling from how I felt before . . . You don't get anything definite *said*, but everyone in the practice knows the difference, the recep-tionist staff, particularly the ones who've been there a long time, are slightly disappointed if you're only a locum or whatever.

In a profession traditionally reluctant to lend its seal of approval to movement between practices, being in transition was not entirely safe. GP locums were expected to change categories, but there was always the possibility that they might never cease being locums. Despite recent challenges to this, the long-term locum may be an anomaly in a profession where 'arrival' is still manifested in being a full-time (senior) partner.

Other non-principals were anxious to ensure that they projected some semblance of stability, both to the practice and to their patients. This retainer explained:

> I work like a *regular* locum, but that's me. I feel that commitment, I am there. When patients ask me 'Are you here for good?' I say 'yes', because that's how I feel. I don't want to feel like a locum coming in a few months a year and then stopping.

Working one session per week, this GP nonetheless saw herself as permanent and stable, providing that continuity of care which was the bedrock of general practice. She was not just 'passing through'. Yet, eighteen months later, that position was becoming increasingly untenable for her, and she was seriously considering opting out of medicine altogether.

Older traditions were giving way to a new wave of young registrars, less prepared to give their all to patients. This young male LIZ EI (London Initiative Zone Educational Initiative) doctor, working part of each week in two different practices, had a cool eye on keeping the pressures of modern medicine at bay:

> When you're working in practices, you tend to get engulfed in things, whereas working as an assistant and maybe job-sharing, there's a little more distance. There are much less pressured ways of doing medicine and look-ing after children. If you're a partner, you're expected to be there, fully taking your share in whatever's done, chairing meetings, being part of management decisions. You just really pull your weight. Whereas as an assistant, you're more like a long-term locum, accepted by the practice and

the patients, who feel quite happy about it. I mean it's quite permanent, which makes everyone feel better about it, but without the same responsibilities. You get the good without the bad.

Although the LIZ EI scheme has recently been disbanded, alternative career pathways, to counter the pressure in general practice, were gradually finding their way into the profession. Working in a practice where no one else was full-time made weaving in one's own flexible style easier. Yet it is important not to exaggerate the degree to which things have changed: the indications were that most GPs who had tasted a more varied professional career were nonetheless prepared to pick up a traditional work life later on. The pull of belonging still held members in its sway.

Discussion

GPs' accounts have shown the many contradictions and paradoxes which surround the subject of flexible working options. A complex picture suggests itself, one dominated as much by the rhetoric of change as change itself. This chapter has argued that those who occupy ambiguous or weakly defined roles may be seen as less safe, less reliable, provoking anxieties about loyalty in a profession where full-time partnership is still the major social category. Despite modest change, (masculine) full-time work still retained its symbolic significance as the unnamed standard, the 'natural', 'right' and 'obvious' path, from which (mainly female) flexible working was a deviation. Yet as Coles (1984) noted, 'People are many things. The mind has many rooms'. Not only was there ambiguity – and anxiety – about blurred boundaries between different kinds of part-time statuses. Women were sometimes ambivalent and defensive about their own attitudes to flexible working; sometimes reproving, sometimes approving. In our speeded-up culture, there is enormous pressure on us to be internally consistent, to think in straight clear lines, to be either superwoman or earth mother, but not both.

What distinguishes locums from retainers, clinical assistants from part-time principals, and non-principals from full-time principals are not merely 'the facts'. Boundaries were also symbolic. Distinctions were weighted with meaning concerning the desirability, or otherwise, of certain behaviours thought to characterise non-principals, particularly women: clock watching, or not doing 'enough'. Women part-timers carried more than their fair share of emotional baggage for any errors. A hefty moral charge underpinned the anxieties, illustrating much wider social processes whereby those who are 'different' accumulate deficits. Separating the reality from the construction is always problematic.

An ideology of commitment

To some extent, the notion of commitment has replaced the more traditional ideology of 24-hour availability to patients. As shown, non-principals' apparent 'lack of commitment' to the practice was the focus of considerable anxiety: indeed, shorter hours and commitment were a contradiction in terms. Women were caught in the trap of offering flexibility but signalling divided loyalties, a lack of ambition, and avoidance of responsibility. Commitment is both a material 'fact' and a symbol of far more potent apprehensions. Like continuity of care, which it closely parallels, it is an ideal, a mobilising metaphor, which articulates deeply held beliefs about belonging in a profession where the role of the full-time partner still signifies stability, order and coherence. It was seen in absolutist terms, as a reification, something which full-timers immutably 'had' and an ideal from which part-timers necessarily deviated. However, notions of appropriateness were fluid and contingent: each GP had his/her own 'bottom line'. Symbols are powerful, Cohen (1985) argues, because they are imprecise. We know generally what they mean, yet they have a large repertoire of alternative meanings.

The ideology also reflects an intense nostalgia for the past, for 'the good old days' of general practice when things were (apparently) simpler, the lines clearer, as well as fears for the future of a profession which, like others, is increasingly being seen as instrumental and technical (see Fournier's chapter in this volume). GPs were trying to articulate a shared coherent vision of general practice in the face of far-reaching changes. The prospect of a profession becoming a 'nation of part-timers', with its implied loss of 'specialness', galvanised anxieties, so that it was easy to lose sight of the fact that 'we're all part-timers in a sense, we go on holiday and we get sick' (full-time female GP). Yet although the framework for delivery of care may be changing quite dramatically, the part-timers and non-principals interviewed still demonstrated an impressive desire to be of service: there was no shortage of dedication.

Layers of significance

In rolling out gender as 'the problem', it is important that this does not obscure the wider socio-economic and political issues in which the flexibility debate is embedded. Part-time women found themselves at the centre of many competing imperatives: personal demands, such as guilt about 'not being there' for their children, and attempts by both sexes to achieve a more balanced lifestyle; professional demands 'not to waste their expensive training', to 'do the job properly'; organisational pressures, such as the increasing fragmentation of tasks in multi-purpose health centres (Armstrong 1988), the decline in home visiting, the growing involvement of nurses, anxieties concerning demands for the profession to become salaried, and, most recent of all, the growth of co-operatives (Ehrlich 1998). Part-time women were also caught in the grip of wider contemporary trends: concerns about the growing feminisation of the workforce (and its inevitable backlash); the disproportionately faster rate of change for women than for men (Thompson and Walker 1989; Reeves and Gallagher 1990); contradictory perceptions about the work ethic itself (*Sunday Times* 1997a,b); and the massive increase in the number of hours worked generally in the labour force (Hochschild 1997; Segal 1998). The personal and the professional could not be syphoned off into separate compartments. Yet, despite some evidence that men are taking more responsibility at home (Segal 1990, 1998; Seidler 1994), the modern dilemma of how to combine career and family is still primarily a woman's problem.

A way forward: expecting homogeneity, valuing difference

The findings suggested that some non-principals were actively shaping their own future, and contesting some of the negative stereotypes about part-time work. The first NANP conference in October 1998 showed doctors taking a more robust attitude towards managing their difference. The possibility that women coming into medicine would do things differently from men, that they would not step into power without problematising or modifying it, may slowly be taking root. At the same time, a strong conservative force was evident, prompting the question: is change going to be liberal but not radical? Will general practice work on a short or long agenda of reform (Lees and Scott 1990; Cockburn 1991)? Putting equal opportunities in place cannot simply be a matter of 'topping up', or rectifying a few wrongs, important though discrete adjustments may be. A longer agenda involves transforming power relations within medicine; an understanding of how structured inequality arose in the first place, and how it continues to be produced and reproduced outside as well as within general practice (Elston 1993); and an appreciation of the way masculinity is embodied in full-time work, to become 'the natural', 'obvious' way of doing things. It also requires a recognition of men's own discomfort with their powerful positions, and some women's disillusionment with the power they may have gained.

Creativity and innovation tend to take place at the margins rather than at the centre. Both men and women will need to work out ways of dealing with, and possibly disagreeing with, one another, and to recognise that role complexity may be both socially enriching and revitalising (Coser 1991). Apprehensions about part-timing are likely to have a comparatively short history as people learn to rub along with each other.

For flexible working to succeed, it means recognising that the varied experiences of women (and men) can contribute positively to a healthy and vibrant profession. Difference can be the 'right' difference if GPs have the ears to hear.

Huxley (1949) recognised half a century ago that 'The good life can only be lived in a society in which tidiness is preached and practised, but not too fanatically, and where efficiency is always haloed, as it were, by a tolerated margin of mess.'

Acknowledgements

I gratefully acknowledge the continued support of the Royal College of General Practitioners in funding the first research grant (October 1996–September 1997), and extending it for a further two years (March 1998–February 2000). The chapter is based on this work.

Notes

1 Retainers are women GPs who wish to devote more time to child care while simultaneously maintaining a foothold in the profession. They must work at least 12 sessions over a year, but not more than four sessions a week.
2 Principals are partners in the practice who share in the capital investment and rewards according to privately negotiated proportions, whereas non-principals do not share the responsibility of running a business.
3 Locums are male or female GPs who are non-principals and who work in practices on an ad hoc basis as required. Like retainers, they have traditionally had few rights – a situation the NANP is attempting to redress.

References

Abbott, A. (1988) *The System of Professions: An Essay on the Division of Expert Labor*, Chicago: University of Chicago Press.
Allen, I. (1992) *Part-time Working in General Practice*, London: Policy Studies Institute.
Ardener, S. (ed.) (1993) *Women and Space: Ground Rules and Social Maps*, Oxford: Berg Publishers.
Armstrong, D. (1988) 'Space and time in British general practice', in M. Lock and D. Gordon (eds) *Biomedicine Examined*, Kluwer Academic Publishers, Dordrecht: Reidel, pp. 207–35.
Baker, M., Williams, J. and Petchey, R. (1995) 'GPs in principle but not in practice: a study of vocationally trained doctors not currently working as principals', *British Medical Journal* 310: 1301–4.
Brooks, F. (1998) 'Women in general practice: responding to the sexual division of labour', *Social Science and Medicine* 47(2): 181–93.
Carter, G. (1998) 'Quality non-principals in a quality NHS', paper given at the First Non-Principals Conference, Norwich.
Chambers, R. and Campbell, I. (1996) 'Gender differences in general practitioners at work', *British Journal of General Practice* 46: 291–3.
Chambers, R. and Maxwell R. (1996) 'Helping sick doctors', *British Medical Journal* 312: 722–3.
Chambers, R., Field, S. and Muller, E. (1998) 'Key points arising from the national workshop: educating GP non-principals', *Education for General Practice* (supplement) 9(l): 112–15.
Cockburn, C. (1991) *In the Way of Women: Men's Resistance to Sex Equality in Organisations*, Basingstoke: Macmillan.
Cohen, A. (1985) *The Symbolic Construction of Community*, London: Routledge.
Coles, R. (1984) in *Higher Education*, 18 July.
Coser, R. (1991) *In Defence of Modernity: Role Complexity and Individual Autonomy*, Stanford, CA: Stanford University Press.
Daly, K.J. (1996) *Families and Time: Keeping Pace in a Hurried Culture*, Thousand Oaks, CA: Sage.
Doctor (1996) 'Survey: women's work', 7 June.
Douglas, M. (1966) *Purity and Danger: An Analysis of the Concepts of Pollution and Taboo*, London: Routledge.
Ehrlich, K. (1998) 'Out of hours, out of the question? Questioning assumptions underlying the current debate about demand for "out of hours" consultations in primary care', paper delivered at the BSA Medical Sociology Conference, York.

Elston, M.A. (1993) 'Woman doctors in a changing profession', in E. Riska and K. Weger (eds) *Gender, Work and Medicine*, London: Sage.

General Practitioner (1996) Flexible working survey, 20 December.

Gilley, J. (1994) '"Lady doctors" take on tokenism', *Young Principal*, September p. 12.

Hayden, J. (1991) 'Women in general practice: time to equalise the opportunities', *British Medical Journal* 303: 733–4.

Hochschild, A. (1997) *The Time Bind: When Work Becomes Home and Home Becomes Work*, New York: Henry Holt.

Horobin, G. (1983) 'Professional mystery: the maintenance of charisma in general medical practice', in R. Dingwall and P. Lewis (eds) *The Sociology of the Professions: Lawyers, Doctors and Others*, Basingstoke: Macmillan.

Huxley, A. (1949) *Prisons. The Carceri Etchings by Piranesi*, London: Trianon Press.

Kleinman, A. (1996) *Writing at the Margins: The Discourse between Anthropology and Medicine*, Berkeley: University of California.

Lees, S. and Scott, M. (1990) 'Equal opportunities: rhetoric or action?', *Gender and Education* 2(3): 333–43.

Lopatea, H.Z. (1993) 'The interweave of public and private: women's challenge to American society', *Journal of Marriage and Family* 55: 176–90.

Lupton, D. (1998) *The Emotional Self*, London: Sage.

Myerson, S. (1997) 'Seven women GPs' perceptions of their strategies and the impact of these on their private and professional lives', *Journal of Management in Medicine* 2(1): 8–14.

NHS Wales Opportunity 2000 (1996) *The Future of General Practice: The Role of Women Doctors*, Conference Report.

Perin, C. (1977) *Everything in Its Place: Social Order and Land Use*, Princeton, NJ: Princeton University Press.

—— (1988) *Belonging in America: Reading between the Lines*, Madison: University of Wisconsin Press.

Pulse (1996) 'Needs of women GPs will be pivotal to solving crisis', 7 December.

Reeves, P. and Gallagher, R. (1990) *Beyond the Second Sex: New Directions in the Anthropology of Gender*, Pittsburgh: University of Pennsylvania Press.

Rout, U. and Rout, J.K. (1993) *Stress and General Practitioners*, Dordrecht: Kluwer.

Segal, L. (1990) *Slow Motion: Changing Masculinities and Changing Men*, London: Virago Press.

—— (1998) 'The F-Word', seminar series at the South Bank, London, October.

Seidler, V. (1994) *Unreasonable Men: Masculinity and Social Theory*, London: Routledge.

Sibley, D. (1995) *Geographies of Exclusion*, London: Routledge.

Sunday Times (1997a) 'Work: the new way to escape family life', 23 April.

Sunday Times (1997b) 'Wife, mother, breadwinner: is the effort killing you?', 1 June.

Thompson, L. and Walker, A.J. (1989) 'Gender in families: women and men in marriage, work, and parenthood', *Journal of Marriage and the Family* 51: 845–71.

West, C. and Zimmerman, D. (1998) 'Doing gender' in K. Myers, C. Anderson and B. Risman (eds) *Feminist Foundations: Towards Transforming Sociology*, Thousand Oaks, CA: Sage, pp. 16–17.

Willows, R. (1997) Personal communication.

Part V

Professionalism and emotion management

12 Mixed feelings

Emotion management in a caring profession

Sharon C. Bolton

When looking at the caring professions,[1] nurses are by far the largest occupational group. Numbering half a million in Britain, they account for two-thirds of the National Health Service (NHS) workforce, and one-third of the health service budget is spent solely on nurses' pay (Labour Research 1997). The sheer size of their numbers and the nature of their 'care work' – within the context of the dramatic recent reforms to the NHS – make nurses an interesting occupational group to study.

To understand a nurse's work – the necessary emotion management skills involved, and how the boundaries surrounding a nurse's ability to provide 'care' are changing – it might be argued that their work should be viewed within the context of a variety of processes: political, managerial and economic. The combined effect of these ongoing processes has been succinctly described as the 'enterprise culture' (du Gay 1992). What this represents are changes that have affected organisations and their members in general, with the public services being the most dramatically influenced. The result is that differences between public service and private sector organisations are gradually being eradicated. This blurring of the boundaries between public welfare services and private commercial ventures can be better understood by examining the foundation of the enterprise culture, its effects on organisations in general, and how the pervading management philosophy attempts to force public sector organisations to emulate their private sector counterparts. Such an examination will, in turn, allow an understanding of the driving force behind the 'new' NHS and give some insight into how management-led 'quality' initiatives have deeply affected the use of nurses' emotion management skills.

Emotional investment is increasingly recognised as an essential, although often under-valued, element of nurses' work. Descriptive terms such as 'emotional labour' and 'sentimental work' are used as a means of stressing its importance (Strauss *et al.* 1982; Smith 1988, 1992; James 1989, 1992, 1993). However, 'care work', as with many other types of work, requires different forms of emotion management, and the use of labels such as 'emotional labour' tend to underestimate its complexity. Throughout a working day nurses, using their emotion management skills, are able to present a variety of 'faces'; perhaps their performances may be better understood if they are classified into four distinct, clearly labelled categories: presentational (emotion management according to general social 'rules'), philanthropic (emotion management given as a 'gift'), prescriptive (emotion management according to organisational/professional rules of conduct) and pecuniary (emotion management for commercial gain). The categorisation of various forms of emotion management, as well as an acknowledgement of the underlying forces which currently act to shape nurses' 'care work', help to display its multi–faceted nature and show how a professional carer's skill lies not only in the accomplishment of technical tasks, but in the creation of the 'correct' emotional climate.

The use of categories such as the 'four principles of emotion management' ('4 Ps') highlights how, as a caring professional, a nurse weaves in and out of different 'emotional zones' (Fineman 1993), drawing upon a variety of 'feeling rules' to help match 'feeling and situation' (Hochschild 1979). The following examples show how nurses appear to move effortlessly from one performance to another: during a social encounter within the workplace they may well perform presentational emotion management; while carrying out technical tasks they are capable of deciding whether to offer philanthropic emotion management as an extra 'gift' to a patient in their care; their training and socialisation as a professional dictate when to perform prescriptive emotion management and, due to the recent 'marketisation' of the NHS, nurses may well perform pecuniary emotion management as a means of producing 'customer contentment'. A working day may involve performing all four principles of emotion management or, depending on the situation and who they are dealing with, the nurse may only need to rely on two or three of the categories.

By recognising the complex nature of nursing work and how both NHS staff and patients are increasingly affected by recent 'reforms', it may be possible to ask: 'who benefits and who pays?' in the changing NHS. Are patients (as consumers) being given 'quality' care or are nurses being asked to use their caring skills to paper over the cracks? It has been noted that in an attempt to provide a 'value-for-money' health service, efficiency is now being measured 'in terms of maximum measurable output for minimum measurable input' (Davidson 1987). The problem is that health care is not so easily quantifiable and, as Ackroyd (1995: 3) suggests, 'minuscule attention has been given to a systematic analysis of the [NHS] reforms in terms of costs and benefits'. One of the aims of this chapter is to attempt just such an analysis. The introduction of a conceptual model such as the '4 Ps' makes it conceivable that something so subjective as emotion management can be opened up to 'systematic analysis' and help promote an understanding of how emotion management may become a valuable organisational commodity. It is envisaged that such an in–depth analysis will act as an acknowledgement of nurses' status as highly skilled emotion managers and, when viewed in the context of attempts to commercialise the provision of health care, will allow a cost–benefit analysis to be applied.

The emotional organisation in the enterprise culture

The political, economic and managerial processes which have contributed greatly to recent organisational change may be classified as the discourse of enterprise (du Gay 1992) and can be traced to recent attempts in Britain to create an 'enterprise culture' in place of a 'dependency culture' (Rose 1994). Perhaps the most pervasive element of the enterprise culture is that of 'consumer power'; a theme introduced by the Conservatives but one which continues to be endorsed by the Labour government. The idea of the enterprise has been pushed so far that local authority housing tenants, National Health Service patients and university students have all now become 'customers', with the various public service charters enforcing their belief in consumer 'rights'. A major theme of the enterprise culture is the notion of the 'sovereignty' of the customer (du Gay 1992), and there is little doubt that both British industry and public services have become much more customer conscious.

The new entrepreneurial culture has seen a substantial increase in managerial power, enabling dramatic changes to occur in both private sector and public service organisations. The motive behind workplace change is said to be the requirements of the more discerning consumer who demands a wide variety of quality products and services. The current consumer is no longer the grateful, passive customer of the Fordist era, but one who now actively shapes supply through their demands (du Gay 1992). This, in turn, has created a need for a new flexible, multi-skilled post-Fordist worker who enables the post-bureaucratic company to respond to the requirements of the volatile market. In effect, the post-industrial worker is seen to be managed by the demands of the customer rather than bureaucratic control measures, and this development rests on management being convinced of the 'good sense of the discourse of enterprise' (du Gay 1992). The discerning customer expects to be satisfied, and management often see that the way to do this is through the application of 'commercial love', hence the increasing recognition of an employee's emotion management skills. In direct contrast to the orthodox view of the rational bureaucracy, we are now presented with the emotional organisation, and it is becoming increasingly accepted that emotion forms a major element of the organisation of the 1990s. The enterprise culture appears to have transformed organisations into 'emotional cauldrons' (Albrow 1992).

Examples of how emotionality finds expression in organisations now abound and, not surprisingly, many of these accounts concern the medical professional (Smith 1988, 1992; James 1989, 1992, 1993; Dent *et al.* 1991; Phillips 1996). The acknowledgement of emotion as a valuable ingredient of organisational life is clearly reflected in changed nursing practice. Traditionally, nursing work was structured around specific tasks. This served two purposes: it gave nurses a claim to base their practice on medical-scientific knowledge, while also allowing them to remain less involved with the patient as a person. Recently, however, 'primary nursing' (Smith 1992; Porter 1994; Savage 1995) has been introduced, which promotes a patient-centred, rather than task-centred, approach to nursing.

The 'new' nursing process is said to counter the previous authoritarian relationship between patient and nurse and allows the patient much more participation in their own healthcare while hospitalised. This is said not only to act as a 're-affirmation of the full humanity of people requiring health care', but also serves to improve the occupational status of nursing by 'rationalising' the concept of care (Smith 1992; Porter 1994). The change in the nurse–patient relationship has been greeted with enthusiasm by nurses, and yet, no matter how 'rationalised' the new process may be, it does require nurses to invest more of themselves emotionally into the job and, despite claims of increased professional status for nurses, many initiatives appear to be management driven.

Emotional investment is not a development unique to the caring professions. Recent research has revealed how many organisations and a wide variety of occupations are now being asked to invest their work with 'feeling'. The 'writing in' of emotion to organisation studies has led to the publication of a wide range of literature on the subject. The recognition, for example, of the importance of research concerning 'commercialization of feeling' (Hochschild 1983), organisation sexuality (Hearn and Parkin 1987), 'the social regulation of feelings' (James 1989), and 'sexuality and the labour market' (Adkins 1995), along with the vast array of management guru literature which encourages managers to use 'instinct' (Peters and Austin 1985; Peters 1987; Kanter 1990), has led to the acceptance that human emotions are an important factor within organisations.

The Weberian portrayal of the passionless bureaucracy where emotion is a by-product, an interference to be locked outside, appears to have changed. It has been explicitly stated that by offering an 'unfolding picture of some of the passions and perturbations of men and women at work' it can be shown how 'organizations are emotional arenas' (Fineman 1993: 8/31). Nevertheless, despite rationality being flogged as a dead horse, the emotional organisation clearly remains a site of purposeful activity oriented to achieving specific goals. This has never been more clearly demonstrated than in the way the organisation of the 1980s and 1990s has come to recognise the value of 'emotion work' – an employee's ability to manage emotion in order to create the 'correct' climate: it has now become a valuable management tool, a means to an end.

Emotional labour: the public face of emotion management

Many recent works have shown a concern for how organisations increasingly appear to seek to regulate an employee's emotion management as part of the labour process. Empirical accounts show that when working in the service sector, with its increasing emphasis upon 'consumerism', in exchange for a wage 'emotional labour' is provided – a vital contribution to the profitable product of customer satisfaction. Emotion management is now classed as another resource, a factor of production to be accounted for when balancing the books. Increasingly, in the absence of adequate financial resources, the human element is being used by management to fill in the gaps: for instance, a Trust hospital's survival relies upon the nurse's ability to keep the 'customer' satisfied. What an in-depth review of much of the existing literature reveals is that the term 'emotional labour'[2] is now common parlance when discussing emotion management within the emotional organisation, whether it is applied to public sector professionals such as nurses (Smith 1988, 1992; James 1989, 1992, 1993) or private sector service organisations like the airline industry (Hochschild 1983; Taylor 1996).

Clearly 'commercial love' is now becoming an essential part of many routine face-to-face jobs (Hochschild 1983), and the employee performs 'emotional labour' in order to create the correct emotional climate and keep the customer satisfied. They are able to accomplish this performance by drawing upon the emotion management skills they have learned as a socialised being. In other words, a lifetime's social training has enabled a person to assess the situation correctly and to produce the expected feeling according to social guidelines: 'a set of shared, albeit often latent rules' (Hochschild 1983: 268). But when this social training is used for the benefit of a commercial organisation and acts of private emotion management 'fall under the sway of large organizations, social engineering and the profit motive', Hochschild would refer to it as the 'trans-mutation of an emotion system' (ibid.: 19). In other words, what was once thought of as non-rational and belonging strictly in the private domain has now been welcomed into the public world of work. Implicit social feeling rules are being replaced by more explicit organisational rules, making emotion manage-ment another form of paid work: in effect, 'emotional labour'.

This 'transmutation' of feeling appears to amount to a crossing of the divide between the public and the private worlds of emotion management. Behind the theory of the appropriation of a person's emotion management system by the 1980s' and 1990s' organisation lies a clear-cut, black-and-white view of the private and public worlds of emotion management. As Wouters (1989) points out in his discussion of Hochschild's *Managed Heart* (1983), every time she describes the 'public face' of emotion management Hochschild appears to be referring to that which is appropriated by capitalism and automatically labels it as 'emotional labour'. It would appear simplistic (and not a little pessimistic) to assume that emotion management is carried out within organisations simply because management, as agents of capital, decide to appropriate it as a 'renew-able resource'. Yet this is the implication when the term 'emotional labour' is used to describe organisational emotion in its various forms.

A new agenda

To understand the multi-faceted nature of organisational life and how the 'texture of affectivity is even more multi-layered and convoluted than that of rationality' (Albrow 1992: 326) a new method of conceptualising emotion management in an organisational setting is required. If the complexities in-volved in organisational life and the contradictions this can bring into actors' lives are to be acknowledged, then a view of organisations needs to be devel-oped which can accept them as being a curious mix of both social arena and

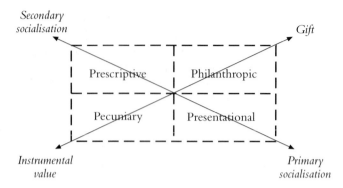

Figure 12.1 A typology of emotion management

rational goal-seeking tool. This also requires a recognition of the various means an organisation employs in order to achieve its ends, while also acknowledging the interference of the subjective experiences of its members. When discussing the 'discovery' of the emotional 'underlife' of an organisation it should not be imagined that rationality has disappeared, rather that rationality and emotion have become intertwined. However, using catch–all phrases such as 'emotional labour' to describe all forms of emotionality within organisations is to assume that the iron cage has taken another prisoner; that the complete 'subjectification of work, involving the saturation of the working body with feelings, emotions and wishes' (Rose 1989: 244) has finally taken place. Surely this neglects the pockets of human vitality within organisations, areas of human activity which have been referred to as 'the space for resistance and misbehaviour' (Thompson and Ackroyd 1995) and the 'unmanaged organisation' (Gabriel 1995). Without recognition of the emotional activity which occurs within these 'spaces' it is impossible fully to understand the emotional organisation.

If the emotional organisation is to be de-constructed there is a need to high-light the different characteristics of various types of organisational emotionality and to assign different forms of workplace emotion to distinct, clearly labelled categories. To attempt to categorise such a subjective experience as emotion into defined categories would appear to be a positivistic pursuit; however, it is in fact a pursuit with the final aim of revealing the lived reality of people's working lives. It is with such an aim in mind that it is proposed that four categories of emotion management be introduced (the '4 Ps'). Mis–describing and 'lumping' together different types of emotion at work, gives little credit to the wealth of a person's experience, their ability to adapt to situations, and their skill in managing situations in order to create the correct emotional climate. Figure 12.1 demonstrates the multi-faceted nature of organisational life and highlights the danger of labelling all performances of emotion management within the workplace under one heading.

Using umbrella terms such as 'emotional labour' to describe all feelings in organisations neglects the workplace as a social setting where it is possible to perform 'equal emotional exchanges' (Hochschild 1979). Emotion management is performed and often exchanged as a 'gift', it is not always sold for a wage. Feelings are 'managed' for a wide variety of reasons: legitimacy, conformity, economy, empathy, and according to vastly differing rules: organisational regulations, professional norms, social guidelines, personal histories. Only a small proportion of these reasons and rules come under the 'sway of large organisations' and are governed by a corporation's profit motive. Often the rules which guide us in the private domain are the same as those we use in an organisation, and often for the same reasons. The divide between the public and the private is never clear-cut, and we form friendships and create different 'emotional zones' within the workplace. It is well documented that work can be both a source of sadness and alienation as well as engagement and humour (Roy 1973; Westwood 1984; Collinson 1992; Hearn 1993), while there are essential elements of our lives which the organisation never captures.

Moreover, although it is important to recognise that the 'experience and construction of emotions has to be placed in the context of the experiences of organizations' (Hearn 1993: 161), this does not automatically label every emotion experienced within an organisation as 'emotional labour'. We may all 'work' on our emotions when present in an organisation, but not always in order to achieve company goals. For instance, nurses may genuinely empathise with a patient rather than present the face of a detached personal carer within the service provider–customer relationship; that is, they perform philanthropic emotion management rather than purely prescriptive. This is not to say that their private feelings have been 'transmutated', rather that their skills are so fine-tuned that they are capable of mixing and managing all forms of emotion management according to rules other than those solely controlled by the organisation.

Mixed feelings: emotion management in a medical setting

The nursing professional has long been recognised for their ability in managing their own and client's feelings in order to create the correct emotional climate. Nurses combine a professionally attained air of detachment (Lawler 1991) with the display of an appropriate 'caring' attitude, thus creating an emotionally controlled atmosphere which helps to eliminate embarrassment at invasive medical procedures but enables the patient still to feel human. Strauss *et al.* (1982: 254) clearly recognise that 'there was more to medical nursing work than its physiological core' when they coined the phrase 'sentimental work' to describe how a nurse 'manages' the emotional climate. Interestingly, they point out there is nothing particularly new about the idea of 'sentimental work', giving the example of 'tender loving care' in recognition of this. However, it is stressed that 'sentimental work' is not only carried out because of humanistic considerations but as a means of getting the 'work done effectively'. The combination of both subjective and objective considerations in the performance of 'sentimental work' means that it can be equated with both 'presentational' and 'prescriptive' emotion management. In some situations 'presentational' or 'philanthropic' emotion management may be performed out of 'humanistic' considerations, as a 'gift' to the patient as a person in a potentially awkward social situation; whilst in another setting 'prescriptive' emotion management may be performed in order to 'get the job done'.

This is where a professional carer's skill lies: a fine-tuned balance between providing the necessary physical and emotional care. However, due to many of these particular accomplishments being associated with the domestic sphere (i.e. feminine qualities of being loving and kind) and the vocational drive to 'care' for people, the required emotion management has never actually been acknowledged as a skill. Many of these vocations are seen as 'women's worlds', the most obvious being nursing. Briggs's (1972) report notes that nursing has retained an inherited image which belongs to the nineteenth century: the vision of Florence Nightingale, acting as surrogate mother, wife and mistress, lingers in many minds when the nursing profession is mentioned. This explains their status being described as 'semi-professionals' (Etzioni 1969), or 'feminine professionals' (Lorentzon 1990). To 'care' is not viewed as a skill, or even in many cases as 'proper work', it is merely seen as a result of innate female nurturing qualities. Quite simply this is what women 'do', it is 'women's work' (Abbott and Wallace 1990; Hugman 1991). National ideology expects nurses 'to care'. When patients are asked to describe a 'good' nurse they rarely mention technical skills, but rather the nurses' demeanour: are they cheerful, considerate and sympathetic, and do they make the patient feel 'at home' (Smith 1992). In other words, the image of the 'good nurse' looks suspiciously like the image of the 'good woman' (Abbott and Wallace 1990; Mackay 1990). Therefore nurses are relegated to semi-professional status without attempts being made to understand the complexities involved in 'caring' and how a vital prerequisite for any nurse is the necessary expertise in emotion management. As Smith (1992: 18) points out: 'managing emotions requires skill over and above "natural" caring qualities, and is different to love'.

Despite the persistent public image of the nurse as an 'angel of mercy' with the virtues of 'unstinting compassion and self-sacrifice' (Salvage 1985: 5), there is increasing acknowledgement of how nurses' emotion management can in fact be viewed as an essential part of their work, with many writers borrowing Hochschild's term 'emotional labour' to stress the point (Smith 1988, 1992; James 1989, 1992, 1993; Dent *et al.* 1991; Phillips 1996). This is despite 'sentimental work' appearing to be an ideal term to describe the emotion management performed by nurses. It takes into account their subjective experience of dealing with patients as people, while also recognising the need to complete tasks according to objective criteria laid down by the organisation. Nevertheless, it is not a term which has 'caught on' and in no way matches Hochschild's 'emotional labour' in the popularity stakes. Dent *et al.* attribute 'sentimental work's' lack of popularity to its interactionist origins and state that 'emotional labour' 'draws attention, in the way the interactionists are unable, to the labour process implications of the managing of emotions and feelings' (Dent *et al.* 1991: 2). However, 'emotional labour' has its own inherent weakness as a descriptive term: its emphasis on the organisation and the 'commercial' often goes too far in the exclusion of the social self. Notwithstanding this weakness, when describing the work of medical professionals, 'emotional labour' remains a favoured conceptual device.

James, in particular, uses the term 'emotional labour' to stress the relationship between emotional and physical labour: 'with both being hard, skilled work requiring experience, affected by immediate conditions, external controls and subject to divisions of labour' (James 1993: 95). The formula produced by James, 'Care = organisation + physical labour + emotional labour', summarises what she sees as the essential components of 'care work'. From her studies of 'nursing the dying', James concludes that 'emotional labour' can be described as 'productive work', 'hard work', 'difficult' and even 'sorrowful'. Emphasising the gender division of emotional labour, James applies the term equally to public service care workers such as nurses and unpaid female domestic workers such as 'housewives'. In doing this, James claims that she is 'using the concept in a broader sense than Russell Hochschild' (1989: 30) and appears to be trying to blur the boundaries between the public and private, showing how emotion management skills are carried from the private domestic sphere into the public world of work. However, although the use of the term 'emotional labour' does stress the 'hard work' involved in some forms of emotion management, ultimately it has led to an over-simplification of a nurse's work and neglects how the professional carer moves between various 'emotional zones'.

When describing the caring relationship between patient and nurse James (ibid.: 21) highlights that 'the expression of emotions is a negotiated process involving a mutual sounding out of what is acceptable'. This surely equates with the idea of 'equal emotional exchange' and allows for 'presentational' and 'philanthropic' emotion management to be performed. Nevertheless, there will be instances when nurses are not free to negotiate their own rate of 'exchange'. Their position in the hierarchy of the division of emotional labour may dictate that nurses perform emotion management (James 1993), or schedules may be set allowing no time for the negotiation of the caring relationship (James 1992). At these times emotion management ceases to be a 'gift' and becomes part of the process of work: 'prescriptive' emotion management carried out according to organisational and professional rules. Despite there being little doubt that the emotion 'work' carried out by nurses who care for the terminally ill is 'demanding and exhausting, and subject to different forms of organisation' (James 1989: 20), it gives little credit to nurses who, through their skilled performance of emotion management, obviously derive satisfaction from their ability to make a difference to the patient's well-being.

Pecuniary emotion management and the National Health Service

Using the conceptual model of the '4 Ps', the above review of care work shows how prescriptive, presentational and philanthropic forms of emotion management are performed, but pecuniary is notably absent. There are indications, however, that the potential for pecuniary emotion management within the public caring services is at last being recognised: Phillips (1996) questions the effects of paying nurses to 'smile'; Savage (1995) warns of the political implications of the named-nurse concept and Smith (1992: 137) notes how 'private health insurance schemes advertise their services through images of smiling nurses'. Clearly, there are early indications that the 'culture of the customer' could have far-reaching effects on the public sector caring services.

A 'factory-like' logic has been introduced into the NHS hospital system (Cousins 1986); talk is now of 'maximum measurable output for minimum measurable input' (Davidson 1987: 50). The onset of the 'quasi-market' has forced hospitals to enter into competition with each other as a means of reducing costs, increasing efficiency and improving quality. The government's rhetorical emphasis on consumer choice means that the survival of a Trust status hospital lies in its ability to keep the 'customer' satisfied. This atmosphere of competition, with the commercial manager at the helm of many Trust hospitals, has led to a new understanding of the association between providing a quality service and survival. Prominence has been given to 'good consumer relations'. The majority of health authorities are now experimenting with quality initiatives such as quality circles and total quality management (TQM), many obviously borrowed directly from the commercial manufacturing industries. And even more managers are being appointed to control the drive for quality (Davidson 1987; Morgan and Murgatroyd 1994).

It has been commonly believed that nurses are outside the 'capitalist mode of production', that they are not subject to de-skilling as described by Braverman, and that the concept of 'surplus value' does not apply to their work (Davies and Rosser 1986). There are signs, however, that this is no longer the case, as NHS managers are now 'constrained to act as capitalists' (Cousins 1986). Traditionally, nurses could be compared to Braverman's (1974) craft worker, within obvious medical restrictions, and according to professional 'implicit feeling rules' (prescriptive emotion management) they are autonomous in their decisions on how to emotionally manage the situation. They are also free to negotiate their own rate of 'exchange' – where, when, how, and if they will perform philanthropic emotion management. In this way, they are able to gain some satisfaction from their skilled performance. As 'jugglers and synthesizers' (Goffman 1961) nurses are able to slide in and out of various 'emotional zones', devising ways of coping with the stress involved in the job as they go: they may share experiences with their colleagues, have a laugh and a joke with the patients, or they may prefer to have a 'quiet day', remaining introverted until they sort themselves out.

However, in the 'new' NHS the nurse, like an assembly line worker, is expected to provide a quality service to more patients in less time while all the time increasingly sophisticated information systems make management's monitoring of nurse's work easier (Harrison and Pollitt 1994). At the same time the Citizen's Charter (1991, 1992) increases consumer expectations by promising a 'value-for-money' health service where both waiting lists and service quality will be dramatically decreased. Nurses, as the people who 'shape the interface' between the patient and the hospital (Burnell and Burnell 1989; Ackroyd 1996), have been given the job of meeting these raised expectations. In effect, on the one hand nurses are being asked to perform much more prescriptive emotion management in order to get the job done under greater time constraints, while on the other hand they now perform pecuniary emotion management as part of a quality drive which views consumer satisfaction as of 'fundamental importance'. In the 'enterprise culture' it is now the consumer who is the 'ultimate authority' (Morgan and Murgatroyd 1994), and the responsibility for quality care has been placed firmly with the individual nurse rather than with the hospital Trust or government (Savage 1995).

A cost–benefit analysis

The illustration of the '4 Ps' shows that when viewing organisations as both social arena and goal-seeking entity it is possible that all forms of emotion management may be performed by organisational actors for a wide variety of reasons. However, as caring professionals working within an increasingly marketised NHS, nurses must be one of the few occupational groups who regularly use all four principles of emotion management in organisations, with pecuniary emotion management only recently becoming an applicable category to nursing. It would appear, therefore, that within the context of recent changes in the NHS, a direct contrast can be made between public sector workers such as nurses and Hochschild's air stewardesses, thus overcoming the original objections to the use of 'emotional labour' to describe their work. However, as mentioned previously, using a blanket term such as 'emotional labour' to describe nursing 'care work' is to ignore its complexities. It also tends to make nurses disappear from view; it disregards their ability to adapt and change according to the needs of the particular situation, while also ignoring the sense of vocation which lies behind much of the caring professional's work.

Only by acknowledging the organisational actor's vast array of emotion management skills can a detailed analysis of the 'emotional organisation' begin, and only by recognising how nurses are able deftly to move from one form of emotion management to another can it be understood how valuable a contribution their emotion management really is.

The question of who benefits from the NHS reforms is not easily answerable. There appears little doubt that medical professionals are paying a price, with nurses being the biggest target for management's cost-cutting and quality initiatives (Davidson 1987; Ackroyd 1995). There have been clear attempts to cut costs through work intensification, casualisation and lowering grade levels (Lloyd and Seifert 1995). Normally this situation would be addressed via collective agreements, but now Trusts employ their staff directly and can set their own terms and conditions. This clearly fits in with the previous Conservative government's policy throughout the public sector: that of de-centralising pay determination, thereby empowering local managers and devolving decision making to levels where public sector unions traditionally have been weaker (Corby 1992). Moreover, the Trust's greatest emphasis has been on the need to change organisational culture so that 'greater priority is given to the needs of customers rather than providers' (ibid.: 36).

This is where an essential contradiction lies. Although the emotion management carried out by nurses has been acknowledged as an important aspect of providing a quality service (this is clear in the high profile given to holistic care), the relational skills nurses use in achieving high standards of care are seen as 'womanly qualities', which as such have no cash value. They are neither acknowledged as essential technical skills nor rewarded in financial or professional terms (Davies and Rosser 1986; Phillips 1996). In fact, despite the hospital Trust continually stressing the need for 'quality care', it is not something that is budgeted for:

> The new managerial tools have allowed the NHS to make very large savings in the name of efficiency and value for money, but we should be aware that they are crude and occasionally misleading instruments and that we may not be able to measure, and therefore, not even be aware of, some of the things we are losing.
>
> (Davidson 1987: 56)

There is little doubt that nurses are at the front line of care, and their emotion management skills do make a difference to how a patient views the health care they have received. By all accounts, it is the 'little things' which make the difference (Smith 1992), and if nurses were to withdraw their 'philanthropic' emotion management and only perform 'prescriptive' emotion management half-heartedly, then clearly this would be of great cost to the patient. Yet a 'go-slow' on emotion management does not seem a realistic option for most nurses. It is in the accomplishment of 'good' patient care that they derive their job satisfaction; research has shown, despite nurses expressing dissatisfaction with their work, rarely is it ever accompanied by 'disaffected behaviour' (Ackroyd 1993). At the heart of the nurse's work is a sense of vocation (Salvage 1985; Ackroyd 1993); unfortunately the 'new' NHS seems able to exploit their sincere drive to 'care' for patients.

Consumers of health care would appear to benefit from the consumerist thread in the 'new' NHS. And yet, despite the Citizen's Charter (1992) claiming to give the citizen 'a real voice', the actual consumer of health care is not the customer. The purchasing power lies with fund-holding GPs and district health authorities, which begs the questions of how much voice the citizen really has. There is little in Labour's recent recommendations for dismantling the internal market and implementing primary care groups (Department of Health December 1997) which heralds a dramatic change in this area. There is also mounting evidence that Patient's Charter league tables, supposedly compiled as a means of auditing quality, contain decidedly 'dodgy' information. In effect, some hospitals are 'fiddling the figures', with nurse managers defending the production of false data by claiming their jobs would be on the line if their units fell below charter standard (Friend 1995). As Harrison and Pollitt (1994: 111) point out: 'Despite the heady rhetoric of the TQM gurus it is hard to see that patients and citizens have more than walk-on parts.'

This leads to the conclusion that, despite decreasing waiting lists and higher patient turnover, neither consumers nor staff truly benefit from the 'new' NHS. It will be interesting to see what the future will bring. It can only be a matter of time before nurses begin to rebel against management 'feeding' from their feelings. As this analysis has shown, 'caring labour' is potentially a source of great satisfaction but it may also become the site of 'tremendously hostile and painful feelings' (Rose 1986: 169). With the increasing 'commercialisation' of the NHS there is less and less chance of nurses gaining job satisfaction and more likelihood that feelings of hostility will increase, thus making the development of 'unmanaged spaces', where 'misbehaviour' may well evolve, more probable. In the light of nurses desperately trying to retain their professional status, along with their popular public image, what forms any resistance may take can only be a matter for conjecture at this stage. However, it is envisaged that with the ability clearly to label emotion management in organisations, it will be possible further to investigate a nurse's work, revealing the truth behind what it is to perform the act of emotion management in the customer-oriented health service of the 1990s.

Notes

1 The caring professions are commonly described as comprising 'social workers, nurses and remedial therapies' (Hugman 1991: 2).
2 The term 'emotional labour' is introduced by Hochschild (1983) in her study *The Managed Heart*, to describe emotion management with a 'profit motive slipped under it'. Her study of air stewardesses highlights how emotion management is being increasingly appropriated by organisations in a 'service-producing society'.

References

Abbott, P. and Wallace, C. (1990) *The Sociology of the Caring Professions*, Basingstoke: The Falmer Press.

Ackroyd, S. (1993) 'Towards an understanding of nurses' attachment to their work: morale amongst nurses in an acute hospital', *Journal of Advances in Health and Nursing Care* 2(3): 23–45.

—— (1995) 'The new management and the professionals: assessing the impact of Thatcherism on the British public services', working paper no. 24, Work–Organization–Economy Working Paper Series, Department of Sociology, Stockholm University.

—— (1996) 'Traditional and new management in the NHS hospital service and their effects on nursing', in K. Soothill, C. Henry and K. Kendrick (eds) *Themes and Perspectives in Nursing*, London: Chapman and Hall.

Adkins, L. (1995) *Gendered Work: Sexuality, Family and the Labour Market*, Buckingham: Open University Press.

Albrow, M. (1992) 'Sine ira et studio – or do organizations have feelings?', *Organization Studies* 13(3): 313–29.

Braverman, H. (1974) *Labor and Monopoly Capital*, New York: Monthly Review Press.

Briggs, A. (1972) *Report of the Committee on Nursing*, London: HMSO.

Burnell, G. and Burnell, A. (1989) *Clinical Management of Bereavement*, New York: Human Sciences Press.

Cabinet Office (July 1991) *The Citizen's Charter*, London: HMSO.

—— (1992) *The Citizen's Charter*, First report, London: HMSO.

Corby, S. (1992) 'Industrial relations developments in NHS Trusts', *Employee Relations* 14(6): 33–44.

Collinson, D.L. (1992) *Managing the Shopfloor: Subjectivity, Masculinity and Workplace Culture*, Berlin: Walter de Gruyter.

Cousins, C. (1986) 'The labour process in the state welfare sector', in D. Knights and H. Willmott (eds) *Managing the Labour Process*, Aldershot: Gower.

Davidson, N. (1987) *A Question of Care: The Changing Face of the National Health Service*, London: Michael Joseph.

Davies, C. and Rosser, J. (1986) 'Gendered jobs in the health service', in D. Knights and H. Willmott (eds) *Gender and the Labour Process*, Aldershot: Gower Publishing.

Dent, M., Burke, W. and Green, R. (1991) 'Emotional labour and renal dialysis: nursing and the labour process', paper presented to the 9th Annual International Labour Process Conference.

Department of Health (December 1997) White Paper, 'New NHS: modern, dependable'.

du Gay, P. (1992) 'The cult(ure) of the customer', *Journal of Management Studies* 29(4): 615–33.

Etzioni, A. (1969) *The Semi-Professions and Their Organization*, New York: The Free Press.

Fineman, S. (1993) *Emotion in Organizations*, London: Sage.

Friend, B. (1995) 'Shallow standards', *Nursing Times*, 12 July, 91(28): 14–15.

Gabriel, Y. (1995) 'The unmanaged organization: stories, fantasies and subjectivity', *Organization Studies* 16(3): 477–501.

Goffman, E. (1961) *Encounters*, New York: Bobbs-Merrill.

Harrison, S. and Pollitt, C. (1994) *Controlling Health Professionals: The Future of Work and Organization in the National Health Service*, Buckingham: Open University Press.

Hearn, J. (1993) 'Emotive subjects: organizational men, organizational masculinities and the (de)construction of emotions', in S. Fineman (ed.) *Emotion in Organizations*, London: Sage.

Hearn, J. and Parkin, W. (1987) *'Sex' at 'Work': The Power and Paradox of Organisation Sexuality*, London: Wheatsheaf Books.

Hochschild, A. (1979) 'Emotion work, feeling rules, and social structure', *American Journal of Sociology* 85(3): 551–75.

—— (1983) *The Managed Heart: Commercialization of Human Feeling*, Berkeley: University of California Press.

Hugman, R. (1991) *Power in Caring Professions*, London: Macmillan.

James, N. (1989) 'Emotional labour: skill and work in the social regulation of feeling', *Sociological Review* 37(1): 15–42.

—— (1992) 'Care = organisation + physical labour + emotional labour', *Sociology of Health and Illness* 14(4): 488–509.

—— (1993) 'Divisions of emotional labour', in S. Fineman (ed.) *Emotion in Organizations*, London: Sage.

Kanter, R. (1990) *When Giants Learn to Dance*, London: Routledge.

Labour Research (1997) 'NHS faces crisis in morale', March.

Lawler, J. (1991) *Behind the Screens: Nursing, Somology, and the Problem of the Body*, Melbourne: Churchill Livingstone.

Lloyd, C. and Seifert, R. (1995) 'Restructuring the NHS: the impact of the 1990 reforms on the management of labour', *Work, Employment and Society* 9(2): 359–78.

Lorentzon, M. (1990) 'Professional status and managerial tasks: feminine service ideology in British nursing and social work', in P. Abbott and C. Wallace (eds) *The Sociology of the Caring Professions*, Basingstoke: The Falmer Press.

Mackay, L. (1990) 'Nursing: just another job?', in P. Abbott and C. Wallace (eds) *The Sociology of the Caring Professions*, Basingstoke: The Falmer Press.

Morgan, C. and Murgatroyd, S. (1994) *Total Quality Management in the Public Sector*, Buckingham: Open University Press.

Parkin, W. (1993) 'The public and the private: gender, sexuality and emotion', in S. Fineman (ed.) *Emotion in Organizations*, London: Sage.

Peters, T. (1987) *Thriving on Chaos*, London: Macmillan.

Peters, T. and Austin, N. (1985) *A Passion for Excellence*, London: Guild Publishing.

Phillips, S. (1996) 'Labouring the emotions: expanding the remit of nursing work?', *Journal of Advanced Nursing* 24: 139–43.

Porter, S. (1994) 'New nursing: the road to freedom?', *Journal of Advanced Nursing* 20: 269–74.

Putman, L. and Mumby, D. (1993) 'Organizations, emotion and the myth of rationality', in S. Fineman (ed.) *Emotion in Organizations*, London: Sage.

Rose, H. (1986) 'Women's work: women's knowledge', in J. Mitchell and A. Oakley (eds) *What is Feminism?*, Oxford: Basil Blackwell.

Rose, M. (1994) 'Skill and Samuel Smiles: changing the British work ethic', in R. Penn, M. Rose and J. Rubery (eds) *Skill and Occupational Change*, Oxford: Oxford University Press.

Rose, N. (1989) *Governing the Soul: The Shaping of the Private Self*, London: Routledge.

Roy, D.F. (1973) 'Banana time: job satisfaction and informal interaction', in G. Salaman and K. Thompson (eds) *People and Organisations*, London: Longman.

Salvage, J. (1985) *The Politics of Nursing*, London: Heinemann Nursing.

Savage, J. (1995) 'Political implications of the named-nurse concept', *Nursing Times* 91(41): 36–7.

Smith, P. (1988) 'The emotional labour of nursing', *Nursing Times* 84(44): 50–1.

—— (1992) *The Emotional Labour of Nursing*, London: Macmillan.

Strauss, A., Fagerhaugh, S., Suczek, B. and Wiener, C. (1982) 'Sentimental work in the technologized hospital', *Sociology of Health and Illness* 4(3): 255–78.

Taylor, S. (1996) 'Something old, something new: investigating emotion in organizations', paper presented to The Future of the Sociology of Work, Employment and Organisations, Grey College, University of Durham, 9 September.

Thompson, P. and Ackroyd, S. (1995) 'All quiet on the workplace front? A critique of recent trends in British industrial sociology', *Sociology* 29(4): 615–33.

Westwood, S. (1984) *All Day Every Day*, London: Pluto Press.

Wouters, C. (1989) 'The sociology of emotions and flight attendants: Hochschild's managed heart', *Theory, Culture and Society* 6: 95–123.

13 The 'fat envelope patient'

Dynamics between the patient, the
doctor and the osteopath in some UK
National Health Service Settings

Richenda Power

'Oh, she's a fat envelope patient.'

On first hearing the term used by a doctor at a meeting I was struck by its
apparent denotation of some quality intrinsic to the patient. There is no such
word in the thesauri for either Medline or Sociofile, though 'difficult' is productive.[1] However, the term does seem to be current: when discussing this
chapter in health care circles, it was understood immediately. A 'fat envelope'
may be developed on behalf of a frequently consulting patient, as at each visit a
record should be made; also, much paper may result from one or two episodes
of illness, or an ongoing situation which the general practitioner (GP) and the
patient decided required further investigation, resulting in reports from numerous specialists and hospital departments. It is unlikely that the term 'fat envelope
patient' would be used to your face, even if you should have such an envelope
or file at the doctor's surgery. Whatever record-keeping line of work with
clients or cases you are in, perhaps an analogous term comes to mind?

I chose the 'fat envelope patient' as a topic for a collection called *Professionalism, Boundaries and the Workplace* because it seems as if often such people (defined solely for the purposes of this chapter by the size, as actually handled, or
suspected size, judged by the case history plus their referral letter, of their envelope or file of medical records) are referred through National Health Service
channels to osteopaths, acupuncturists, homoeopaths, masseurs, herbalists and
so on. The reasons for this are probably multiple and beyond the scope of this
chapter. My concern here is with the emotional dynamics that arise in the
three-way relationships that develop as they attend for treatment in Health
Service settings or via Health Service contracts with previously 'unofficial' health
care practitioners.

Such formal relationships have only been developed generally in Britain in
the 1990s. Peters's (1994) discussion 'Sharing responsibility for patient care',
based on a few years work and audit at the Marylebone Health Centre, raised
the topic of referral, which we might consider the initiation of such relationships by doctors:

> Typical problems arise in the process of referral . . . Too many could signal
> 'I don't understand what you do', though they might also indicate 'I am

trying to discover your limits', or 'I can't deal with x, y, z. I hope you can'. It could also suggest the organisation or individual GP is overstrained or that for some other reason GPs are not 'gate-keeping' adequately. Impossible referrals are sometimes made; not always unwittingly: perhaps when a GP feels disempowered, de-skilled, passive/aggressive, or over-optimistic.

(Peters 1994: 183)

This seems an honest admission of *feelings* on the part of the GP. However, in the following paragraph he wrote: 'Even where an extended team is available, "fat envelope" patients still confound practitioners' attempts to cure them. Several types of multi-consulter can be recognised' (ibid.: 183), mentioning the 'consumer', the 'desperate mechanic', the 'heartsink' patient and the 'iatrogenic multi-consulter'. Peters commented on the 'heartsink': 'These patients always have *thick files of notes*, having previously been referred to every available resource because either they or their GP was driven to desperation by their problem' (ibid.: 184, emphasis added). He suggests that

> better teamwork, a clearly agreed management plan and a clear key worker is more likely *to contain these patients' distress* (see Gerrard and Riddell 1988), and undoubtedly these patients with *persistently unorganised illness*, who are often chronically depressed or anxious, or with problems of daily living, do need help to become less dependent on multi-consulting.
>
> (ibid.: 184, emphases added)

While Peters, himself both a medical doctor and an osteopath, does acknowledge that ' "unorganised illness" to a conventional practitioner' might be 'a recognisable syndrome on which the appropriate CP [his abbreviation for 'complementary practitioner'] can exert specific therapeutic leverage',[2] the way in which the typology is presented says more about a medical gaze, with allied notions about specific 'professional' tasks, than anything particular to the patients themselves. Could it be that the *GP's* sight of the bursting envelope of referral letters, radiological reports, blood tests, etc. triggers their fear of bursting with the feelings the patient seems to produce in them? Are these then 'stuck' to the patient so that somehow the patient is held responsible? That this seems to be the case is borne out by a brief perusal of other doctors' typologies (see Gerrard and Riddell 1988; Asher 1995; Hammond 1996).

It seems strange that the generation of paperwork becomes a label that cleaves to the patient. Not all record-keeping situations would be negatively construed: consider the academic with a long list of publications, or someone with a busy bank account! When I mentioned writing this chapter to one GP she thought some research on the 'thin envelope patient' would be fascinating too. Does this speak of a feeling of being underused and undepended upon by those who merely register and are then never seen? This resonates with a discussion held with naturopaths on the topic of 'failure', some of which focused on 'the patient who only came once' (Power 1998). Does this suggest an optimum amount of, and style of, consultations, with organisable symptoms, as 'ideal' patient behaviour?

'Not according to the terms and times prescribed . . .'

For those who do not conveniently fit an 'ideal' patient role the following passage by Doris Lessing may resonate:

> June was not well. Our questions brought out of her that this was nothing new; she hadn't been too good 'for quite a time'. Symptoms? 'I dunno, just feel bad, you know what I mean.'
>
> She had stomach pains and frequent headaches. She lacked energy – but energy cannot be expected of a Ryan. She 'jst didn't feel good anywhere at all – it comes and goes, reely.'
>
> This affliction was not only June's; it was known to a good many of us.
>
> Vague aches and pains; indispositions that came and went, but not according to the terms and times prescribed by the physicians; infections that would go through the community like an epidemic, but not with an epidemic's uniformity – they demonstrated their presence in different symptoms with every victim; rashes that did not seem to have any cause; nervous diseases that could end in bouts of insanity or produce tics or paralyses; tumours and skin diseases; aches and pains that 'wandered' about the body; new diseases altogether that for a time were categorised with the old ones for lack of information, until it became clear that these were new diseases; mysterious deaths; exhaustions and listlessness that kept people lying about or in bed for weeks and caused relatives and even themselves to use the words 'malinger' and 'neurotic', and so on, but then, suddenly vanishing, released the sufferers from criticism and self-doubt.
>
> (Lessing 1981: 155–6)

The narrator voices ideas and feelings possibly quite close to the subjective experience of the 'fat envelope patient'. Several features are salient for a sociological reading: 'energy cannot be expected of a Ryan' suggests that the narrator's place is other than working class and Irish; however, the narrator is also probably not a physician, as the shared experience of suffering in 'terms and times not prescribed' is stressed. Nevertheless, despite this difference, 'relatives and even themselves' use the words 'malinger' and 'neurotic'. Certainly the experience of 'criticism and self-doubt' are routinely described by 'fat envelope patients'. One hospital consultant asked whether I was 'going the rounds' when I attended his department as a patient, because I mentioned a previous investigation in another setting, as if I was pursuing 'a career' (Herzlich 1973). Patients arrive saying things such as 'I know I'm a hopeless case' as if it is their fault, but perhaps also as a challenge. Others apologise by prefacing their histories with 'well, I may be paranoid, but . . .' or 'I'm a hypochondriac . . .', probably soliciting reassurance and perhaps a contradiction of another professional opinion.

Although these labels are never, or hardly ever, said directly to the patient, they seem to evolve within certain health professional–patient relationships. Some osteopaths have written about referred patients in an NHS hospital setting 'often lacking commitment and motivation, ungrateful, and taking very little responsibility for their own wellbeing' (Huzzey and Summers 1995: 4), thus exposing their own notions of 'ideal' patient behaviour. It is emotionally demanding to be in a caring profession when the caring appears to 'fail' and one has been unable to help, or one's intervention appears to have made things worse. Perhaps, for the majority of practitioners, rewards come from the satisfaction of the happy customers and their recommendations. Much of the language of health care delivery and its quantification in terms of 'outcomes' is based on discrete categories of disease that can be identified in order to apply specific approaches to its management or cure (see Bowling 1991 and 1995 for useful discussions). A body that does not attract easily inscribed formulae of care and outcome poses a challenge to the managing system and its workers. In the context of changes in the organisation of health care delivery by the Conservative government in Britain from 1989 there was both a shift in terms of doctors' accountability (for example in new management structures and the legal requirement for audit) and their range of choices as 'gatekeepers' to other health care services for referral (see Allsop 1995). On the one hand a sense of autonomy has been diminished; on the other, they may have more power over local hospitals and health centres (public and private, including 'alternative') than they had previously. During the same period of change the status of osteopaths and chiropractors has altered from being seen at worst as 'quackery', to state recognition with legislation to agree the formation of independent state registers (osteopathy 1993; chiropractic 1994), while avoiding any mention of formal relationships with the NHS. Nevertheless there has been a busy production of literature within the osteopathic profession regarding the negotiation and establishment of such. Further changes in Britain are afoot as I write (late 1998), under the auspices of the Labour government, with the formation of primary care groups, which will alter the balance of power and responsibility again.

A participant observer's account

I was employed at a non-fund-holding general practice from early 1991, initially via 'Health Promotion' funding, for one afternoon a week, as an osteopath. General practitioners could refer patients to me; I assessed their 'suitability' for osteopathy and continued to see them at my discretion, keeping the appointment book myself. I was paid for by the local Family Practitioner Committee at first, and subsequently by the Family Health Services Association (FHSA) which funded 70 per cent of my costs, in a similar way to other staff. The other source of health service work has been through a contract with the FHSA at a privately run natural health centre, whereby GPs from all over the borough[3] could refer patients through for acupuncture, homoeopathy, massage or osteopathy; again, the patients were seen free at the point of service, but the practitioners were paid their normal fees for private work. There are differences between these frames which may affect the relationships that develop between the osteopath, the patient and the referring doctor, which I shall bring out later.

A sequence of fictionalised vignettes is presented, after which a discursive reflection on possible theoretical explanations is offered. Writing illustrative examples has been a most agonising process as a participant/observer. At first I tried 'fictionalising' specific interactions from the different settings mainly with the preservation of the anonymity of the *patient* in mind. But when I read the narratives back to myself there were still too many contextual features. I recalled Harrison and Lyon's (1993) discussion of ethical issues in the use of autobiography in sociological research:

> The value of autobiography lies precisely in that it can clarify the extent to which the domains of the private and personal, in the sense of subjective understandings of self and others in time and place, operate *across* rather than within separate spheres. It is precisely its possibilities for bringing private understandings and emotions about the private and the public into the public arena as textual narratives that raises ethical questions about the use of autobiography for the researcher.
>
> (Harrison and Lyon 1993: 103)

I hope that what I have tried to do here respects privacy and avoids exploitation and betrayal. I welcome further suggestions as how best to do this. My story is interwoven with others', who also have feelings, and different views to my own, whether they are patients or professionals. So, in addition to the removal of names, specific symptoms, ages and so on of the patients, I decided also not to locate them in their specific settings but to discuss differences between 'the frames' in a more general way after the vignettes. This is my view, as a practitioner, who is also trained in social science. It is in no way an end point to be cited as a general case or a 'truth'.

A. wanted another opinion because of continuing pain following an accident. Possible litigation was being explored. On examination I considered that some form of arthritis might be present. The doctor ordered numerous tests, all of which came back negative. Subsequently A. was referred to me, and attended from time to time as they felt necessary. The trigger would usually be the recurrence of intolerable pain. A. was embarrassed about returning – A. felt too often – and with what seemed like multiple complaints. A. talked about the doctor's apparent despair about not being able to help, nor to have diagnosed. Sometimes A. felt that the doctor did not believe them. A. did not give up in the search for diagnosis and help. I felt helpless often in the face of A.'s pain and would discuss what little input I might offer to give some temporary relief. This patient persisted in requesting further investigations and referrals and received some diagnoses eventually. The diagnostic labelling seemed to be a source of some psychological relief, perhaps from ideas such as being a nuisance to the practice, or that the pain was entirely stress-related or imagined.

B. was referred for joint and muscular pain which had not responded well to physiotherapy. There was a complex medical history, with numerous current conditions all being treated pharmacologically. Working with a patient on a lot of medication is unpredictable because their tissue responses may be either dampened down or over-reactive to physical treatment such as massage, which stimulates the circulation of blood and lymph. (I had been criticised for even working collaboratively by one naturopathic colleague, particularly on these grounds, as well as the philosophical differences between medicine and 'nature cure' – see Power 1994.) The doubts about whether it was clinically appropriate for me to work with B. were somehow mitigated by our first conversations when a major recent loss was mentioned. I felt that at the very least I could probably assist with some relaxation techniques and exercises which could be learned and practised at home, along with some gentle massage (a different approach to the previous physiotherapy). B. also began to visit a specialist counsellor. During the time I worked with B. they suffered from several further medical problems. There was anxiety about these and their investigation, and B. sometimes felt hopeless about going on generally. I felt as if continuity in support was of value.

C. had a very long history of previous intervention by physiotherapists, osteopaths, masseurs, and numerous investigations including X-rays, MRI scans, as well as orthopaedic and neurological opinions. There was an air of hopelessness about this patient that came over in a diffident and self-deprecating manner. There was almost constant daily pain. I always feel extremely challenged when such a patient attends: at least if osteopathy has not been tried before, there's always a slim hope that it may 'do the trick', if only because a fresh mind comes to the case history-taking and the examination, and has the advantage of hindsight in knowing what didn't work before. (As I write this it is clear I am exhibiting a 'cure' mentality which my naturopathic colleagues might criticise.) However, this case is perhaps a type, that is not fully diagnosed; the missing pieces – if the practitioner perhaps avoids being totally driven by the 'frame' of the referral letter, and takes a fresh history, gaining perhaps a fuller context – may begin to make sense. But how the practitioner communicates diplomatically with the referring GP, but ensures that they are heard, is a major issue.

Dynamics

Practising alone in private practice there usually evolves a one-to-one relationship with the patient. Things are more complex when a third party is involved, especially with the long histories of antagonism that lie between doctors and osteopaths as professional groups. Co-operation is very new territory, and for both the dyadic relationship they normally enjoy with patients is shifted. In the simplest sense this has implications for where 'power' lies. Why and how this may be different again for an osteopath than for hospital consultants, physiotherapists or nurses is worth considering.

The rate of referral of 'the fat envelope patient' appeared to differ between the settings, being about 10 per cent within the GP surgery compared with possibly as high a rate as 50 per cent at the natural health centre. This is not a scientific enumeration, based as it is on handling the actual envelope(s) in the setting of the GP surgery, and guessing the size from the complexity of the case history taken by myself in the other, the natural health centre. In fact, until the measurement of envelopes is done in every case, the guesses may well say more about my bias, in the face of what I personally and professionally found 'difficult' in both senses of the word.

A. can be thought of as one of the 'fat envelope patients' with an undiagnosed illness. A. persistently sought other opinions and is quite likely to have initiated the doctor's referral for osteopathy. Active involvement on A.'s part was evident throughout. A. was highly motivated to follow any instructions that might help, realistic about the situation, and also able to appreciate the GP's feelings of helplessness mixed with concern. However, any ideas that the symptoms could be psychogenic or stress related were rejected.

Some GPs were happy for me to continue seeing such patients, saying I kept the 'heartsink' patients going. Communication with the GPs was important for me, to know that continued contact with the patient was endorsed, while mutually acknowledging the chronic unresolvable undiagnosed nature of the problems. However, I privately disagreed with some of the doctors' statements about some such patients being 'somatisers', feeling it more my role as an osteopath to be the patient's *advocate* in acknowledging that something was physically wrong, and an ally in their search for knowledge. My primary commitment is to believe the patient, as part of my sense of 'professional-self'. This sort of evolution of trust with the patient is potentially subversive of both the doctor and of certain medical frames. This may flatter me and give me a sense of a privileged position (see Morris 1995), and a dangerous sense of professional pride. This was further vindicated by A.'s eventual diagnosis, the achievement of the labels vindicating my position of belief.

In B.'s case, it seemed clear that the referring GP's remit was 'holistic' in that they were well aware of multiple levels of disease and distress going on. This felt like shared knowledge, so I felt the agenda was to work with 'the whole person' in ways I saw to be relevant. The GP's referral and my reception of that matched well, with an acknowledgement on both sides that this was a 'difficult' patient in the sense of the *complexity* involved.

C. perhaps comes closest to Peters's description of the patient whose 'GP was driven to desperation', and probably knows it. Feelings of being unwanted and useless seemed to emanate from this individual and it was easy to react by rushing into 'rescuer' mode, only to have every therapeutic suggestion rebutted, and then to start feeling angry. C. would attract the label 'difficult' in its two meanings, as *complex* and *awkward*. The challenge with such a patient is to pace oneself, as the desire to rush in and rescue where others have 'failed', is great; the desire is to make the healthy and healing therapeutic relationship where others have rejected. Writing this I am struck by a parallel with the temptation faced by foster parents to do it better than the 'birth parents'.

(I realise I have not mentioned another category, the patient the GP has found perplexing, who appears straightforward to an osteopath/naturopath's perceptions, where, as Peters put it above, there is a 'recognisable syndrome', amenable to such approaches. This sometimes seems like a 'miracle cure' to the GP, and their reaction will depend upon their experience of, understanding of and fantasies about the other practitioner. Sometimes an osteopath is thought to have 'healing hands' in a rather esoteric sense, which feels difficult to the practitioner who has slogged hard for four years full-time to qualify. Receiving the words 'healing' or 'magic hands' from the referring GP sets off a resonance with the belittling of knowledges 'learned at mother's knee' or thought to derive from 'feminine intuition'. Getting other health professionals to watch what one does, or even to have osteopathic work done to them, is a good way of disabusing them of 'miracle' fantasies.)

By elaborating on my feelings and temptations during such cases I am sketching a picture of the potential for the development of some interesting dynamics between three people in certain contexts. I shall now tackle issues of 'professionalism', 'boundaries' and 'workplace' in a more systematic and abstract way.

Professionalism is an abstract concept in process of definition and redefinition within both medicine (see Stacey 1992) and osteopathy (GCRO 1993). The latter publication on *Competences Required for Osteopathic Practice* (known as 'CROP' – GCRO 1993) includes, as part of 'Competence to evaluate the patient': 'Establish a relationship with the patient and anyone accompanying him/her' (ibid.: 11), part of which includes '[to] Have a method of dealing with *difficult patients*' (ibid.: 12). No specific definition of such a patient is given and the further information to which the practitioner is directed is mainly to do with care in the provision of information, issues of informed consent and other matters of a potentially legal nature. A long footnote is appended to the use of the word 'contract' which is claimed to be intended 'not . . . in a strong legal sense, but more in its therapeutic meaning', which is interpreted to include the 'involvement of both the osteopath and the patient' (ibid.: 24). However, it is subsequently acknowledged that 'misunderstandings can occur' and that 'The practical reality is that in the relationship the osteopath assumes greater authority, and therefore has greater responsibility for detecting and resolving such misunderstandings (ibid.: 24). By implication this uses the second meaning of 'difficult', a possibly complaining or demanding unhappy patient, or dissatisfied customer, but perhaps moves some way to recognising the *relationship* as problematic, not the *patient*.

It has been normal for patients to come to osteopaths when they felt that doctors did not know what they were doing, or were unable to help, so, perhaps historically, osteopaths have attracted that category of the 'difficult', and habitually evolved subversive relationships that question what has gone before and reassess previous diagnoses, treatments and relationships. In any gathering of alternative practitioners it is usual to hear boasting anecdotes of diagnoses which doctors missed. These are perhaps the sorts of shoring-up, confidence-building stories that form part of the rhetoric that helped such professions survive this century in the face of an apparent monopoly of medicine. Within the broader context of statutory funding and the necessity of purchasers' decisions it does not seem to make for easy territory. The recent osteopathic literature (for example GCRO 1994; Weeks 1996; Sharp 1998) has emphasised the development of a view of the osteopath as part of the primary health care team.

Doctors are equally aware of the antagonisms of our histories, and this may render the gratitude for 'keeping the heartsink patient' from their door a mixed blessing emotionally, not to mention financially, as the pressures for accountability for spending allocation increase. So while extreme gratitude is expressed, clinical resentment and indeed jealousy may also be felt and sometimes admitted, not only for being able to 'do something for' the difficult patient, but for the privilege of having half an hour to spend with them, compared with the GP's seven minutes, if lucky.

While some doctors have welcomed the help offered to the 'heartsink', others wondered why I didn't work 'more like a physio' perhaps, for example setting a limit of six sessions available to any one patient, but this may also have referred to the remit of care. The atmosphere of rationing I found difficult to deal with as it was a new experience, being unnecessary in private practice where the patients decide how much contact they wish to have. Bell (a psychotherapist) has spoken of

> The Stock Market of Health, primed with the day-to-day anxiety of survival, is a vision, not an ennobling one of man realising himself [sic], but one of the alienation of health-workers from each other and also from themselves as agents of human value. They become totally 'commoditised' and exchange on the Market is their only hope of survival. This is not likely to lead to much co-operation in the provision of health.
>
> (Bell 1996: 56)

The use by GPs of an analogy with physiotherapy spoke to me more of the difficulties doctors and managers might have in reconciling themselves to the relatively autonomous position that osteopaths hold vis-à-vis other health professionals. If we take a Weberian model of competition between professional groups, perhaps osteopaths and chiropractors come close in some areas (not pharmacology or surgery!) to potential usurpation of the general practitioner's territory, in terms of their bodies of knowledge, the applicability of that knowledge and their skills, their status and clinical autonomy, despite the 'official' rhetoric about the narrow musculoskeletal remit that gained the recent legislative successes. As a small piece of evidence of a contested territory, it is not clear where ultimate responsibility lies should litigation occur in these situations where osteopaths receive referrals via health service contracts.

Beyond issues of overlapping knowledge and skill bases is that of the contemporary emphasis on the personal qualities looked for in the professional-self. Some time ago Stacey (1988) wrote about the development within general practice of a view of the quality of the doctor–patient relationship as intrinsically therapeutic. Studies of doctor recruitment (Allen 1997) noted that the personal qualities of empathy and sensitivity were most highly rated for the choice of GP trainees. In co-operative situations where two or more important dyadic relationships evolve with the patient, there is the potential for major emotional involvement between all parties. These are considered in Figure 13.1.

Boundaries

There are then several 'boundaries' that can be discussed: central to this discussion are those of the remits of knowledge and skill felt to 'belong' to different types of health professional; there are also those of human relationships and the emotions involved. It is difficult to separate these out in practice where they feel intimately related. Such matters are not unique to osteopaths, for example see Fox's discussions of similar conflicts in nursing, arising particularly around the 'ethic of advocacy for the patient' (Theis cited by Fox 1989: 61).

Contrasts may be drawn between the three case vignettes from the initiation of referral, through the fantasy and reality checking of the individuals involved via the process of treatment. A. initiated the referral. The GP agreed to this, and later expressed gratitude, linked to their own feelings of relief that something could be done despite the lack of diagnosis. The patient, however, did not always feel believed, so there was more pull for myself into advocacy of the patient, potentially against the GP. In B.'s case there was mutual recognition between the GP and the osteopath that the case was complex and multi-levelled, and a 'whole person' approach was relevant. This felt like an even relationship between myself and the GP as peers, valuing each other. For C. there was an element of testing of the practitioner, to which Peters referred. From his list, I would suggest that the 'I can't deal with . . .' overlaps with 'I am trying to discover your limits' type of impetus for referral. We could precis the motive colloquially as sending a 'crock' to the 'quack'. However understandable as an avoidance of waste of finance in 'impossible' referrals, the lists that the purchasers are endlessly trying to evolve of matches between 'conditions' and 'therapies' are anathema to the philosophy of care on which naturopaths and osteopaths used to be raised. We were not trained to think solely in terms of organised illnesses anyway, but to work with 'the whole person' and sometimes to 'be with the patient in their pain' (see Hawkins and Shohet 1989, ch. 13) and to attempt to make sense *with the patient* of the meaning of their illness. In this case we should be welcoming the 'fat envelope'. One medical herbalist endorsed my suspicion that a high percentage of challenges were sent our way, but said it was not that a miracle was done if change was effected, but that often the patient learned to 'listen' to their body.

The patient who is referred may feel the doctor has come to the end of their tether and that they cannot bear to see them any more, so they have been sent 'beyond the pale'. Alternatively, they might feel specially valued by a referral to an osteopath, that they have been considered 'worth it' both in terms of the continuing possibility of help, another opinion, and the expense. We can consider Goffman's work on stigma, which suggests 'that an individual's sense of worth is likely to be affected by judgements made about the worth of the body' (in Shilling 1993: 186).

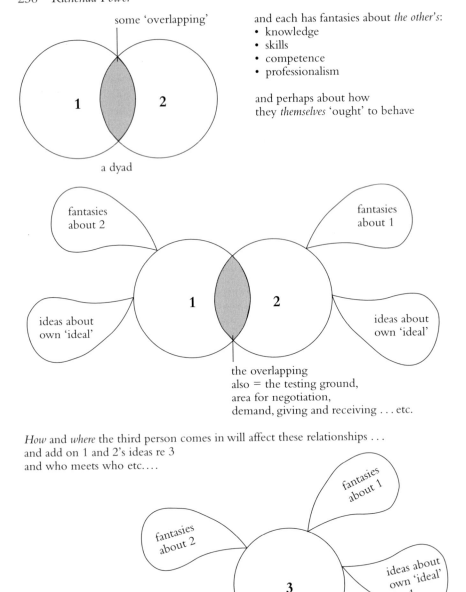

some 'overlapping'

1   2

a dyad

and each has fantasies about *the other's*:
• knowledge
• skills
• competence
• professionalism

and perhaps about how
they *themselves* 'ought' to behave

fantasies
about 2

fantasies
about 1

ideas about
own 'ideal'

1   2

ideas about
own 'ideal'

the overlapping
also = the testing ground,
area for negotiation,
demand, giving and receiving . . . etc.

How and *where* the third person comes in will affect these relationships . . .
and add on 1 and 2's ideas re 3
and who meets who etc. . . .

fantasies
about 1

fantasies
about 2

ideas about
own 'ideal'
for 1

3

ideas about
own 'ideal'
for 2

Figure 13.1 Important emotional relationships

The workplace

The relationships between myself as osteopath and the referred patients and their GPs differed also according to the context of our meeting. The 'frames' are compared and contrasted in Table 13.1.

Organising my experiences retrospectively has been therapeutic in itself as it has made me think more clearly about intensely lived experiences that mattered deeply to me personally and professionally, as a practitioner coming 'out of the margins'. Bell's (1996) pessimistic view makes me consider retrospectively that at the GP surgery I worked with exceptional people who to a large extent shared a vision of 'whole' human needs; this must have been true, or co-operation would not have been possible, nor would my work have been called for in the first place. I do not wholly share Hoag's (another psychotherapist) view of the GP surgery as a 'deviant frame', but her systematic analysis of her experience providing three-days-a-week psychotherapy in general practice has influenced me and assisted my identification of features of differences between the two settings. She concludes that 'Part of the therapist's work within the GP surgery

Table 13.1 Considering differences in the 'frame': the workplace

Workplace	GP practice	Natural health centre
how I feel as practitioner	quack in the doctors' den	at home in my space
how this affects me	over-eager to please, more clinical compromises	more relaxed
time	30 mins per patient	1 hr consultation; 45 mins subsequently
length of treatment	controlled by me, but discussed, and modified	set format of 6, then review, up to 12
equipment	couch lacks face hole, smaller space	couch for osteopathy, enough space
information about the patient from GP	full access to patient's medical records	referral letter from GP
communication with GPs	in the corridor, the kitchen, in each other's rooms	systematised via the contract: letters, phone
boundaries	potential for blurring, e.g. friendship and work	clearly maintained, formal, isolated
advantages	I am personally known; referrals are likely to match	I maintain more sense of clinical autonomy, which may feel safer for the patients
disadvantages	dangers to confidentiality; work involves intense relationships with many people	may be used for the 'difficult' patients

is, undoubtedly, to establish and maintain a working alliance with the surgery staff as well as with her patients' (Hoag 1992: 427). This is true, but it is also extremely satisfying to feel like part of a team rather than an outpost to whom the doubly 'difficult' may be despatched.

Material for sociology

The brief outlines above may serve as a series of suggestions of opportunities in new and changing fields of work which I trust will be 'plowed and plotted in different ways' (Lévy-Zumwalt's 1988 comment on distinctions and tensions between literary and anthropological folklorists) by social researchers of various persuasions. The developing body of work in the sociology of the emotions inspired by Hochschild's (1983) study of emotion management by flight attendants is promising, as is sociologists' shift in the conceptualisation of medicine away from an archetypal profession to its 'proletarianisation' (Annandale 1998).

Acknowledgements

I wish to thank all the patients and the staff (medical, nursing and managerial) who have enabled me to have these experiences. Also, thanks are due to Judith Allsop for inviting me to share some initial sociological thoughts about 'working as an osteopath in a GP surgery' to the Health Research Group seminar series, South Bank University, 19 June 1995, where the audience raised pertinent and thought-provoking questions, particularly Anne Murcott. Thanks also to Gwynnedd Somerville for a series of invaluable conversations about 'the frame'. Thank you Mark Corson and Sophie Raitz, clinical tutors at the British School of Osteopathy, for reading and commenting on the draft chapter. I thank the Open University Research Fund for support to complete this chapter for publication.

Notes

1 'Difficult' was broken down by Medline, searched in early 1997, to 'Difficult . . . to assess; . . . to classify; . . . to cure; . . . to diagnose; . . . to manage.'
2 I don't feel comfortable with the metaphor of 'leverage', which sounds rather like the mechanical removal of bicycle tyres, and is used specifically in manipulation!
3 A borough is an administrative tier of local government in Britain.

References

Allen, I. (ed.) (1997) *Choosing Tomorrow's Doctors*, London: The Policy Studies Institute and St George's Hospital Medical School.
Allsop, J. (1995) 'Shifting spheres of opportunity: the professional powers of general practitioners within the British National Health Service', in T. Johnson, G. Larkin and M. Saks (eds) *Health Professions and the State in Europe*, London: Routledge, pp. 75–85.

Annandale, E. (1998) *The Sociology of Health and Medicine: A Critical Introduction*, Cambridge: Polity Press.

Asher, R. (1995) 'Malingering', in B. Davey, A. Gray and C. Seale (eds) *Health and Disease: A Reader*, 2nd edn, Buckingham: Open University Press, pp. 157–60.

Bell, D. (1996) 'Primitive mind of state', *Journal of the Association of Psychoanalytic Psychotherapy*, pp. 45–57.

Bowling, A. (1991) *Measuring Health*, Buckingham: Open University Press.

—— (1995) *Measuring Disease*, Buckingham: Open University Press.

Fox, R. (1989) *The Sociology of Medicine: A Participant Observer's View*, Englewood Cliffs, NJ: Prentice Hall.

The General Council and Register of Osteopaths [GCRO] (1993) *Competences Required for Osteopathic Practice*, Reading: GCRO.

—— (1994) *Osteopaths – Part of the Health Care Team* (video), Reading: GCRO.

Gerrard, T. and Riddell, J. (1988) 'Difficult patients: black holes and secrets', *British Medical Journal* 297: 20–7, August, pp. 530–2.

Hammond, P. (1996) 'There are five categories of heartsinkers, each with their own delightful idiosyncracies. Which one are you?', in 'The Tabloid', *The Independent*, 22 October: 3.

Harrison, B. and Lyon, S. (1993) 'A note on ethical issues in the use of autobiography in sociological research', *Sociology* 27(1): 101–9.

Hawkins, P. and Shohet, R. (1989) *Supervision in the Helping Professions: An Individual, Group and Organisational Approach*, Milton Keynes: Open University Press.

Herzlich, C. (1973) *Health and Illness: A Social Psychological Analysis*, trans. D. Graham, London and New York: European Association of Experimental Psychology and Academic Press.

Hoag, L. (1992) 'Psychotherapy in the general practice surgery: considerations of the frame', *British Journal of Psychotherapy* 8(4): 417–29.

Hochschild, A. (1983) *The Managed Heart*, London: University of California Press.

Huzzey, E. and Summers, P. (1995) 'Practising "osteopathy" in an NHS Trust hospital: the experiences of registered osteopaths', in 'Reading matters', *OAGB Newsletter* May: 4.

Lessing, D. (1981) *The Memoirs of a Survivor*, London: Picador, pp. 155–6.

Lévy-Zumwalt, R. (1988) *American Folklore Scholarship. A Dialogue of Dissent*, Indianapolis: Indiana University Press.

Morris, S. (1995) '"A very privileged position": complementary therapists receiving NHS oncology referrals', unpublished paper presented at the British Sociological Association Medical Sociology annual conference 22–24 September, University of York.

Peters, D. (1994) 'Sharing responsibility for patient care: doctors and complementary practitioners', in S. Budd and U. Sharma (eds) *The Healing Bond*, London: Routledge, pp. 171–92.

Power, R. (1994) '"Only nature heals": a discussion of therapeutic responsibility from a naturopathic point of view', in S. Budd and U. Sharma (eds) *The Healing Bond*, London: Routledge, pp. 193–213.

—— (1998) 'Failure in clinical practice: what does this mean?', in V. Olgiati, L. Orzack and M. Saks (eds) *Professions, Identity, and Order in Comparative Perspective*, Onati, Spain: The International Institute for the Sociology of Law, pp. 197–215.

Sharp, G. (1998) 'Osteopaths in business. Which NHS contract?', *The Osteopath* 1(8): 12–13.

Shilling, C. (1993) *The Body and Social Theory*, London: Sage.

Stacey, M. (1988) *The Sociology of Health and Medicine*, London: Unwin Hyman.

—— (1992) *Regulating British Medicine*, Chichester: John Wiley.

Weeks, D. (1996) 'NHS interface study', *The General Council and Register of Osteopaths Limited News Bulletin*, April: 12–13.

14 Emotions, boundaries and medical care

The use of complementary medicine by people with cancer

Steve Killigrew

Introduction

This chapter will investigate the therapeutic relationships between health care professionals, complementary therapists and people with cancer.

There have only been modest improvements in prognosis in the common cancers over the last two decades (Price and Sikora 1995: 10). Alongside this are reports of increasing numbers of patients using complementary therapies to address the psychological and emotional impact of cancer, often without the knowledge of health care professionals (Burke and Sikora 1992). Coupled with this is evidence that 'fighting spirit', an empowered mental outlook, can be a positive influence on well-being and prognosis (Moorey and Greer 1989), even in advanced breast cancer (Speigel 1989; Burch 1997).

There are many institutions or settings where people with cancer can go. Those patients wishing to use complementary medicine (CM) alongside their medical treatment may find them available in some form at their cancer centre (White 1998) but, more significantly, at institutions outside the National Health Service (Weir *et al.* 1995).

In keeping with the theme of this book there are several boundary points which will be theorised and then examined empirically. These boundary points are:

1 the implicit hierarchy of knowledge, skill and status between the physician, complementary therapist and patient;
2 the emotional dimensions of cancer and the relative significance attributed to the emotions in the illness experience of cancer;
3 the relationship between the use of complementary therapies and patient empowerment in the context of cancer;
4 the different frontiers and forms of communication between the patient and practitioner in the various institutions and settings.

The primary focus will be to examine these boundaries by studying the use of complementary therapies from the viewpoint of people with cancer.

This patient-centredness is akin to that of Richenda Power's chapter in this book, albeit with a different methodology and aims. There are shared concerns about patient advocacy, particularly in terms of self-care strategies, the emotional needs of patients, ownership of the body and the role of holism in health care.

Previous research carried out by the author has demonstrated a clear demarcation between lay and professional attitudes regarding the place of complementary therapies in cancer, notably in relation to the significance attached to emotional, psychospiritual and quality of life issues (Killigrew 1994, 1995).

The rationale for the present study came about as a result of the growing burden placed upon cancer services in the United Kingdom by government reforms impacting upon oncology centres in the Health Service as embodied in a series of Department of Health White Papers.[1] Coupled with this is the growing advocacy of patients and self-help groups who are aware of their rights as set out by the Patient's Charter, with its developments in clinical accountability, access to information, the right of informed consent to treatments, and more accessible channels of complaint and litigation. Therefore cancer centres are being squeezed from above by government policy and from below by the increasing demands of more assertive patients and self-help groups.[2]

The first half of the chapter will survey the literature on complementary therapy use among people with cancer.

The second half of the chapter will attempt to look at a small-scale cross-sectional study in terms of the broader perspective and will make recommendations which may be of interest to health care professionals, managers, academics in medical anthropology and health care policy, as well as to people with cancer and their carers.

Background: doctors, patients and cancer

Patient management has traditionally been based upon the Parsonian model of compliance and hierarchy. Parsons's model (1952) describes how the doctor takes the lead in returning the ill patient back to health when a cure is achieved. This model has never had any empirically verified place in cancer care. The natural history of cancers and their inherent ability to metastasise means that in place of cure there is remission, disease-free intervals and palliation of unpleasant or painful symptoms. These, not cure, are more prevalent outcomes of cancer treatment. So if the Parsonian model is tested to destruction by cancer care, what is there in its place?

Cancer and therapeutic relationships

It has often been stated to me by patients that the ingrained, unempathic disposition which informs and limits the interpersonal approach of many clinicians in the cancer field towards their patients is a professionally created boundary. This delineation allows minimal scope for the discussion of issues such as emotional or psychospiritual support which people with cancer may require. This, in theory at least, would appear to be in contrast to the nature of the type of therapeutic relationship found in many complementary therapies. In these therapeutic relationships, which are commonly informed by holism, there is the potential for exploration of such psychosocial and psychospiritual issues (Mitchell and Cormack 1998). The holistic framework may facilitate an openness of communication in the therapeutic relationship which integrates more readily with lay perceptions of illness than does the strictly biomedical approach used by many cancer clinicians.

As Angela Hall (1992) concludes in her review of lay beliefs about cancer, there are at least three identifiable areas where the differences between lay and professional views about cancer have serious implications. First, cancer patients can be confused between which model to internalise: 'they can be torn between belief and disbelief and therefore subject to internal conflict' (Hall 1992: 137). Second, people who hold onto idiosyncratic beliefs can experience conflict with their clinicians. For example, those with cancer who wish to use a complementary therapy despite its value being undermined or dismissed by their doctors, are rejecting biomedicine's presumed ownership of their bodies. Third, people with cancer avoid discussion with important others either to avert apportioning blame or because they may side against the patient and alongside the clinician. These factors point to the potential for emotional conflicts and isolation from medical and social support when it is most needed.

The NHS and cancer care

Within the wider political context of recent government health policy initiatives there are other managerially driven undertakings which impact upon the NHS, not least in cancer treatment. These include ideas and methods from outside the traditional health care system, such as quality assurance, clinical audit, standardisation of care via written protocols, evidence-based practice and interdisciplinary networking.

Concurrently there are a number of moves which herald a change from traditional precedence-based approaches where 'the doctor knew best' towards evidence-based approaches where continual research and audit is conducted into all aspects of clinical work. It is in this environment that patients are now managed, rather than cared for, and health care professionals have an increasing amount in common with production line workers.

Prompted by the initiatives towards a more accountable health care system, and armed with increased expectations, people with cancer are forming new strata within the health care system as a whole. These include not only localised patient self-help groups, but also informational resources such as national telephone helplines and internet websites, as well as informal peer networks and support systems. Clearly such resources exist in response to patients' needs which are not met by the NHS.

Complementary medicine in oncology 1980–98

As Fulder (1996) and Trevelyan and Booth (1994: 3–5) have identified, the holistic, qualitative and vitalist approaches and philosophies in health care have been challenging those of the reductionist, quantitative and mechanistic persuasion for centuries. In the last two decades this contest for hearts and minds has had considerable intensity in the area of cancer care.

In the 1980s the British Medical Association saw non-orthodox therapies as 'quackery' and a 'flight from science' (BMA 1986). This response from the medical profession had been necessitated by the significant rise in the numbers of both practitioners and users of unconventional or alternative therapies since the 1970s (Sharma 1992). Cancer patients, often in the advanced or untreatable stages of disease, are among this growing user group.

In 1980 Penny Brohn co-founded the Bristol Cancer Help Centre (BCHC), which offered a range of non-orthodox therapies to patients across the United Kingdom. This institution was the outcome of her own personal experiences in exploring non-biomedical approaches to the treatment of malignant disease (Brohn 1987). Most controversially, the Bristol programme sought to educate cancer patients through a series of residential workshops on nutritional therapy, macrobiotic cooking, self-hypnosis techniques, counselling, art therapy and spiritual healing (ibid.: 33–158). The aim at Bristol was, and still is, to educate and empower people with cancer to be self-caring; the approach was described by Weir *et al.* (1995) as 'radical holistic'.

In 1990 Bagenal and McElwain published a report following a joint research programme between the BCHC and the Imperial Cancer Research Fund (ICRF). According to the results those attending the BCHC fared two to three times worse than those receiving conventional treatment only. The researchers were at a loss to explain why. The media reported it as a clear victory for biomedicine over its non-orthodox 'rivals'. *The Times* (9 September 1990) covered the findings in fatalistic terms: 'orthodox medicine last week won a victory so total, so devastating over its alternative competitors that for many the argument will be over'. The curious question emerged: why, if these therapies were unproven in their clinical effectiveness, were they so powerfully dangerous to cancer patients?

Given the controversy over the results, plus the psychological impact upon those who had or were attending the BCHC, the findings were examined in detail by an independent review panel. They identified the reasons for the results of the study, a seriously flawed methodology and incompatible patient selection criteria (the BCHC group had many more people with advanced cancers), thereby explaining and fatally undermining the findings. Patients have campaigned to put the record straight and have described their outrage at being used as 'pawns' by a medical profession keen to undermine public credibility in complementary medicine (Carlisle 1992; Lloyd 1992).

In the wake of the BCHC/ICRF controversy a survey of 415 cancer patients was carried out by Downer *et al.* (1994). Despite its relatively small sample size and cross-sectional nature this study represents the start of a fresher, more objective evaluation of the subject by medical researchers. Their study found that 16 per cent of cancer patients in the study used some form of complementary therapy. More commonly users were younger, well-educated women, but there was representation in the user group from across the demographic spectrum. The most popular therapies were healing, visualisation, vitamins, herbalism and, interestingly, the Bristol Cancer Help Centre programme. These findings are broadly in line with other larger studies examining the general use of complementary therapies in industrial societies, such as Ooijendick's (1980) Dutch study of over 4,000 adults and Thomas's (1991) UK study. Respondents in Downer *et al.*'s (1994) study were also sent a series of psychological profile tests to complete.

The data generated showed that those using CM demonstrated higher levels of:

1   satisfaction with its use and a higher level of dissatisfaction with conventional treatments, compared to those people with cancer who used just orthodox methods;
2   anxiety compared to the standard users;
3   internal locus of control, indicating a belief in their own inherent healing capabilities.

Interviews also detected that many people with cancer used more therapies than indicated by the questionnaire data.

The study also looked at the patients' motivation for accessing complementary therapies. It acknowledged that along with the general growth in interest in complementary therapies during the 1970s and 1980s there appeared to be a general dissatisfaction with the increasingly technical approach to medicine, coupled with the growing 'unrealisable expectations' placed upon biomedicine.

Downer's group also identified those complementary therapies which cancer patients considered not to be appropriate. Restricted cancer-beating diets and herbalism, in particular, were identified. It may be that the dissatisfaction with diets is a remnant of the discredited BCHC/ICRF findings, where nutritional therapy was highlighted as unproven, dangerous quackery. It may also be that radical changes in diet can cause considerable social and psychological problems as well as unnecessary emaciation.[3] However, weight loss is a very common problem for people with cancer, particularly those in the advanced stages of the disease. As Downer points out, this group may be overly represented in the CM user group as they are more likely to seek help elsewhere when conventional treatment options are proving unsuccessful or increasingly limited in scope.

Downer concludes by stating that patients benefit psychologically from accessing CM, they are more hopeful and optimistic, as well as being more anxious. They go on to recommend that clinicians need to be more aware of the more commonly used therapies and not under-estimate the value of a positive 'feel good factor' among people with cancer. Booth (1993) considers that the denial of access to CM, where it may be effective and appropriate for people with cancer, is unethical.

Complementary therapies in oncology: current debates

The longest-running debate in professional circles about the use of CM in oncology is that of its unproven effect on prognosis. Despite the controversy surrounding the flawed study carried out at the BCHC there has, until recently, been no concrete refutation of the alleged harm for people with cancer.

In January 1998, Risberg *et al.* published the results of a longitudinal ethno-graphic study of cancer patients using what they term as non-proven therapies (NPT) in Norway after a five-year follow-up study. The study found higher levels of uptake of NPT than other studies, at between 17.4 per cent and 27.3 per cent. Of these three-quarters used spiritual/faith healing. Risberg also con-cluded that cross-sectionally designed studies will under-estimate the numbers of patients using NPT. Although the maximum number of users at any one point in the study was 27.3 per cent, over the five-year period as a whole no fewer than 45 per cent of people with cancer used an NPT at some stage, much higher than any previous finding. Significantly for the debate surrounding prog-nosis, there was no statistically detectable effect on survival either positively or negatively when people with cancer used NPT.

Risberg's study also concluded that measures other than survival were more applicable to measuring the benefits of NPTs for people with cancer, for exam-ple those in relation to the emotional aspects of cancer and quality of life. The study also emphasises the increased accuracy obtained in longitudinal studies as compared with cross-sectional methods. This may go some way to explain the higher levels of uptake detected in this study.

Another long-standing and continuing debate was addressed by an editorial in a leading international oncology journal. In it the 'attractive nuisance' value of unorthodox therapies as perceived by many cancer clinicians were reviewed and discussed, as were the implications for an open and trustworthy doctor–patient relationship (Durant 1998). The author acknowledges that many patients combine both approaches, albeit in a concealed form. The editorial concludes that 'Handling the complexities associated with unorthodox cancer therapies, no doubt, will continue to be most challenging in this era of excessive expectation and growing anti-science' (ibid.: 1998).

It is unclear how fostering self-care, empowerment, hope and a positive mental attitude in people living in the shadow of cancer equates as 'anti-science'. It may equally be viewed as the genuine needs of patients being left unaddressed by the adherence to a biomedical model which has more to do with fostering and affirming professional identity than acknowledging or meeting patients' needs.

As medical sociologist Mike Saks suggests, another shift is currently being played out, in the medical field at least, by the increasing impact of vitalist and holistic models (such as those of complementary therapies) upon the fabric of the health care system:

8

18   *Steve Killigrew*

Consideration of the position of the alternatives to medicine is of much interest not only because of its topicality, but also because it raises the question of the extent to which popular, consumer-based demand in an increasing market-orientated society can diminish established patterns of professional dominance.

(Saks 1994: 84)

Correspondingly, Fallowfield's studies (1990; Fallowfield and Clarke 1991) indicate that quality-of-life issues have often been excluded from cancer care by the narrowly defined paradigm of medical science.

The study: aims, rationale and methodology

The methodology used in the study described here combines qualitative and quantitative methods in an ethnomedical approach. Data were derived from a questionnaire and semi-structured interviews.

The primary aims of the research project were:

1   to examine the relationship between CM and oncology;
2   to focus on patients' views using an ethnomedical methodology;
3   to review the literature on patients' use of CM in cancer self-care to assess and evaluate potential benefits and risks;
4   to produce an evidence-based strategy regarding the use of complementary therapies by people with cancer.

Locating the study

In the spring of 1997 the management team of a cancer unit approached the author to conduct an investigation into the role that complementary medicine may have in the patient services at the unit. This was to be one element in a wide-ranging review of services locally in response to government White Papers, (most significantly) the Calman–Hine Report (1995), and growing numbers of patient-driven local projects. These different initiatives coincidentally shared the ideas of patient centredness, rapid access to clinical expertise as well as the rationalisation and modernisation of care pathways in cancer care within the NHS as a whole.

Results of the survey: quantitative data analysis

Two hundred questionnaires were distributed to patients at an oncology unit over a four-month period: 148 were returned, a 74 per cent response. Of these, 19 were incomplete, 16 partially and there were 3 blanks. The data set is therefore 145 (= 100 per cent).

Forty patients (27.6 per cent) had used complementary therapies (commonly more than one) at some time in the past. Table 14.1 shows a rank ordering of popularity.

Table 14.1 Previous use of complementary therapies by people with cancer

Therapy	Percentage	Number/145
Yoga	12.6	18
Relaxation and visualisation	11.7	17
Aromatherapy	9.7	14
Counselling	8.3	12
Healing	6.9	10
Hypnotherapy	6.9	10
Reflexology	5.5	8
Acupuncture	4.1	6
Herbalism	4.1	6
Homeopathy	1.4	2
Art therapy	0.7	1
Other: osteopathy, vitamin injection,		
crystal healing, massage	3.4	5

N.b. some used more than one therapy.

Table 14.2 Current use of complementary therapies by cancer patients

Therapy	Percentage	Number/145
Relaxation and visualisation	8.3	12
Yoga	6.2	9
Herbalism	4.1	6
Counselling	3.5	5
Healing	3.5	5
Aromatherapy	2.8	4
Homeopathy	0.7	1
Hypnotherapy	0.7	1
Reflexology	0.7	1
Art therapy	0.7	1
Shiatsu	0.7	1
Acupuncture	0	0

There were 19 patients (13 per cent) who were using CM at the time of the study. Table 14.2 gives them in rank order.

From the responses to these questions we can tell that while one in four respondents (40 out of 145, 27.6 per cent) had used complementary medicine at some stage in the past, only one in eight (19 out of 145, 13.1 per cent) were using them following their diagnosis of cancer. This reduction may be explained in a number of ways. First, people with cancer may be wary of using non-authorised forms of care given the seriousness of their condition, a view not supported by the interview data. A second explanation may be that the financial expense and time-consuming aspects of CM may prove prohibitive to those regularly attending the oncology unit. Third, this cross-sectional data may well under-estimate the actual levels of use as indicated by Risberg's larger, longitudinal and more methodologically complex Norwegian study (Risberg *et al.* 1998).

Yoga and relaxation and visualisation are the two most popular among both the past and current user groups. Aromatherapy, hypnotherapy and acupuncture show marked falls in use. There is evidence that in the case of aromatherapy some therapists working from a framework of the beautician rather than a therapist may be reluctant to treat people with cancer. Although there may be some limited circumstances where this applies, in the main there is no empirical evidence for a blanket ban on aromatherapy. One of the interviewees was refused an aromatherapy massage at a health spa because she had cancer.

In both the Downer *et al.* (1994) and Risberg *et al.* (1998) studies it was found that healing, i.e. spiritual healing or laying-on of hands, was the most popular therapy. This contrasts with the present study, where it was moderately popular but only half as popular as yoga and relaxation and visualisation.

Although only one in eight of the people with cancer currently use CM, nearly three-quarters (107 out of 145, 73 per cent) of the respondents felt that there is a role for CM alongside modern medicine. Correspondingly two-thirds of respondents (87 out of 145, 60 per cent) felt that CM could be of significant benefit to people with cancer, and two-thirds (97 out of 145, 66.9 per cent) felt that CM should be available at the cancer unit. More than three-quarters of the respondents felt that staff at the unit should be available to advise them about CM (113 out of 145, 77.9 per cent) and that they would benefit from having information on availability and cost of CM locally.

This grand increase from one in eight currently using CM to three out of four favouring easier access and greater information represents what Sharma (1992) describes as the 'halo effect', namely that the level of expressed support for, and positive interest in CM far exceeds the reported level of use, as in this present set of data.

The large difference described as the halo effect can be analysed and explained in several ways. First, by the fact that CM is predominantly to be found in the private health sector and is therefore, due to time and financial constraints, outside the scope of many sections of society. This may be the most pertinent explanation. If it is, then CM is currently under-supplied by health care delivery systems such as the NHS. This explanation can also be used to identify the underlying social forces responsible for the growth in the use of CM over the last three decades, where demand, in the form of the halo effect, continually exceeds supply. Other explanations may include those of Ros Coward (1989), who sees that CM benefits from the generally uncritical and positive impression attributed to everything 'natural' by advertisers, marketing organisations and the media. Alternatively the difference may be due to the methodological bias inherent in ethnographic studies, where respondents may be keen to give the answers that they believe the researcher is seeking. This explanation is also related to the findings of Cornwell's (1984) study, where she identified two strands of ethnographic discourse, private and public narratives. The former, more intimate and personal, took place between insiders, close family and friends;

Table 14.3 Rank ordering of preferences for payment of CM by people with cancer

Option	Percentage	Number/145
NHS funding	42.8	62
Special charity	26.9	39
Users pay	15.2	22
Other★	3.4	5

★ options offered by respondents were: subsidised payment, lottery grant and/or tax on tobacco firms.

the latter, more formal and reserved, characterised wider discussions, including those with researchers and other outsiders. The halo may therefore be a methodological mirage projected by the public narrative of informants.

The respondents were also asked about how CM should be paid for. They were given a choice, presented in rank order in Table 14.3.

Most patients preferred that CM should, like other treatments in the NHS, be free at the point of use. Even so, less than half saw this as their first choice.

Patient interview data

The aim of the interviews was to complement the quantitative questionnaire data with some ethnographic, qualitative material in order to examine in greater depth the assumptions which emerge from the first part of the study.

This qualitative data was obtained from five sources:

1   written data in an open comments section of the questionnaire. This was completed by 46 of the 145 respondents (31.7 per cent);
2   two randomly selected groups of people attending the oncology unit;
3   a focus group meeting with a cancer patient self-help group who encourage the use of complementary therapies (16 patients);
4   a cancer patient who had recently obtained a first class honours degree in psychology and had researched patients' attitudes in a similar area;
5   patients training in relaxation and visualisation techniques seen by the researcher.

When the material was analysed, concerning the use of CM by oncology patients who ranged from ardent users to occasional participants, four domains were identified.

The implicit hierarchy of knowledge, skill and status between the physician, complementary therapist and patient

The responses in this area were consistently that CM should be used alongside the conventional biomedical approach. A comment from one retired engineer was:

Really, y'know we should . . . we should be looking to find ways of utilising the best from both, using them synergistically.

Patients were also aware of the current uncertainty about asking their hospital doctors about complementary medicine. They wanted to be appropriately informed but were reticent to make enquiries for fear of attracting the disapproval of the clinical staff, which could, in the patients' eyes, prove detrimental to the treatment they received. As one woman who used aromatherapy and visualisation explained:

> You'd like to ask but . . . you think it might be wise just to keep quiet about it . . . you know . . . keep it to yourself.

Patients are also able to detect some discrepancy between the primary and secondary care sectors in the NHS in relation to different attitudes towards the use of CM. This is at odds with the NHS aims for cancer care and its goal of a seamless and standardised service with channels of communication and administration between different sectors of the health and social services, and where regional variations in care and resources are eliminated.

Patients viewed the role of CM in oncology as embodying a continuity of care after the active treatment phase comes to an end. For many interviewees the diagnosis of cancer casts a long shadow, often exceeding the duration of treatment. As one informant put it:

> These therapies, as well as other helpful agencies, help the client to move toward a reasonable quality of life . . . for however long that might be.

Improving information for patients at the end of a treatment programme and better networking between official institutions, such as the cancer unit, and unofficial bodies, for example self-help groups, could be of benefit here. Many unofficial bodies and informal cancer patient support groups make significant use of CM already and have been doing so for some time.

Complementary medicine, oncology and the emotional dimensions of cancer

Many interviewees commented on the lack of consideration taken by health care professionals of the emotional and psychospiritual aspects of their overall condition and well-being. This typical quote comes from a woman in her forties:

> When you get the diagnosis of cancer you don't take it in at first. Then you get the shock and the stress. You need support and I think complementary therapies can help this.

Similarly a retired mechanical engineer in his early sixties commented:

> The complementary therapies may help with the feelgood factor in the longer term.

Another interviewee, a woman involved with organising the complementary therapies provided by a self-help group, commented:

> The problem with medicine as far as cancer is concerned is that it promises so much in terms of breakthroughs and magic bullets, it is always jam tomorrow. But what about help now? That's where we believe complementary therapies come in. Giving people the possibility of help and support right here and now!

These comments indicate that complementary therapies fill in those areas where the current cancer service does not appear to address patients' emotional, quality-of-life issues adequately.

If the 'New NHS' is to become more patient-centred, the long-standing taboo areas such as the emotional, psychosocial and psychospiritual dimensions of cancer can no longer be justifiably excluded from the agenda of health care providers. Department of Health reports such as that of Calman–Hine (1995) emphasise the support of people with cancer as well as treatment. One of the Calman–Hine report's General Principles states that: 'In recognition of the impact that screening, diagnosis and treatment of cancer have on patients, families and their carers, psychosocial aspects of cancer should be considered at all stages' (ibid.: 6) and 'The services of the cancer unit should include palliative medical consultation, access to counselling and other forms of psychological help' (ibid.: 13).

In its identification of outcome measures Calman–Hine goes yet further:

> Clearly survival is a most important outcome and it is data which is normally collected by registries. However, in providing high quality cancer care, survival is by no means the only outcome of importance. Patients are interested in the quality as well as the quantity of their survival and it is likely that different patterns of care will be associated with differences in quality of life.
>
> (ibid.: Appendix B, 3.1)

Although Calman–Hine is helpful in emphasising that quality-of-life considerations need to be formally addressed by the Health Service, it provides little practical elaboration on the manner and wherewithal to do so. The evidence from talking with cancer patients concurs with the philosophy of care put forward by Calman–Hine but goes further, in stating that CM may provide a significant strand in the support network necessary in promoting quality of survival.

Patients viewed the role of CM in oncology as containing the opportunity to talk about the social, psychological, and spiritual dimensions of the illness experience. A respondent who had just finished a treatment programme of combined chemotherapy and radiotherapy said:

> How do you cure isolation? How do you cure the fact that you are not feeling yourself? . . . A friend at work has had the throat cancer and . . . you know the worst thing is not the treatment or wanting to die or anything like that . . . it's asking questions like are you supposed to get this side effect, are you supposed to feel like this? . . . The anxiety . . . confused, frightening . . . isolated . . . you feel very much alone. Just the contact . . . the physical contact is important . . . apart from the benefits of the massage itself . . . it's important . . . I work with the elderly and giving them a hand massage makes them feel special for that fifteen minutes or so . . . it is important . . . it fights the feelings of isolation.

The benefits of CM for cancer patients are commonly reported in these intangible, qualitative and psychospiritual terms. It re-emphasises the divide between the priorities and lay-values of those people with cancer and the scientism underpinning the value system of professional cancer carers.

Patients believed that the holistic framework of most complementary therapies enabled a non-judgemental and open-minded approach to these issues in which there is a more shared and empathic value system shared by both the patient and the practitioner. It therefore represents a different type of therapeutic context and interpersonal relationship than the one they have with their cancer doctors and other health care professionals (Mitchell and Cormack 1998).

Engel (1997) has explored the problems and contradictions inherent in being scientific in the human domain:

> Medicine has come full circle. From the beginning those interested to understand what distinguishes being 'sick' from being 'well' have never not known the importance of verbal exchange as a primary source of the data needed for that task. Nor have those 'scientifically minded' ever not known the limitations imposed by the frailty of human memory and therefore the inherent unreliability of that means of data acquisition. Indeed the imperative to exclude from science the human domain has rested to no small degree on that reality.
>
> (Engel 1997: 527)

Engel was one of the first clinicians to espouse the psychosocial model in health care. He has now shifted his position and makes the case for moving medicine from a biomedical to a biopsychosocial framework.

People with cancer: CM empowerment and self-care

Patients viewed the role of CM in oncology as a means of expanding sources of potential support. A comment typical of several made by patients in this area was spoken by one middle-aged woman who had just finished radiotherapy:

> We need supportive counselling by a specialist . . . Someone with specialist knowledge about cancer, cancer treatment, complementary therapies and

other things that might be helpful when you finish coming to the hospital every day and you are on your own . . . At least you feel like you are on your own.

Another female respondent undergoing treatment commented:

> Other complementary therapies would at least help the patient to relax and maybe even feel as though they had some control over their own situation. Surgery, radiotherapy and chemotherapy are all very frightening treatments, and complementary therapies may at least help the patient to deal with these situations in a more positive way.

Patients viewed the role of CM in oncology as a function of patient choice. They acknowledge that not all people with cancer want to be empowered or self-caring but information on CM should be offered to all patients in an unbiased manner to enable individuals to make their own informed choice.

Doctors, patients, CM and the limits of the therapeutic relationship in biomedicine

Several patients made the observation that doctors were not best placed to advise or counsel patients about the possibilities of using complementary therapies. The retired engineer commented typically:

> Doctors are too biased towards orthodox medicine . . . they couldn't recommend that [i.e. CM] . . . it goes against their training. You would need someone neutral to advise you.

Clearly patients view their specialists as highly qualified but with a narrower view of support than their own. The professional adherence to a biomedical model limits the scope of their role, in the eyes of their patients. It also significantly influences the form and content of communication between cancer patient and clinician.

Patients viewed the role of CM in oncology as identifying deficiencies in the current service provision, where staff are perceived of as being too busy regularly to spend time with patients, or listening and supporting their psychosocial and psychospiritual needs. One gentleman in his late middle age commented:

> I mean . . . don't get me wrong . . . the staff at the Royal are all very good and that but . . . there's little time to talk . . . too busy. It needs someone to be up-front, available.

The hospital staff, of all grades, tend to be aware of this but also acknowledge that they are under time pressure in an environment where there are only a few minutes allocated to each patient in order for resources to meet the pressures placed on the service.

One woman in her mid–fifties added that she had told no one of her distress following diagnosis for many weeks; not until she was discharged from hospital could she deal with her own emotional reactions well enough to be more open with family and friends:

> When I was in hospital having my treatment I did not really want to know. I wanted to get it over with and get home . . . I'm a lot better now, that was a very strange reaction to me . . . Usually if someone's got a problem I would want to sit and talk with them and discuss about it regardless.

For this patient, use of relaxation techniques and aromatherapy in her work with old people influenced her decision to use it herself only after the cancer treatment had been completed.

Patients expressed the view that the role of CM in oncology required more objective clarification and a more open attitude among clinicians, so that the fear of being ridiculed by their doctors is removed. As a business woman in her thirties commented:

> I am an individual and I have the right to individualised treatment. I want to be able to fully discuss all the options with someone qualified. I do not want to be seen as awkward or a crank. In my job I am used to taking responsibility for my decisions but here I'm just supposed to be passive and to wait to be told what to do. I am using relaxation and visualisation because it gives me a role, something to do that helps me with my disease.

Discussion and conclusions

The aims of the project, which included the examination of CM in cancer care from the patients' viewpoint, have largely been met. The intention of developing an evidence-based approach to integrating CM into the cancer unit requires more discussion, effort and networking for the medium and longer term. Suffice it to say that, on the basis of the study and the evidence from the literature review, the unit is about to commence a staff education programme as well as forging improved links with various local cancer self-help groups.

While acknowledging the limited scope of the survey there are clear conclusions which can be drawn in context with other studies and the wider literature previously reviewed in this chapter.

Lay and professional boundaries: the implications of differing perspectives regarding the role of CM in oncology

In examining the use of complementary therapy by people with cancer, the data produced strongly suggest that ideological differences do exist between the health care professions and the lay population whom they serve. These differences highlight questions about who decides what are the important issues in cancer care and around the types of useful techniques and approaches. The boundary line is highlighted not only by the uptake of CM by cancer patients but also by the general perception gleaned from them, concerning the need for greater attention to emotional/affective support, quality-of-life issues, self-care strategies and informed and unbiased choices for people with cancer.

The interviews and questionnaire data presented in the study are in broad agreement with other empirical research in this field. The present study, along with those carried out by Risberg *et al.* (1997), Downer *et al.* (1994) and White (1998), indicates that there is already a well-established role for complementary medicine in oncology. However, as Lewith (1996) correctly indicates, while CM does not cure cancer, it does have a role in the management of the toxic side-effects of cancer treatment and in the emotional support of people with cancer. None of the respondents or informants in this present study viewed CM as a panacea or miracle cure, nor as an alternative to their hospital treatments. They did see it as beneficial in helping people with cancer deal with the consequences and psychosocial and psychospiritual correlates that follow a diagnosis of cancer. Hall (1992) points out that these differences in beliefs can result in significant problems of communication between patient and clinician. Although, as Lewith comments:

> It is quite clear, however, that more enlightened cancer specialists are beginning to use a variety of complementary therapies in conjunction with conventional medicine. These may be used to alleviate the adverse reactions from conventional chemotherapy, or may be directed at the spiritual and emotional well-being of the individual cancer patient.
>
> (Lewith 1996: 242)

Alongside the actual therapeutic techniques employed in CM, people with cancer identified as a valuable element the additional time to talk afforded in these longer sessions.

From the questionnaire data in particular it is evident that perceptions of the role of CM in cancer care are not universal and do vary from patient to patient. Informal discussions with staff from oncology units across the country indicate that there are also wide variations in their views concerning the utility of CM in cancer care. The implications of Calman–Hine and its promise of uniformity of cancer care in all centres means that CM presents an interesting dilemma for the Health Service. Some centres are beginning to assimilate CM into the care pathways they provide, while others still view CM as incompatible with clinical science (Weir *et al.* 1995; White 1998). How can such polarised and contradictory views be resolved within the context of Calman–Hine's drive towards modernisation and standardisation of cancer services across England and Wales?

Modernisation of cancer services: patterns of care, CM and quality of life for people with cancer

In the arena of cancer care, this present study and the coherence from other similar studies indicate that one element in the modernisation of cancer services would be a rationalisation of the strategy for and clarification of the role of CM, with particular reference to self-care, patient empowerment and quality-of-life issues for people with cancer.

This study, along with other similar findings, suggests that acknowledging these roles for CM in oncology could have a significant effect upon the emotional care and quality of life for people with cancer – not least in respect of the all-important level of trust between people with cancer and the clinical staff in oncology units – by bringing discussion of the subject out into the open for unprejudiced examination and discussion. Correspondingly this would require meeting the educational needs of staff that such an initiative implies.

The new challenge is one of being scientific in the human domain, or conversely of being humane in a clinical one. As Engel (1997: 521) states, 'It is the challenge – yet the reward – of the physician to empathically make meaningful connections between the patient's life history and presenting problems to diagnose the problems which the patient presents.'

Engel proposes that the biomedical ideology needs modernising, and thereby the health services will follow suit. Engel proposes a biopsychosocial model. Others, this author included, would simply call such a proposal holistic, integrated health care.

In talking to people with cancer it emerges from them that clinicians need to acknowledge more readily that many people with cancer may fear the consequences of orthodox treatment options as much as the growing presence of the tumour itself. One way forward may be to identify ways in which empathy and trust replaces fear and suspicion between patients and clinicians. Ideally appropriate empowerment, informed consent and self-care strategies can be integrated alongside the need for narrow compliance with purely physical, often highly toxic, treatments. There would also appear to be a strong case for a review of why treatment outcome is measured solely by prognosis to the exclusion of other considerations, such as the associated quality of life and emotional adjustment to diagnosis and treatment.

The evidence clearly indicates that the use of complementary therapies by significant numbers of people with cancer is now an established feature of the clinical landscape in oncology.

Cancer holds a deep personal meaning for each individual it afflicts, often with a psychosocial and psychospiritual dimension to the disease alongside its pathological structure. Cancer is simultaneously subjective, for those people who have it, and objective, for those who study and treat it. There is much invaluable objective clinical evidence about cancer, yet the important questions concerning how this knowledge affects the lives of people with cancer is poorly researched and understood. It is in this sense that the meaning assigned by the patient is important, and this in turn is dependent upon how information is communicated. The current attempts at modernising the NHS may have to mean more than re-inventing such notions as patients as informed consumers, more even than the current emphasis upon evidence-based practice, for when was medical science and clinical theory not based upon evidence?[4]

There are ethical and clinical reasons for challenging the treatment of cancer within a biomedical framework, primarily in terms of emphasising a view of patients as knowing subjects rather than passive objects. The move being taken by many people with cancer towards complementary medicine is evidence of a shift towards the development of a more integrative, humanistic model of health care incorporating quality-of-life assessment, the nature of healing and healers, psychosocial and psychospiritual support, within a wider-ranging conceptual gaze, perhaps one such as holism.

Notes

1 The most recent and relevant White Papers to the present topic are *The New NHS* (DoH 1997), *Our Healthier Nation* (DoH 1998), and *A Policy Framework for Commissioning Cancer Services* (Calman–Hine 1995). These are discussed in more detail later in the main text.
2 See Kelleher (1995) for a detailed account of this growing medical phenomenon.
3 The commonly used macrobiotic diets would not appeal to all family members, for instance, are easy to 'fail' or transgress, leading to a sense of failure, and tend to be heavily criticised, even opposed by dieticians in the health service.
4 The point about evidence-based practice is that much is tried without sound evidence and that much fundamental evidence exists which is not utilised. National and local databases would help dissemination, but even then, keeping up with new data is difficult within the constraints and demands of busy clinical practice.

References

Bagenal, F.S. and McElwain, T.J. (1990) 'The survival of patients with breast cancer attending the Bristol Cancer Help Centre', *The Lancet* 336(8715): 606–10.
Booth, B. (1993) 'Healthy alternatives?', *Nursing Times* 89(17): 34–6.
British Medical Association [BMA] (1986) *Alternative Therapy*, BMA Report, London: BMA.
—— (1993) *Complementary Medicine; New Approaches to Good Practice*, Oxford and New York: Oxford University Press.
Brohn, P. (1987) *The Bristol Programme: An Introduction to the Holistic Therapies Practised by the Bristol Cancer Help Centre*, London: Century.
Burch, R. (1997) 'Alive and kicking', *Nursing Times* 93(9): 26–9.
Burke, C. and Sikora, K. (1992) 'Cancer – the dual approach', *Nursing Times* 88(38): 62–5.
Calman, K. and Hine, D. (1995) *A Policy Framework for Commissioning Cancer Services: A Report by the Expert Advisory Group on Cancer to the Chief Medical Officers of England and Wales*, Department of Health and The Welsh Office.
Carlisle, D. (1992) 'Healing the haven', *Nursing Times* 87(16): 18–19.
Cornwell, J. (1984) *Hard Earned Lives: Accounts of Health and Illness from East London*, London and New York: Tavistock.
Coward, R. (1989) *The Whole Truth; The Myth of Alternative Medicine*, London: Faber and Faber.
Department of Health [DoH] (1997) *The New NHS*, London: HMSO.
—— (1998) *Our Healthier Nation*, London: HMSO.
Downer, S.M., Cody, M.M., Mcluskey, P., Wilson, P.D., Arnott, S.J., Lister, T.A. and Slevin, M.L. (1994) 'Pursuit and practice of complementary therapies by cancer patients receiving conventional treatment', *British Medical Journal* 309: 86–9.

Durant, J.R. (1998) 'Alternative medicine: an attractive nuisance', *Journal of Clinical Oncology* 16(1): 1–2.

Engel, G.L. (1997) 'From biomedical to biopsychosocial: being scientific in the human domain', *Psychosomatics* 38(6): 521–8.

Fallowfield, L. (1990) *The Quality of Life: The Missing Measurement in Health Care*, London: Souvenir Press.

Fallowfield, L. and Clarke, A. (1991) *Breast Cancer*, London: Tavistock/Routledge.

Fulder, S. (1996) *The Handbook of Alternative and Complementary Therapies*, 3rd edn, Oxford: Oxford Medical Publishing.

Hall, A. (1992) 'Lay beliefs about the causes of cancer', in T. Heller, L. Bailey and S. Pattison (eds) *Preventing Cancers*, Buckingham: Open University Press, pp. 132–8.

Kelleher, D. (1995) 'Self-help groups and their relationship to medicine', in J. Gabe, D. Kelleher and G. Williams (eds) *Challenging Medicine*, London and New York: Routledge, pp. 104–17.

Killigrew, S.G. (1994) 'The paradox of cancer treatment', *The Therapist* 2(2): 32–3.

—— (1995) 'Towards a self care strategy for cancer patients?', *Radiography Today* 61(692): 17–19.

Lewith, G. (1996) 'Cancer: complementary therapies', *Medicine* 4: 242–6.

Lloyd, A. (1992) 'Rebuilding the centre', *Nursing Times* 88(26): 16–17.

Mitchell, A. and Cormack, M. (1998) *The Therapeutic Relationship in Complementary Health Care*, London: Churchill Livingstone.

Moorey, S. and Greer, S. (1989) *Psychological Therapy for Patients with Cancer*, Oxford: Heinemann.

Ooijendick, W.T.M. (1980) *What is Better?* London: Threshold Foundation.

Parsons, T. (1952) *The Social System*, London: Routledge and Kegan Paul.

Price, P. and Sikora, K. (1995) *Treatment of Cancer*, London: Chapman and Hall Medical.

Risberg, T., Lund, E., Wist, E., Kaasa, S. and Wilsgard, T. (1998) 'Cancer patients' use of nonproven therapy; a five year follow-up study', *Journal of Clinical Oncology* 16(1): 6–12.

Saks, M. (1994) 'The alternatives to medicine', in J. Gabe, D. Kelleher and G. Williams (eds) *Challenging Medicine*, London and New York: Routledge, pp. 84–103.

Sharma, U. (1992) *Complementary Medicine Today: Practitioners and Patients*, London and New York: Routledge.

Speigel, D. (1989) 'Effects of psychological treatment on survival of patients with metastatic breast cancer', *The Lancet* 298: 291–3.

Thomas, K.J. (1991) 'Use of non-orthodox and conventional health care in Great Britain', *British Medical Journal* 302(26): 207–10.

The Sunday Times (1990) 'Chaos creeps up on science as two medicines collide', 9 September 1990: 3.4.

Trevelyan, J. and Booth, B. (1994) *Complementary Medicine for Nurses, Midwives and Health Visitors*, Basingstoke and London: Macmillan.

Weir, M.W., Zollman, C. and Addington-Hall, J. (1995) 'Developing psychosocial services for people with cancer: a review of six centres', *Journal of Cancer Care* 4: 3–10.

White, P.W. (1998) 'Complementary medicine treatment of cancer; a survey of provision', *Complementary Therapies in Medicine* 6: 10–13.

15 Conclusion

Nigel Malin

The individual chapters of this book collectively present perspectives on how professionalism and professional boundaries have been re-defined. These examples have been drawn largely from health and social welfare fields and are based upon recent research. The suggestion of Abbott (1988) that a way of thinking about professional work is as something that is defined and re-defined through continuous struggle between occupational groups is as valid now as it was then. Professionalism is viewed as a shifting phenomenon, with the values and attributes of professionals subject to change and struggle. The discourse of enterprise (du Gay 1992) referred to continuously has contributed to profound organisational change, impacting upon professional workplace practices in both public and private sectors.

Earlier 'inclusivist' analyses of professions, which identified common traits in initially different professional settings, now give way to alternative perspectives concerned with the impact of commercialisation and consumerist values. As Anleu (1992: 24) has pointed out, writers in this field in the first half of the century 'conceptually distinguished professions from non-professions by identifying their core defining characteristics', which most frequently included 'formal education and entry requirements; a monopoly over an esoteric body of knowledge and associated skills; autonomy over the terms and conditions of practice; collegial authority; a code of ethics; and, commitment to a service ideal'.

Hugman (1991: 104), writing on caring professions, from a contemporary perspective, claimed professionalism is limited by the success in gaining power over such factors as an area of knowledge and associated autonomy, rather than limited by the intrinsic nature of those factors. The social service ethos of professionalism outlined by Marshall (1939) centred around providing a service on the basis of need rather than ability to pay. This concept, as opposed to individualistic notions of service based upon payment, underpinned the social consensus that formed the basis of the post-war welfare state. Individuals were guaranteed certain rights on the basis of citizenship and these rights were delivered by professionals employed in health care, education and social welfare. In recent decades, competing definitions of professionalism emerged stressing the need to have managerial and entrepreneurial skills. Hanlon (1998) writes that this professionalism normally emphasises three factors: first, technical ability – this will allow one to practise in the profession but it will not guarantee advancement nor success; second, managerial skill – this is the ability to manage other employees, the ability to balance budgets and the capacity to manage and satisfy clients; third, the ability to bring in business and/or act in an entrepreneurial way. Hugman (1998) has reviewed the changing boundaries of formal and informal care relationships and the extent to which the marketisation of social welfare has transformed professional workers into functional operatives and citizens into quasi-consumers.

An implication central to this line of argument is the encouragement of client empowerment, and the notion of profitability taking precedence over serving clients in need. Keeping the paying client happy gives the client a powerful voice in determining a professional service and tailors the service more to the needs of selective clients rather than a total population. Customer power (or lack of) as influencing professional boundaries and practices has been taken up as a main theme in several chapters (for example 2, 3, 7, 12). One view is that as part of enterprise culture the current consumer is no longer the grateful passive customer but actively shaping supply through demands. This may apply more to British industry than to public health and welfare provision. For instance, market assumptions of self-actualising consumers requiring social care have falsely presumed a level of power and assertion that is not evident. There is, however, a perception that contemporary culture has produced a need for the professional worker to be multi-skilled and more flexible to the demands of consumers.

Changes in professionalism are depicted as a response to managerialism and commercialism, but they also need to be seen as a response to a quite oppositional set of pressures from service users, feminists and black workers, and from a range of radical movements which have challenged the whole basis of expert professionalism. This follows Giddens's (1991: 14–34) suggestion that one of the basic characteristics of high modernity is that individuals no longer simply 'trust' expert systems. An emphasis on reflexivity and experientialism encourages individuals to question and learn from their interaction with society, thereby altering knowledge. Some occupational groups challenge notions of professionalism and deliberately espouse a philosophy of client empowerment, including the use of shared identification as a resource to abnegate hierarchical practitioner–client relations (see, for instance, chapter 2). User self-advocacy creates a direct challenge to professionally controlled features of an organisation.

Enterprise culture has altered boundary contours both to limit and expand the knowledge base and expertise of professional groups. This has applied to politically vulnerable or semi-professions, such as nursing, teaching and social work, where the root basis of knowledge and accompanying expertise has required affirmation. Attempts by the state to control public sector costs have involved reform and restructuring to make such groups of professionals accountable and to enforce financial and managerial discipline upon them. This has led to professionals moving to become expert within new spheres of knowledge, competing for ownership of different areas and viewing that which might be considered their protected knowledge base. The constitution of the independent field of professional knowledge, with its social, historical and economic contingencies, has been a neglected area of study – see, for instance, chapter 4. The argument here is that the professional project involves not only an occupational group appropriating a field as its exclusive area of jurisdiction and expertise but also the making of this field into a legitimate area of knowledge and intervention. The means is through creating a boundary between itself and other groups, and between itself and the lay public. Larson (1990: 83) argued that the one central function of professions (or their counterparts) in most advanced societies was that of 'organising the acquisition and certification of expertise in broad functional areas, on the basis of formal educational qualifications held by individuals'.

The nursing profession is an example where development of speciality expertise has become an inevitable consequence of pressures within society, technology complexity and consumer demand. This is seen as the culmination of a gradual process of professionalisation (Scott 1998), as well as a response to changes including marketisation and regulation of health care in the late twentieth century.

There is no doubt that current socio-economic restructuring challenges and gives opportunities to professionals and experts to re-assess their knowledge. It pressurises different groups to legitimise their cultural capital, credentialism being a conventional strategy of social closure. Notwithstanding the significance of this, any proposed expansion of the state role directed towards greater transparency, openness and regulation is likely to force the question of who legitimises working practices and behaviour of professionals – an expanded state, commercial or lay regulation or self-regulation?

References

Abbott, A. (1988) *The System of Professions*, London: University of Chicago Press.
Anleu, S. (1992) 'The professionalisation of social work? A case study of three organisational settings', *Sociology* 26(1): 23–43.
du Gay, P. (1992) 'The culture of the customer', *Journal of Management Studies* 29(4): 615–33.
Giddens, A. (1991) *Modernity and Self-Identity*, Cambridge: Polity Press.
Hanlon, G. (1998) 'Professionalism as enterprise: service class politics and the redefinition of professionalism', *Sociology* 32(1): 43–63.
Hugman, R. (1991) *Power in Caring Professions*, Basingstoke: Macmillan.
—— (1998) *Social Welfare and Social Value: The Role of Caring Professions*, Basingstoke: Macmillan.
Larson, M. (1990) 'In the matter of experts and professionals, or how impossible it is to leave nothing unsaid', in R. Torstendahl and M. Burrage (eds) *The Formation of Professions: Knowledge, State and Strategy*, Sage, London, pp. 24–50.
Marshall, T. (1939) 'The recent history of professionalism', *Canadian Journal of Economics and Political Science* 5: 325–40.
Scott, C. (1998) 'Specialist practice: advancing the profession?', *Journal of Advanced Nursing* 28(3): 554–62.

Index